Medical Statistics

A Guide to Data Analysis and Critical Appraisal

Medical Statistics

A Guide to Data Analysis and Critical Appraisal

Jennifer Peat

Associate Professor, Department of Paediatrics and Child Health, University of Sydney and Senior Hospital Statistician, Clinical Epidemiology Unit, The Children's Hospital at Westmead, Sydney, Australia

Belinda Barton

Head of Children's Hospital Education Research Institute (CHERI) and Psychologist, Neurogenetics Research Unit, The Children's Hospital at Westmead, Sydney, Australia

Foreword by Martin Bland, Professor of Health Statistics at the University of York

Blackwell
Publishing

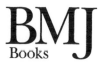

First edition 2005

Library of Congress Cataloging-in-Publication Data

Peat, Jennifer K.
    Medical statistics: a guide to data analysis and critical appraisal / by Jennifer
Peat and Belinda Barton. – 1st ed.
        p. ; cm.
    Includes bibliographical references and index.
    ISBN-13: 978-0-7279-1812-3
    ISBN-10: 0-7279-1812-5
    1. Medical statistics.   2. Medicine–Research–Statistical methods.
I. Barton, Belinda. II. Title.
    [DNLM: 1. Statistics–methods.   2. Research Design.   WA 950 P363m 2005]
R853.S7P43 2005
610′.72′7–dc22   2005000168

A catalogue record for this title is available from the British Library

Set in 9.5/12pt Meridien & Frutiger by TechBooks, New Delhi, India
Printed and bound in Harayana, India by Replika Press Pvt Ltd

Commissioning Editor: Mary Banks
Editorial Assistant: Mirjana Misina
Development Editor: Veronica Pock
Production Controller: Debbie Wyer

For further information on Blackwell Publishing, visit our website:
http://www.blackwellpublishing.com

The publisher's policy is to use permanent paper from mills that operate a sustainable
forestry policy, and which has been manufactured from pulp processed using acid-free
and elementary chlorine-free practices. Furthermore, the publisher ensures that the text
paper and cover board used have met acceptable environmental accreditation standards.

Contents

Foreword

Most research in health care is not done by professional researchers, but by health-care practitioners. This is very unusual; agricultural research is not done by farmers, and building research is not done by bricklayers. I am told that it is positively frowned upon for social workers to carry out research, when they could be solving the problems of their clients. Practitioner-led research comes about, in part, because only clinicians, of whatever professional background, have access to the essential research material, patients. But it also derives from a long tradition, in medicine for example, that it is part of the role of the doctor to add to medical knowledge. It is impossible to succeed in many branches of medicine without a few publications in medical journals. This tradition is not confined to medicine. Let us not forget that Florence Nightingale was known as 'the Passionate Statistician' and her greatest innovation was that she collected data to evaluate her nursing practice. (She was the first woman to become a fellow of the Royal Statistical Society and is a heroine to all thinking medical statisticians.)

There are advantages to this system, especially for evidence-based practice. Clinicians often have direct experience of research as participants and are aware of some of its potential and limitations. They can claim ownership of the evidence they are expected to apply. The disadvantage is that health-care research is often done by people who have little training in how to do it and who have to do their research while, at the same time, carrying on a busy clinical practice. Even worse, research is often a rite of passage: the young researcher carries out one or two projects and then moves on and does not do research again. Thus there is a continual stream of new researchers, needing to learn quickly how to do it, yet there is a shortage of senior researchers to act as mentors. And research is not easy. When we do a piece of research, we are doing something no one has done before. The potential for the explorer to make a journey which leads nowhere is great.

The result of practitioner-led research is that much of it is of poor quality, potentially leading to false conclusions and sub-optimal advice and treatment for patients. People can die. It is also extremely wasteful of the resources of institutions which employ the researchers and their patients. From the researchers' point of view, reading the published literature is difficult because the findings of others cannot be taken at face value and each paper must be read critically and in detail. Their own papers are often rejected and even once published they are open to criticism because the most careful refereeing procedures will not correct all the errors.

When researchers begin to read the research literature in their chosen field, one of the first things they will discover is that knowledge of statistics is essential. There is no skill more ubiquitous in health-care research. Several of my former medical students have come to me for a bit of statistical advice, telling me how they now wished they had listened more when I taught them. Well, I wish they had, too, but it would not have been enough. Statistical knowledge is very hard to gain; indeed, it is one of the hardest subjects there is, but it is also very hard to retain. Why is it that I can remember the lyrics (though not, my family assures me, the tunes) of hundreds of pop songs of my youth, but not the details of any statistical method I have not applied in the last month? And I spend much of my time analysing data.

What the researchers need is a statistician at their elbow, ready to answer any questions that arise as they design their studies and analyse their data. They are so hard to find. Even one consultation with a statistician, if it can be obtained at all, may involve a wait for weeks. I think that the most efficient way to improve health-care research would be to train and employ, preferably at high salaries, large numbers of statisticians to act as collaborators. (Incidentally, statisticians should make the ideal collaborators, because they will not care about the research question, only about how to answer it, so there is no risk of them stealing the researcher's thunder.) Until that happy day dawns, statistical support will remain as hard to find as an honest politician. This book provides the next best thing.

The authors have great experience of research collaboration and support for researchers. Jenny Peat is a statistician who has co-authored more than a hundred health research papers. She describes herself as a 'research therapist', always ready to treat the ailing project and restore it to publishable health. Belinda Barton brings the researcher's perspective, coming into health research from a background in psychology. Their practical experience fills these pages. The authors guide the reader through all the methods of statistical analysis commonly found in the health-care literature. They emphasise the practical details of calculation, giving detailed guidance as to the computation of the methods they describe using the popular program SPSS. They rightly stress the importance of the assumptions of methods, including those which statisticians often forget to mention, such as the independence of observations. Researchers who follow their advice should not be told by statistical referees that their analyses are invalid. Peat and Barton close each chapter with a list of things to watch out for when reading papers which report analysis using the methods they have just described. Researchers will also find these invaluable as checklists to use when reading over their own work.

I recently remarked that my aim for my future career is to improve the quality of health-care research. 'What, worldwide?', I was asked. Of course, why limit ourselves? I think that this book, coming from the other side of the world from me, will help bring that target so much closer.

Martin Bland,
Professor of Health Statistics, University of York,
August 2004

Acknowledgements

We extend our thanks to our colleagues and to our hospital for supporting this project. We also thank all of the students and researchers who attended our classes and provided encouragement and feedback. We would also like to express our gratitude to our friends and families who inspired us and supported us to write this book. In addition, we acknowledge the help of Dr Andrew Hayen, a biostatistician with NSW Health who helped to review the manuscript and contributed his expertise.

Introduction

Statistical thinking will one day be as necessary a qualification for efficient citizenship as the ability to read and write.
H.G. WELLS

Anyone who is involved in medical research should always keep in mind that science is a search for the truth and that, in searching for the truth, there is no room for bias or inaccuracy in statistical analyses or their interpretation.

Analysing the data and interpreting the results are the most exciting stages of a research project because these provide the answers to the study questions. However, data analyses must be undertaken in a careful and considered way by people who have an inherent knowledge of the nature of the data and of their interpretation. Any errors in statistical analyses will mean that the conclusions of the study may be incorrect[1]. As a result, many journals ask reviewers to scrutinise the statistical aspects of submitted articles and many research groups include statisticians who direct the data analyses. Analysing data correctly and including detailed documentation so that others can reach the same conclusions are established markers of scientific integrity. Research studies that are conducted with integrity bring personal pride, contribute to a successful track record and foster a better research culture.

In this book, we provide a guide to conducting and interpreting statistics in the context of how the participants were recruited, how the study was designed, what types of variables were used, what effect size was found and what the *P* values mean. We also guide researchers through the processes of selecting the correct statistic and show how to report results for publication or presentation. We have included boxes of SPSS and SigmaPlot commands in which we show the window names with the commands indented. We do not always include all of the tables from the SPSS output but only the most relevant information. In our examples, we use SPSS version 11.5 and SigmaPlot version 8 but the messages apply equally well to other versions and other statistical packages.

We have separated the chapters into sections according to whether data are continuous or categorical in nature because this classification is fundamental to selecting the correct statistics. At the end of the book, there is a glossary of terms as an easy reference that applies to all chapters and a list of useful Web sites. We have written this book as a guide from first principles with explanations of assumptions and how to interpret results. We hope that both novice statisticians and seasoned researchers will find this book a helpful guide to working with their data.

In this era of evidence-based health care, both clinicians and researchers need to critically appraise the statistical aspects of published articles in order to judge the implications and reliability of reported results. Although the peer review process goes a long way to improving the standard of research literature, it is essential to have the skills to decide whether published results are credible and therefore have implications for current clinical practice or future research directions. We have therefore included critical appraisal guidelines at the end of each chapter to help researchers to review the reporting of results from each type of statistical test.

There is a saying that 'everything is easy when you know how' – we hope that this book will provide the 'know how' and make statistical analysis and critical appraisal easy for all researchers and health-care professionals.

References

1. Altman DG. Statistics in medical research. In: Practical statistics for medical research. London: Chapman and Hall, 1996; pp 4–5.

CHAPTER 1

Data management: preparing to analyse the data

There are two kinds of statistics, the kind you look up and the kind you make up.
REX STOUT

Objectives

The objectives of this chapter are to explain how to:
- create a database that will facilitate straightforward statistical analyses
- devise a data management plan
- ensure data quality
- move data between electronic spreadsheets
- manage and document research data
- select the correct statistical test
- critically appraise the quality of reported data analyses

Creating a database

Creating a database in SPSS and entering the data is a relatively simple process. First, a new file can be opened using the *File → New → Data* commands at the top left hand side of the screen. The SPSS data editor has two different screens called the Data View and Variable View screens. You can easily move between the two views by clicking on the tabs at the bottom left hand side of the screen.

Before entering data in Data View, the characteristics of each variable need to be defined in Variable View. In this screen, details of the variable names, variable types and labels are stored. Each row in Variable View represents a new variable. To enter a variable name, simply type the name into the first field and default settings will appear for the remaining fields. The Tab or the arrow keys can be used to move across the fields and change the default settings. The settings can be changed by pulling down the drop box option that appears when you double click on the domino on the right hand side of each cell. In most cases, the first variable in a data set will be a unique identification number for each participant. This variable is invaluable for selecting or tracking particular participants during the data analysis process.

The Data View screen, which displays the data values, shows how the data have been entered. This screen is similar to many other spreadsheet packages. A golden rule of data entry is that the data for each participant should occupy one row only in the spreadsheet. Thus, if follow up data have been collected from the participants on one or more occasions, the participants' data should be an extension of their baseline data row and not a new row in the spreadsheet. An exception to this rule is for studies in which controls are matched to cases by characteristics such as gender or age or are selected as the unaffected sibling or a nominated friend of the case and therefore the data are naturally paired. The data from matched case-control studies are used as pairs in the statistical analyses and therefore it is important that matched controls are not entered on a separate row but are entered into the same row in the spreadsheet as their matched case. This method will inherently ensure that paired or matched data are analysed correctly and that the assumptions of independence that are required by many statistical tests are not violated. Thus, in Data View, each column represents a separate variable and each row represents a single participant, or a single pair of participants in a matched case-control study, or a single participant with follow-up data.

Unlike Excel, it is not possible to hide rows or columns in either Variable View or Data View in SPSS. Therefore, the order of variables in the spreadsheet should be considered before the data are entered. The default setting for the lists of variables in the drop down boxes that are used when running the statistical analyses are in the same order as the spreadsheet. It is more efficient to place variables that are likely to be used most often at the beginning of the data file and variables that are going to be used less often at the end.

After the information for each variable has been defined in Variable View, the data can be entered in the Data View screen. Before entering data, the details entered in the Variable View can be saved using the commands shown in Box 1.1.

Box 1.1 SPSS commands for saving a file

SPSS Commands
Untitled – SPSS Data Editor
    File → Save As
Save Data As
    Enter the name of the file in File name
Click on Save

After saving the file, the name of the file will replace the word *Untitled* at the top left hand side of the Data View screen. Data entered into the Variable View can be also saved using the commands shown in Box 1.1. It is not possible to close a data file in SPSS Data Editor. The file can only be closed by opening a new data file or by exiting the SPSS program.

Variable names

If data are entered in Excel or Access before being exported to SPSS, it is a good idea to use variable names that are accepted by SPSS to avoid having to rename the variables. In SPSS, each variable name has a maximum of eight characters and must begin with an alphabetic character. In addition, each variable name must be unique. Some symbols such as @, # or $ can be used in variable names but other symbols such as %, > and punctuation marks are not accepted. Also, SPSS is not case sensitive and capital letters will be converted to lower case letters.

Types of variables

Before conducting any statistical tests, a formal, documented plan that includes a list of questions to be answered and identifies the variables that will be used should be drawn up. For each question, a decision on how each variable will be used in the analyses, for example as a continuous or categorical variable or as an outcome or explanatory variable, will need to be made.

Table 1.1 shows a classification system for variables and how the classification influences the presentation of results. A common error in statistical analyses is to misclassify the outcome variable as an explanatory variable or to misclassify an intervening variable as an explanatory variable. It is important that an intervening variable, which links the explanatory and outcome variable because it is directly on the pathway to the outcome variable, is not treated as an independent explanatory variable in the analyses[1]. It is also important that an alternative outcome variable is not treated as an independent risk factor. For example, hay fever cannot be treated as an independent risk factor for asthma because it is a symptom that is a consequence of the same allergic developmental pathway.

Table 1.1 Names used to identify variables

Variable name	Alternative name/s	Axis for plots, data analysis and tables
Outcome variables	Dependent variables (DVs)	y-axis, columns
Intervening variables	Secondary or alternative outcome variables	y-axis, columns
Explanatory variables	Independent variables (IVs) Risk factors Exposure variables Predictors	x-axis, rows

In part, the classification of variables depends on the study design. In a case-control study in which disease status is used as the selection criterion, the explanatory variable will be the presence or absence of disease and the outcome variable will be the exposure. However, in most other observational and experimental studies such as clinical trials, cross-sectional and cohort studies, the disease will be the outcome and the exposure will be the explanatory variable.

In SPSS, the measurement level of the variable can be classified as nominal, ordinal or scale under the *Measure* option in Variable View. The measurement scale used determines each of these classifications. Nominal scales have no order and are generally category labels that have been assigned to classify items or information. For example, variables with categories such as male or female, religious status or place of birth are nominal scales. Nominal scales can be string (alphanumeric) values or numeric values that have been assigned to represent categories, for example 1 = male and 2 = female.

Values on an ordinal scale have a logical or ordered relationship across the values and it is possible to measure some degree of difference between categories. However, it is usually not possible to measure a specific amount of difference between categories. For example, participants may be asked to rate their overall level of stress on a five-point scale that ranges from no stress, mild stress, moderate stress, severe stress to extreme stress. Using this scale, participants with severe stress will have a more serious condition than participants with mild stress, although recognising that self-reported perception of stress may be quite subjective and is unlikely to be standardised between participants. With this type of scale, it is not possible to say that the difference between mild and moderate stress is the same as the difference between moderate and severe stress. Thus, information from these types of variables has to be interpreted with care.

Variables with numeric values that are measured by an interval or ratio scale are classified as scale variables. On an interval scale, one unit on the scale represents the same magnitude across the whole scale. For example, Fahrenheit is an interval scale because the difference in temperature between 10 °F and 20 °F is the same as the difference in temperature between 40 °F and 50 °F. However, interval scales have no true zero point. For example, 0 °F does not indicate that there is no temperature. Because interval scales have an arbitrary rather than a true zero point, it is not possible to compare ratios.

A ratio scale has the same properties as nominal, ordinal, and interval scales, but has a true zero point and therefore ratio comparisons are valid. For example, it is possible to say that a person who is 40 years old is twice as old as a person who is 20 years old and that a person is 0 year old at birth. Other common ratio scales are length, weight and income.

While variables in SPSS can be classified as scale, ordinal or nominal values, a more useful classification for variables when deciding how to analyse data is as categorical variables (ordered or non-ordered) or continuous variables.

These classifications are essential for selecting the correct statistical test to analyse the data. However, these classifications are not provided in Variable View by SPSS.

The file **surgery.sav**, which contains the data from 141 babies who underwent surgery at a paediatric hospital, can be opened using the *File → Open → Data* commands. The classification of the variables as shown by SPSS and the classifications that are needed for statistical analysis are shown in Table 1.2.

Table 1.2 Classification of variables in the file surgery.sav

Variable label	Type	SPSS measure	Classification for analysis decisions
ID	Numeric	Scale	Not used in analyses
Gender	String	Nominal	Categorical/non-ordered
Place of birth	String	Nominal	Categorical/non-ordered
Birth weight	Numeric	Scale	Continuous
Gestational age	Numeric	Ordinal	Continuous
Length of stay	Numeric	Scale	Continuous
Infection	Numeric	Scale	Categorical/non-ordered
Prematurity	Numeric	Scale	Categorical/non-ordered
Procedure performed	Numeric	Nominal	Categorical/non-ordered

Obviously, categorical variables have discrete categories, such as male and female, and continuous variables are measured on a scale, such as height which is measured in centimetres. Categorical values can be non-ordered, for example gender which is coded as 1 = male and 2 − female and place of birth which is coded as 1 = local, 2 = regional and 3 = overseas. Categorical variables can also be ordered, for example, if the continuous variable length-of-stay was re-coded into categories of 1 = 1–10 days, 2 = 11–20 days, 3 = 21–30 days and 4 = >31 days, there is a progression in magnitude of length of stay.

Data organisation and data management

Prior to beginning statistical analysis, it is essential to have a thorough working knowledge of the nature, ranges and distributions of each variable. Although it may be tempting to jump straight into the analyses that will answer the study questions rather than spend time obtaining seemingly mundane descriptive statistics, a working knowledge of the data often saves time in the end by avoiding analyses having to be repeated for various reasons.

It is important to have a high standard of data quality in research databases at all times because good data management practice is a hallmark of scientific integrity. The steps outlined in Box 1.2 will help to achieve this.

Box 1.2 Data organisation

The following steps ensure good data management practices:
- Use numeric codes for categorical data where possible
- Choose appropriate variable names and labels to avoid confusion across variables
- Check for duplicate records and implausible data values
- Make corrections
- Archive a back-up copy of the data set for safe keeping
- Limit access to sensitive data such as names and addresses in working files

It is especially important to know the range and distribution of each variable and whether there are any outlying values or outliers so that the statistics that are generated can be explained and interpreted correctly. Describing the characteristics of the sample also allows other researchers to judge the generalisability of the results. A considered pathway for data management is shown in Box 1.3.

Box 1.3 Pathway for data management before beginning statistical analysis

The following steps are essential for efficient data management:
- Obtain the minimum and maximum values and the range of each variable
- Conduct frequency analyses for categorical variables
- Use box plots, histograms and other tests to ascertain normality of continuous variables
- Identify and deal with missing values and outliers
- Re-code or transform variables where necessary
- Re-run frequency and/or distribution checks
- Document all steps in a study handbook

The study handbook should be a formal documentation of all of the study details that is updated continuously with any changes to protocols, management decisions, minutes of meetings, etc. This handbook should be available for anyone in the team to refer to at any time to facilitate considered data collection and data analysis practices. Suggested contents of data analysis log sheets that could be kept in the study handbook are shown in Box 1.4.

Data analyses must be planned and executed in a logical and considered sequence to avoid errors or misinterpretation of results. In this, it is important that data are treated carefully and analysed by people who are familiar with their content, their meaning and the interrelationship between variables.

Box 1.4 Data analysis log sheets

Data analysis log sheets should contain the following information:
- Title of proposed paper, report or abstract
- Author list and author responsible for data analyses and documentation
- Specific research questions to be answered or hypotheses tested
- Outcome and explanatory variables to be used
- Statistical methods
- Details of database location and file storage names
- Journals and/or scientific meetings where results will be presented

---

Before beginning any statistical analyses, a data analysis plan should be agreed upon in consultation with the study team. The plan can include the research questions that will be answered, the outcome and explanatory variables that will be used, the journal where the results will be published and/or the scientific meeting where the findings will be presented.

A good way to handle data analyses is to create a log sheet for each proposed paper, abstract or report. The log sheets should be formal documents that are agreed to by all stakeholders and that are formally archived in the study handbook. When a research team is managed efficiently, a study handbook is maintained that has up to date documentation of all details of the study protocol and the study processes.

Documentation

Documentation of data analyses, which allows anyone to track how the results were obtained from the data set collected, is an important aspect of the scientific process. This is especially important when the data set will be accessed in the future by researchers who are not familiar with all aspects of data collection or the coding and recoding of the variables.

Data management and documentation are relatively mundane processes compared to the excitement of statistical analyses but, nevertheless, are essential. Laboratory researchers document every detail of their work as a matter of course by maintaining accurate laboratory books. All researchers undertaking clinical and epidemiological studies should be equally diligent and document all of the steps taken to reach their conclusions.

Documentation can be easily achieved by maintaining a data management book for each data analysis log sheet. In this, all steps in the data management processes are recorded together with the information of names and contents of files, the coding and names of variables and the results of the statistical analyses. Many funding bodies and ethics committees require that all steps in data analyses are documented and that in addition to archiving the data, both the data sheets and the records are kept for 5 or sometimes 10 years after the results are published.

In SPSS, the file details, variable names, details of coding etc. can be viewed by clicking on Variable View. Documentation of the file details can be obtained and printed using the commands shown in Box 1.5. The output can then be stored in the study handbook or data management log book.

Box 1.5 SPSS commands for printing file information

SPSS Commands
Untitled – SPSS Data Editor
    File → Open Data
        surgery.sav
    Utilities → File Info
Output – SPSS Viewer
    File → Print
    Click OK
    (to view File Info on screen, double click on the output on the RHS and use
        the down arrow key to scroll down)

The following output is produced:

```
                    List of variables on the working file
Name                                                             Position

ID        ID                                                         1
          Measurement Level: Scale
          Column Width: 8   Alignment: Right
          Print Format: F5
          Write Format: F5


GENDER    Gender                                                     2
          Measurement Level: Nominal
          Column Width: 5   Alignment: Left
          Print Format: A5
          Write Format: A5


PLACE     Place of birth                                             3
          Measurement Level: Nominal
          Column Width: 5   Alignment: Left
          Print Format: A5
          Write Format: A5


BIRTHWT   Birth weight                                               4
          Measurement Level: Scale
          Column Width: 8   Alignment: Right
```

```
                 Print Format: F8
                 Write Format: F8

GESTATIO    Gestational age                                          5
            Measurement Level: Ordinal
            Column Width: 8  Alignment: Right
            Print Format: F8.1
            Write Format: F8.1

LENGTHST    Length of stay                                           6
            Measurement Level: Scale
            Column Width: 8  Alignment: Right
            Print Format: F8
            Write Format: F8

INFECT      Infection                                                7
            Measurement Level: Scale
            Column Width: 8  Alignment: Right
            Print Format: F8
            Write Format: F8

            Value     Label

                1     No
                2     Yes

PREMATUR    Prematurity                                              8
            Measurement Level: Scale
            Column Width: 8  Alignment: Right
            Print Format: F8
            Write Format: F8

            Value     Label

                1     Premature
                2     Term

SURGERY     Procedure performed                                      9
            Measurement Level: Nominal
            Column Width: 8  Alignment: Right
            Print Format: F5
            Write Format: F5

            Value     Label

                1     Abdominal
                2     Cardiac
                3     Other
```

This file information can be directly printed from SPSS or exported from the SPSS output viewer into a word processing document using the commands shown in Box 1.6. From a word processing package, the information is easily printed and stored.

> **Box 1.6** SPSS commands for exporting file information into a word document
>
> *SPSS Commands*
> *Output – SPSS Viewer*
>   *Click on 'File Information' on the LHS of the screen*
>   *File → Export*
> *Export Output*
>   *Use Browse to indicate the directory to save the file*
>   *Click on File Type to show Word/RTF file (*.doc)*
>   *Click OK*

Importing data from Excel

Specialised programs are available for transferring data between different data entry and statistics packages (see Useful Web sites). Many researchers use Excel or Access for ease of entering and managing the data. However, statistical analyses are best executed in a specialist statistical package such as SPSS in which the integrity and accuracy of the statistics are guaranteed. Importing data into SPSS from Access is not a problem because Access 'talks' to SPSS so that data can be easily transferred between these programs. However, exporting data from Excel into SPSS requires a few more steps using the commands shown in Box 1.7.

> **Box 1.7** SPSS commands for opening an Excel data file
>
> *SPSS Commands*
> *Untitled – SPSS Data Editor*
>   *File → Open → Data*
> *Open File*
>   *Click on 'Files of type' to show 'Excel (*.xls)'*
>   *Click on your Excel file*
>   *Click Open*
> *Opening Excel Data Source*
>   *Click OK*

The commands shown in Box 1.7 have the disadvantage that they convert numerical fields to string fields and may lose the integrity of any decimal places, etc. The data then have to be reformatted in SPSS, which is feasible for a limited number of variables but is a problem with larger data sets. As an alternative, the commands shown in Box 1.8 will transport data from Excel to SPSS more effectively. These commands take a little longer and require more patience, but the formatting of the data fields and the integrity of the database will be maintained in SPSS. For numeric values, blank cells in Excel or Access are converted to the system missing values, that is a full stop, in SPSS.

Box 1.8 SPSS commands for importing an Excel file

SPSS Commands
Untitled – SPSS Data Editor
    File → Open Database › New Query
Database Wizard
    Highlight Excel Files / Click Add Data Source
ODBC Data Source Administrator - User DSN
    Highlight Excel Files / Click Add
Create New Data Source
    Highlight Microsoft Excel Driver (.xls)*
    Click Finish
ODBC Microsoft Excel Setup
    Enter a new data name in Data Source Name (and description if required)
    Select Workbook
Select Workbook
    Highlight .xls file to import
    Click OK
ODBC Microsoft Excel Setup
    Click OK
ODBC Data Source Administrator - User DSN
    Click OK
Database Wizard
    Highlight new data source name (as entered above) / Click Next
    Click on items in Available Tables on the LHS and drag it across to the
        Retrieve Fields list on the RHS / Click Next / Click Next
    Step 5 of 6 will identify any variable names not accepted by SPSS (if names
        are rejected click on Result Variable Name and change the
        variable name)
    Click Next
    Click Finish

Once in the SPSS spreadsheet, features of the variables can be adjusted in Variable View, for example by changing the width and column length of string variables, entering the labels and values for categorical variables and checking that the number of decimal places is appropriate for each variable. Once data quality is ensured, a back up copy of the database should be archived at a remote site for safety. Few researchers ever need to resort to their archived copies but, when they do, they are an invaluable resource.

The spreadsheet that is used for data analyses should not contain any information that would contravene ethics guidelines by identifying individual participants. In the working data file, names, addresses, dates of birth and any other identifying information that will not be used in data analyses should be removed. Identifying information that is required can be re-coded and de-identified, for example, by using a unique numerical value that is assigned to each participant.

Missing values

Data values that have not been measured in some participants are called missing values. Missing values create pervasive problems in data analyses. The seriousness of the problem depends largely on the pattern of missing data, how much is missing, and why it is missing[2].

Missing values must be treated appropriately in analyses and not inadvertently included as data points. This can be achieved by proper coding that is recognised by the software as a system missing value. The most common character to indicate a missing value is a full stop. This is preferable to using the implausible value of 9 or 999 that has been commonly used in the past. If these values are not accurately defined as missing values, statistical programs can easily incorporate them into the analyses, thus producing erroneous results. Although these values can be predefined as system missing, this is an unnecessary process that is discouraged because it requires familiarity with the coding scheme and because the analyses will be erroneous if the missing values are inadvertently incorporated into the analyses.

For a full stop to be recognised as a system missing value, the variable must be formatted as numeric rather than a string variable. In the spreadsheet **surgery.sav**, the data for place of birth are coded as a string variable. The command sequences shown in Box 1.9 can be used to obtain frequency information of this variable:

Box 1.9 SPSS commands for obtaining frequencies

SPSS Commands
surgery – SPSS Data Editor
        Analyze → Descriptive Statistics→ Frequencies
Frequencies
        Highlight 'Place of birth' and click into Variable(s)
        Click OK

Frequency table

Place of Birth

		Frequency	Per cent	Valid per cent	Cumulative per cent
Valid	.	9	6.4	6.4	6.4
	L	90	63.8	63.8	70.2
	O	9	6.4	6.4	76.6
	R	33	23.4	23.4	100.0
	Total	141	100.0	100.0	

Since place of birth is coded as a string variable, the missing values are treated as valid values and included in the summary statistics of valid and cumulative percentages shown in the Frequency table. To remedy this, the syntax shown in Box 1.10 can be used to re-code place of birth from a string variable into a numeric variable.

Box 1.10 Recoding a variable into a different variable

SPSS Commands
surgery – SPSS Data Editor
      Transform → Recode → Into Different Variables
Recode into Different Variables
      Highlight 'Place of birth' and click into Input Variable → Output Variable
      Enter Output Variable Name as place2,
      Enter Output Variable Label as Place of birth recoded/ Click Change
      Click Old and New Values
Recode into Different Variables: Old and New Values
      Old Value→Value=L, New Value→Value=1/Click Add
      Old Value→Value=R, New Value→Value=2/Click Add
      Old Value→Value=O, New Value→Value=3/Click Add
      Click Continue
Recode into Different Variables
      Click OK (or 'Paste/Run →All')

The paste command is a useful tool to provide automatic documentation of any changes that are made. The paste screen can be saved or printed for documentation and future reference. Using the *Paste* command for the above re-code provides the following documentation.

RECODE

  place

  ('L'=1) ('R'=2) ('O'=3) INTO place2

  VARIABLE LABELS place2 'Place of birth recoded'.

EXECUTE .

After recoding, the value labels for the three new categories of place2 that have been created can be added in the Variable View window. In this case, place of birth needs to be defined as 1 = Local, 2 = Regional and 3 = Overseas. This can be added by clicking on the Values cell and then double clicking on the grey domino box on the right of the cell to add the value labels. Similarly, gender which is also a string variable can be re-coded into a numeric variable, gender2 with Male = 1 and Female = 2. After re-coding variables, it is important to also check whether the number of decimal places is appropriate. For categorical variables, no decimal places are required. For continuous variables, the number of decimal places must be the same as the number that the measurement was collected in.

A useful function in SPSS to repeat recently conducted commands is the *Dialog Recall* button. This button recalls the most recently used SPSS commands conducted. The *Dialog Recall* button is the fourth icon at the top left hand side of the Data View screen or the sixth icon in the top left hand side of the SPSS Output Viewer screen.

Using the *Dialog Recall* button to obtain *Frequencies* for place2, which is labelled Place of birth recoded, the following output is produced.

Frequencies

Place of Birth Recoded

		Frequency	Per cent	Valid per cent	Cumulative per cent
Valid	Local	90	63.8	68.2	68.2
	Regional	33	23.4	25.0	93.2
	Overseas	9	6.4	6.8	100.0
	Total	132	93.6	100.0	
Missing	System	9	6.4		
Total		141	100.0		

The frequencies in the table show that the recoding sequence was executed correctly. When the data are re-coded as numeric, the nine babies who have missing data for birthplace are correctly omitted from the valid and cumulative percentages.

When collecting data in any study, it is essential to have methods in place to prevent missing values in, say, at least 95% of the data set. Methods such as restructuring questionnaires in which participants decline to provide sensitive information or training research staff to check that all fields are complete at the point of data collection are invaluable in this process. In large epidemiological and longitudinal data sets, some missing data may be unavoidable. However, in clinical trials it may be unethical to collect insufficient information about some participants so that they have to be excluded from the final analyses.

If the number of missing values is small and the missing values occur randomly throughout the data set, the cases with missing values can be omitted from the analyses. This is the default option in most statistical packages and the main effect of this process is to reduce statistical power, that is the ability to show a statistically significant difference between groups when a clinically important difference exists. Missing values that are scattered randomly throughout the data are less of a problem than non-random missing values that can affect both the power of the study and the generalisability of the results. For example, if people in higher income groups selectively decline to answer questions about income, the distribution of income in the population will not be known and analyses that include income will not be generalisable to people in higher income groups.

In some situations, it may be important to replace a missing value with an estimated value that can be included in analyses. In longitudinal clinical trials, it has become common practice to use the last score obtained from the participant and carry it forward for all subsequent missing values. In other studies, a mean value (if the variable is normally distributed) or a median value (if the variable is non-normal distributed) may be used to replace missing values. These solutions are not ideal but are pragmatic in that they maintain the study power whilst reducing any bias in the summary statistics. Other more complicated methods for replacing missing values have been described[2].

Outliers

Outliers are data values that are surprisingly extreme when compared to the other values in the data set. There are two types of outliers: univariate outliers and multivariate outliers. A univariate outlier is a data point that is very different to the rest of the data for one variable. An outlier is measured by the distance from the remainder of the data in units of the standard deviation, which is a standardised measure of the spread of the data. For example, an IQ score of 150 would be a univariate outlier because the mean IQ of the population is 100 with a standard deviation of 15. Thus, an IQ score of 150 is 3.3 standard deviations away from the mean whereas the next closest value may be only 2 standard deviations away from the mean leaving a gap in the distribution of the data points.

A multivariate outlier is a case that is an extreme value on a combination of variables. For example, a boy aged 8 years with a height of 155 cm and a weight of 45 kg is very unusual and would be a multivariate outlier. It is important to identify values that are univariate and/or multivariate outliers because they can have a substantial influence on the distribution and mean of the variable and can influence the results of analyses and thus the interpretation of the findings.

Univariate outliers are easier to identify than multivariate outliers. For a continuously distributed variable with a normal distribution, about 99% of scores are expected to lie within 3 standard deviations above and below the mean value. Data points outside this range are classified as univariate outliers. Sometimes a case that is a univariate outlier for one variable will also be a univariate outlier for another variable. Potentially, these cases may be multivariate outliers. Multivariate outliers can be detected using statistics called leverage values or Cook's distances, which are discussed in Chapter 5, or Mahalanobis distances, which are discussed in Chapter 6.

There are many reasons why outliers occur. Outliers may be errors in data recording, incorrect data entry values that can be corrected or genuine values. When outliers are from participants from another population with different characteristics to the intended sample, they are called contaminants. This happens for example when a participant with a well-defined illness is inadvertently included as a healthy participant. Occasionally, outliers can be excluded from the data analyses on the grounds that they are contaminants or biologically implausible values. However, deleting values simply because they are outliers is usually unacceptable and it is preferable to find a way to accommodate the values without causing undue bias in the analyses.

Identifying and dealing with outliers is discussed further throughout this book. Whatever methods are used to accommodate outliers, it is important that they are reported so that the methods used and the generalisability of the results are clear.

Choosing the correct test

Selecting the correct test to analyse data depends not only on the study design but also on the nature of the variables collected. Tables 1.3–1.6 show the types of tests that can be selected based on the nature of variables. It is of paramount importance that the correct test is used to generate P values and to estimate the size of effect. Using an incorrect test will inviolate the statistical assumptions of the test and may lead to bias in the P values.

Table 1.3 Choosing a statistic when there is one outcome variable only

Type of variable	Number of times measured in each participant	Statistic	SPSS menu
Binary	Once	Incidence or prevalence and 95% confidence interval (95% CI)	Descriptive statistics; Frequencies
	Twice	McNemar's chi-square Kappa	Descriptive statistics; Crosstabs
Continuous	Once	Tests for normality	Non-parametric tests; 1 sample K-S Descriptive statistics; Explore
		One sample t-test	Compare means; One-sample t-test
		Mean, standard deviation (SD) and 95% CI	Descriptive statistics; Explore
		Median and inter-quartile (IQ) range	Descriptive statistics; Explore
	Twice	Paired t-test	Compare means; Paired-samples t-test
		Mean difference and 95% CI	Compare means; Paired-samples t-test
		Measurement error	Compare means; Paired-samples t-test
		Mean-versus-differences plot	Graphs; Scatter
		Intraclass correlation coefficient	Scale; Reliability Analysis
	Three or more	Repeated measures ANOVA	General linear model; Repeated measures

Table 1.4 Choosing a statistic when there is one outcome variable and one explanatory variable

Type of outcome variable	Type of explanatory variable	Number of levels of the categorical variable	Statistic	SPSS menu
Categorical	Categorical	Both variables are binary	Chi-square Odds ratio or relative risk Logistic regression Sensitivity and specificity Likelihood ratio	Descriptive statistics; Crosstabs Descriptive statistics; Crosstabs Regression; Binary logistic Descriptive statistics; Crosstabs Descriptive statistics; Crosstabs
Categorical	Categorical	At least one of the variables has more than two levels	Chi-square Chi-square trend Kendall's correlation	Descriptive statistics; Crosstabs Descriptive statistics; Crosstabs Correlate; Bivariate
Categorical	Continuous	Categorical variable is binary	ROC curve Survival analyses	Graphs; ROC curve Survival; Kaplan-Meier
Categorical	Continuous	Categorical variable is multi-level and ordered	Spearman's correlation coefficient	Correlate; Bivariate
Continuous	Categorical	Explanatory variable is binary	Independent samples t-test Mean difference and 95% CI	Compare means; Independent-samples t-test Compare means; Independent-samples t-test
Continuous	Categorical	Explanatory variable has three or more categories	Analysis of variance	Compare means; One-way ANOVA
Continuous	Continuous	No categorical variables	Regression Pearson's correlation	Regression; Linear Correlate; Bivariate

Table 1.5 Choosing a statistic for one or more outcome variables and more than one explanatory variable

Type of outcome variable/s	Type of explanatory variable/s	Number of levels of categorical variable	Statistic	SPSS menu
Continuous—only one outcome	Both continuous and categorical	Categorical variables are binary	Multiple regression	Regression; Linear
Continuous—only one outcome	Categorical	At least one of the explanatory variables has three or more categories	Two-way analysis of variance	General linear model; Univariate
Continuous—only one outcome	Both continuous and categorical	One categorical variable has two or more levels	Analysis of covariance	General linear model; Univariate
Continuous—outcome measured more than once	Both continuous and categorical	Categorical variables can have two or more levels	Repeated measures analysis of variance Auto-regression	General linear model; Repeated measures Times series; Auto-regression
No outcome variable	Both continuous and categorical	Categorical variables can have two or more levels	Factor analysis	Data reduction: Factor

Table 1.6 Parametric and non-parametric equivalents

Parametric test	Non-parametric equivalent	SPSS menu
Mean and standard deviation	Median and inter-quartile range	Descriptive statistics; Explore
Pearson's correlation coefficient	Spearman's or Kendall's correlation coefficient	Correlate; Bivariate
One sample sign test	Sign test	SPSS does not provide this option but a sign test can be obtained by computing a new constant variable equal to the test value (e.g. 0 or 100) and using non-parametric test; 2 related samples with the outcome and computed variable as the pair
Two sample t-test	Wilcoxon rank sum test	Non parametric tests; 2 related samples
Independent t-test	Mann-Whitney U or Wilcoxon Rank Sum test	Non-parametric tests; 2 independent samples
Analysis of variance	Mann-Whitney U test	Non-parametric tests; K independent samples
Repeated measures analysis of variance	Friedmans ANOVA test	Nonparametric tests; K independent samples

Sample size requirements

The sample size is one of the most critical issues in designing a research study because it affects all aspects of interpreting the results. The sample size needs to be large enough so that a definitive answer to the research question is obtained. This will help to ensure generalisability of the results and precision around estimates of effect. However, the sample has to be small enough so that the study is practical to conduct. In general, studies with a small sample size, say with less than 30 participants, can usually only provide imprecise and unreliable estimates.

Box 1.11 provides a definition of type I and type II errors and shows how the size of the sample can contribute to these errors, both of which have a profound influence on the interpretation of the results.

In each chapter of this book, the implications of interpreting the results in terms of the sample size of the data set and the possibilities of type I and type II errors in the results will be discussed.

Golden rules for reporting numbers

Throughout this book the results are presented using the rules that are recommended for reporting statistical analyses in the literature[3–5]. Numbers are usually presented as digits except in a few special circumstances as indicated

Box 1.11 Type I and type II errors

Type I errors
- are false positive results
- occur when a statistical significant difference between groups is found but no clinically important difference exists
- the null hypothesis is rejected in error

Type II errors
- are false negative results
- a clinical important difference between groups does exist but does not reach statistical significance
- the null hypothesis is accepted in error
- usually occur when the sample size is small

in Table 1.7. When reporting data, it is important not to imply more precision than actually exists, for example by using too many decimal places. Results should be reported with the same number of decimal places as the measurement, and summary statistics should have no more than one extra decimal place. A summary of the rules for reporting numbers and summary statistics is shown in Table 1.7.

Table 1.7 Golden rules for reporting numbers

Rule	Correct expression
In a sentence, numbers less than 10 are words	In the study group, eight participants did not complete the intervention
In a sentence, numbers 10 or more are numbers	There were 120 participants in the study
Use words to express any number that begins a sentence, title or heading. Try and avoid starting a sentence with a number	Twenty per cent of participants had diabetes
Numbers that represent statistical or mathematical functions should be expressed in numbers	Raw scores were multiplied by 3 and then converted to standard scores
In a sentence, numbers below 10 that are listed with numbers 10 and above should be written as a number	In the sample, 15 boys and 4 girls had diabetes
Use a zero before the decimal point when numbers are less than 1	The P value was 0.013

Continued

Rule	Correct expression
Do not use a space between a number and its per cent sign	In total, 35% of participants had diabetes
Use one space between a number and its unit	The mean height of the group was 170 cm
Report percentages to only one decimal place if the sample size is larger than 100	In the sample of 212 children, 10.4% had diabetes
Report percentages with no decimal places if the sample size is less than 100	In the sample of 44 children, 11% had diabetes
Do not use percentages if the sample size is less than 20	In the sample of 18 children, 2 had diabetes
Do not imply greater precision than the measurement instrument	Only use one decimal place more than the basic unit of measurement when reporting statistics (means, medians, standard deviations, 95% confidence interval, inter-quartile ranges, etc.) e.g. mean height was 143.2 cm
For ranges use 'to' or a comma but not '-' to avoid confusion with a minus sign. Also use the same number of decimal places as the summary statistic	The mean height was 162 cm (95% CI 156 to 168) The mean height was 162 cm (95% CI 156, 168) The median was 0.5 mm (inter-quartile range −0.1 to 0.7) The range of height was 145 to 170 cm
P values between 0.001 and 0.05 should be reported to three decimal places	There was a significant difference in blood pressure between the two groups ($t = 3.0$, $df = 45$, $P = 0.004$)
P values shown on output as 0.000 should be reported as <0.0001	Children with diabetes had significantly lower levels of insulin than control children without diabetes ($t = 5.47$, $df = 78$, $P < 0.0001$)

Formatting the output

There are many output formats available in SPSS. The format of the frequencies table obtained previously can easily be changed by double clicking on the table and using the commands *Format → TableLooks*. To obtain the output in the format below, which is a classical academic format with no vertical lines and minimal horizontal lines that is used by many journals, highlight Academic 2 under *TableLooks Files* and click OK. The column widths and other features can also be changed using the commands *Format → Table Properties*. By clicking on the table and using the commands *Edit → Copy objects*, the table can be copied and pasted into a word file.

Place of Birth Recoded

		Frequency	Per cent	Valid per cent	Cumulative per cent
Valid	Local	90	63.8	68.2	68.2
	Regional	33	23.4	25.0	93.2
	Overseas	9	6.4	6.8	100.0
	Total	132	93.6	100.0	
Missing	System	9	6.4		
Total		141	100.0		

SPSS help commands

SPSS has two levels of extensive help commands. By using the commands *Help → Topics → Index*, the index of help topics appears in alphabetical order. By typing in a keyword, followed by enter, a topic can be displayed. Listed under the Help command is also Tutorial, which is a guide to using SPSS, and Statistics Coach, which is a guide to selecting the correct test to use.

There is also another level of help that explains the meaning of the statistics shown in the output. For example, help can be obtained for the above frequencies table by doubling clicking on the left hand mouse button to outline the table with a hatched border and then single clicking on the right hand mouse button on any of the statistics labels. This produces a dialog box with *What's This?* at the top. Clicking on *What's This?* provides an explanation of the highlighted statistical term. Clicking on *Cumulative Percent* gives the explanation that this statistic is the per cent of cases with non-missing data that have values less than or equal to a particular value.

Notes for critical appraisal

When critically appraising statistical analyses reported in the literature, that is when applying the rules of science to assess the validity of the results from a study, it is important to ask the questions shown in Box 1.12. Studies in which

Box 1.12 Questions for critical appraisal

Answers to the following questions are useful for checking the integrity of statistical analyses:
- Have details of the methods and statistical packages used to analyse the data been reported?
- Are the variables classified correctly as outcome and explanatory variables?
- Are any intervening or alternative outcome variables mistakenly treated as explanatory variables?
- Are missing values and outliers treated appropriately?
- Is the sample size large enough to avoid type II errors?

outliers are treated inappropriately, in which the quality of the data is poor or in which an incorrect statistical test has been used are likely to be biased and to lack scientific merit.

References

1. Peat JK, Mellis CM, Williams K, Xuan W. Confounders and effect modifiers. In: Health science research. A handbook of quantitative methods. Crows Nest, Australia: Allen and Unwin, 2001; pp 90–104.
2. Tabachnick BG, Fidell LS. Missing data. In: Using multivariate statistics (4th edition). Boston, MA: Allyn and Bacon, 2001; pp 58–65.
3. Stevens J. Applied multivariate statistics for the social sciences (3rd edition). Mahwah, NJ: Lawrence Erlbaum Associates, 1996; p. 17.
4. Peat JK, Elliott E, Baur L, Keena V. Scientific writing: easy when you know how. London: BMJ Books, 2002; pp 74–76
5. Lang TA, Secic M. Rules for presenting numbers in text. In: How to report statistics. Philadelphia, PA: American College of Physicians, 1977; p. 339.

CHAPTER 2

Continuous variables: descriptive statistics

It is wonderful to be in on the creation of something, see it used, and then walk away and smile at it.

LADY BIRD JOHNSON, U.S. FIRST LADY

Objectives

The objectives of this chapter are to explain how to:
- test whether a continuous variable has a normal distribution
- decide whether to use a parametric or non-parametric test
- present summary statistics for continuous variables
- decide whether parametric tests have been used appropriately in the literature

---

Before beginning statistical analyses of a continuous variable, it is essential to examine the distribution of the variable for skewness (tails), kurtosis (peaked or flat distribution), spread (range of the values) and outliers (data values separated from the rest of the data). If a variable has significant skewness or kurtosis or has univariate outliers, or any combination of these, it will not be normally distributed. Information about each of these characteristics determines whether parametric or non-parametric tests need to be used and ensures that the results of the statistical analyses can be accurately explained and interpreted. A description of the characteristics of the sample also allows other researchers to judge the generalisability of the results. A typical pathway for beginning the statistical analysis of continuous data variables is shown in Box 2.1.

Box 2.1 Data analysis pathway for continuous variables

The pathway for conducting the data analysis of continuous variables is as follows:
- conduct distribution checks
- transform variables with non-normal distributions or re-code into categorical variables, for example quartiles or quintiles
- re-run distribution checks for transformed variables
- document all steps in the study handbook

Statistical tests can be either parametric or non-parametric. Parametric tests are commonly used when a continuous variable is normally distributed. In general, parametric tests are preferable to non-parametric tests because a larger variety of tests are available and, as long as the sample size is not very small, they provide approximately 5% more power than rank tests to show a statistically significant difference between groups[1]. Non-parametric tests can be a challenge to present in a clear and meaningful way because summary statistics such as ranks are less familiar to many people than summary statistics from parametric tests. Summary statistics from parametric tests such as means and standard deviations are always more readily understood and more easily communicated than the equivalent rank statistics from non-parametric tests.

The pathway for the analysis of continuous variables is shown in Figure 2.1.

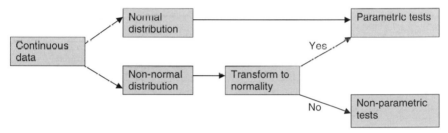

Figure 2.1 Pathway for the analysis of continuous variables.

Skewness, kurtosis and outliers can all distort a normal distribution. If a variable has a skewed distribution, it is sometimes possible to transform the variable to normality using a mathematical algorithm so that the outliers in the tail do not bias the summary statistics and P values, or the variable can be analysed using non-parametric tests.

If the sample size is small, say less than 30, outliers in the tail of a skewed distribution can markedly increase or decrease the mean value so that it no longer represents the centre of the data. If the estimate of the centre of the data is inaccurate, then the mean values of two groups will look more alike or more different than the central values actually are and the P value to estimate their difference will be correspondingly reduced or increased. It is important to avoid this type of bias.

Exploratory analyses

The file **surgery.sav** contains data from 141 babies who were referred to a paediatric hospital for surgery. The distributions of three continuous variables in the data set that is birth weight, gestational age and length of stay can be examined using the commands shown in Box 2.2.

Box 2.2 SPSS commands to obtain descriptive statistics and plots

SPSS Commands
surgery – SPSS Data Editor
        Analyze → Descriptive Statistics → Explore
Explore
        Highlight variables Birth weight, Gestational age, and Length of stay and
            click into Dependent List
Explore
        Click on Statistics
Explore: Statistics
        Click on Outliers
        Click Continue
Explore
        Click on Plots
Explore: Plots
        Boxplots – Factor levels together (default)
        Descriptive – untick Stem and leaf (default), tick Histogram and tick
            Normality plots with tests
        Click Continue
Explore
        Click on Options
Explore: Options
        Missing Values – tick Exclude cases pairwise
        Click Continue
Explore
        Click OK

In the Options menu in Box 2.2, *Exclude cases pairwise* is selected. This option provides information about each variable independently of missing values in the other variables and is the option that is used to describe the entire sample. The default setting for Options is *Exclude cases listwise* but this will exclude a case from the data analysis if there is missing data for any one of the variables entered into the *Dependent List*. The option *Exclude cases listwise* for the data set **surgery.sav** would show that there are 126 babies with complete information for all three continuous variables and 15 babies with missing information for one or more of the three variables. The information for these 126 babies would be important for describing the sample if multivariate statistics that only includes babies without missing data are planned. The characteristics of these 126 babies would be used to describe the generalisability of a multivariate model but not the generalisability of the sample.

Explore

Case Processing Summary

	Cases					
	Valid		Missing		Total	
	N	Per cent	*N*	Per cent	*N*	Per cent
Birth weight	139	98.6%	2	1.4%	141	100.0%
Gestational age	133	94.3%	8	5.7%	141	100.0%
Length of stay	132	93.6%	9	6.4%	141	100.0%

The Case Processing Summary table shows that two babies have missing birth weights, eight babies have missing gestational age and nine babies have missing length of stay data. This information is important if bivariate statistics will be used in which as many cases as possible are included. The Descriptives table shows the summary statistics for each variable. In the table, all statistics are in the same units as the original variables, that is in grams for birth weight, weeks for gestational age and days for length of stay. The exceptions are the variance, which is in squared units, and the skewness and kurtosis values, which are in units that are relative to a normal distribution.

Descriptives

			Statistic	Std. error
Birth weight	Mean		2463.99	43.650
	95% confidence	Lower bound	2377.68	
	interval for mean	Upper bound	2550.30	
	5% trimmed mean		2452.53	
	Median		2425.00	
	Variance		264845.7	
	Std. deviation		514.632	
	Minimum		1150	
	Maximum		3900	
	Range		2750	
	Inter-quartile range		755.00	
	Skewness		0.336	0.206
	Kurtosis		−0.323	0.408
Gestational age	Mean		36.564	0.1776
	95% confidence	Lower bound	36.213	
	interval for mean	Upper bound	36.915	
	5% trimmed mean		36.659	
	Median		37.000	

Continued

Descriptives (*Continued*)

			Statistic	Std. error
	Variance		4.195	
	Std. deviation		2.0481	
	Minimum		30.0	
	Maximum		41.0	
	Range		11.0	
	Inter-quartile range		2.000	
	Skewness		−0.590	0.210
	Kurtosis		0.862	0.417
Length of stay	Mean		38.05	3.114
	95% confidence	Lower bound	31.89	
	interval for mean	Upper bound	44.21	
	5% trimmed mean		32.79	
	Median		27.00	
	Variance		1280.249	
	Std. deviation		35.781	
	Minimum		0	
	Maximum		244	
	Range		244	
	Inter-quartile range		21.75	
	Skewness		3.212	0.211
	Kurtosis		12.675	0.419

Normal distribution

A normal distribution such as the distribution shown in Figure 2.2 is classically a bell shaped curve, that is bilaterally symmetrical. If a variable is normally distributed, then the mean and the median values will be approximately equal.

If a normal distribution is divided into quartiles, that is four equal parts, the exact position of the cut-off values for the quartiles is at 0.68 standard deviation above and below the mean. Other features of a normal distribution are that the area of one standard deviation on either side of the mean as shown in Figure 2.2 contains 68% of the values in the sample and the area of 1.96 standard deviations on either side of the mean contains 95% of the values. These properties of a normal distribution are critical for understanding and interpreting the output from parametric tests.

If a variable has a skewed distribution, the mean will be a biased estimate of the centre of the data as shown in Figure 2.3. A variable that has a classically skewed distribution is length of stay in hospital because many patients have a short stay and few patients have a very long stay. When a variable has a skewed distribution, it can be difficult to predict where the centre of the data lies or the range in which the majority of data values fall.

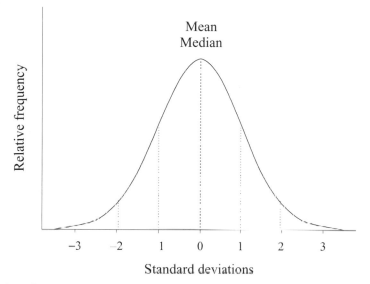

Figure 2.2 Characteristics of a normal distribution.

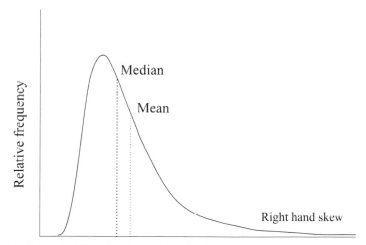

Figure 2.3 Characteristics of a skewed distribution.

For a variable that has a positively skewed distribution with a tail to the right, the mean will usually be larger than the median as shown in Figure 2.3. For a variable with a negatively skewed distribution with a tail to the left, the mean will usually be lower than the median because the distribution will be a mirror image of the curve shown in Figure 2.3. These features of non-normal distributions are helpful in estimating the direction of bias in critical appraisal of studies in which the distribution of the variable has not been taken into account when selecting the statistical tests.

There are several ways of testing whether a continuous variable is normally distributed. Many measurements such as height, weight and blood pressure may be normally distributed in the community but may not be normally distributed if the study has a selected sample or a small sample size. In practice, several checks of normality need to be undertaken to gain a good understanding of the shape of the distribution of each variable in the study sample. It is also important to identify the position of any outliers to gain an understanding of how they may influence the results of any statistical analyses.

The proximity of the mean to the median can indicate possible skewness. A quick informal check of normality is to examine whether the mean and the median values are close to one another. From the Descriptives table, the differences between the median and the mean can be summarised as shown in Table 2.1. The per cent difference is calculated as the difference between the mean and the median as a percentage of the mean.

Table 2.1 Comparisons between mean and median values

Variable	Mean – median	Per cent difference	Interpretation
Birth weight	2464.0 – 2425.0 = 39.0 g	1.5%	Values almost identical, suggesting a normal distribution
Gestational age	36.6 – 37.0 = –0.4 month	1.1%	Values almost identical, suggesting a normal distribution
Length of stay	38.1 – 27.0 = 11.1 days	29.1%	Discordant values, with the mean higher than the median indicating skewness to the right

In Table 2.1, the differences between the mean and median values of birth weight and gestational age are small, suggesting a normal distribution but the large difference between the mean and median values for length of stay suggests that this variable has a non-normal distribution.

An inherent feature of a normal distribution is that 95% of the data values lie between -1.96 standard deviation and $+1.96$ standard deviations from the mean as shown in Figure 2.2. That is, most data values should lie in the area that is approximately two standard deviations from the mean. Thus, a good approximate check for normality is to double the standard deviation of the variable and then subtract and also add this amount to the mean value. This will give an estimated range in which 95% of the values should lie. The estimated range should be slightly within the actual range of data values, that is the minimum and maximum values. The estimated 95% range for each variable is shown in Table 2.2.

For birth weight and gestational age, the estimated 95% range is within or close to the minimum and maximum values from the Descriptives table. However, for length of stay, the estimated 95% range is not a good approximation

Table 2.2 Calculation of 95% range of variables

Variable	Calculation of range (mean ± 2 SD)	Estimated 95% range	Minimum and maximum values
Birth weight	2464 ± (2 × 514.6)	1434 to 3494	1150 to 3900
Gestational age	36.6 ± (2 × 2.0)	32.6 to 40.6	30.0 to 41.0
Length of stay	38.1 ± (2 × 35.8)	−33.5 to 109.7	0 to 244

of the actual range because the estimated lower value is invalid because it is negative and the estimated upper value is significantly below the maximum value. This is a classical indication of a skewed distribution. If the two estimated values are much less than the actual minimum and maximum values, as in this case, the distribution is usually skewed to the right. If the two estimated values are much higher than the actual minimum and maximum values, the distribution is usually skewed to the left.

A rule of thumb is that a variable with a standard deviation that is larger than one half of the mean value is non-normally distributed, assuming that negative values are impossible[2]. Thus, the mean length of stay of 38.1 days with a standard deviation almost equal to its mean value is an immediate alert to evidence of non-normality.

Skewness and kurtosis

Further information about the distribution of the variables can be obtained from the skewness and kurtosis statistics in the Descriptives table. In SPSS, a perfectly normal distribution has skewness and kurtosis values equal to zero. Skewness values that are positive indicate a tail to the right and skewness values that are negative indicate a tail to the left. Values between −1 and +1 indicate an approximate bell shaped curve and values from −1 to −3 or from +1 to +3 indicate that the distribution is tending away from a bell shape. Any values above +3 or below −3 are a good indication that the variable is not normally distributed.

The Descriptives table shows that the skewness values for birth weight and gestational age are between −1 and 1 suggesting that the distributions of these variables are within the limits of a normal distribution. However, the high skewness value of 3.212 for length of stay confirms a non-normal distribution with a tail to the right.

A kurtosis value above 1 indicates that the distribution tends to be pointed and a value below 1 indicates that the distribution tends to be flat. As for skewness, a kurtosis value between −1 and +1 indicates normality and a value between −1 and −3 or between +1 and +3 indicates a tendency away from normality. Values below −3 or above +3 indicate certain non-normality. For birth weight and gestational age, the kurtosis values are small and are not a cause for concern. However, for length of stay the kurtosis value is 12.675, which indicates that the distribution is peaked in a way that is not consistent with a bell shaped distribution.

Further tests of normality are to divide skewness and kurtosis values by their standard errors as shown in Table 2.3. In practice, dividing a value by its standard error produces a critical value that can be used to judge probability. A critical value that is outside the range of -1.96 to $+1.96$ indicates that a variable is not normally distributed. The critical values in Table 2.3 confirm that birth weight has a normal distribution with critical values for both skewness and kurtosis below 1.96 and gestational age is deviating from a normal distribution with values outside the critical range of ±1.96. Length of stay is certainly not normally distributed with large critical values of 15.22 and 30.25.

Table 2.3 Using skewness and kurtosis statistics to test for a normal distribution

	Skewness (SE)	Critical value (skewness/SE)	Kurtosis (SE)	Critical value (kurtosis/SE)
Birth weight	0.336 (0.206)	1.63	−0.323 (0.408)	−0.79
Gestational age	−0.590 (0.210)	−2.81	0.862 (0.417)	2.07
Length of stay	3.212 (0.211)	15.22	12.675 (0.419)	30.25

Extreme values and outliers

By requesting outliers in *Analyze* → *Descriptive Statistics* → *Explore*, the five largest and five smallest values of each variable and the case numbers or data base rows are shown in the Extreme Values table. Outliers and extreme values that cause skewness must be identified. However, the values printed in the Extreme Values table are the minimum and maximum values in the data set and these may not be influential outliers.

Extreme Values

			Case number	Value
Birth weight	Highest	1	5	3900
		2	54	3545
		3	16	3500
		4	50	3500
		5	141	3500
	Lowest	1	4	1150
		2	103	1500
		3	120	1620
		4	98	1680
		5	38	1710

Continued

			Case number	Value
Gestational age	Highest	1	85	41.0
		2	11	40.0
		3	26	40.0
		4	50	40.0
		5	52	40.0[a]
	Lowest	1	2	30.0
		2	79	31.0
		3	38	31.0
		4	4	31.0
		5	117	31.5
Length of stay	Highest	1	121	244
		2	120	211
		3	110	153
		4	129	138
		5	116	131
	Lowest	1	32	0
		2	33	1
		3	12	9
		4	22	11
		5	16	11

[a] Only a partial list of cases with the value 40.0 are shown in the table of upper extremes.

Statistical tests of normality

By requesting normality plots in *Analyze → Descriptive Statistics → Explore*, the following tests of normality are obtained:

Tests of Normality

	Kolmogorov–Smirnov[a]			Shapiro–Wilk		
	Statistic	*df*	Sig.	Statistic	*df*	Sig.
Birth weight	0.067	139	0.200*	0.981	139	0.056
Gestational age	0.151	133	0.000	0.951	133	0.000
Length of stay	0.241	132	0.000	0.643	132	0.000

*This is a lower bound of the true significance.
[a] Lilliefors significance correction.

The Tests of Normality table provides the results of two tests: a Kolmogorov–Smirnov statistic with a Lilliefors significance correction and a Shapiro–Wilk statistic. A limitation of the Kolmogorov–Smirnov test of normality without the Lilliefors correction is that it is very conservative and is sensitive to extreme values that cause tails in the distribution. The Lilliefors significance correction renders this test a little less conservative. The Shapiro–Wilk test has more statistical power to determine a non-normal distribution than the Kolmogorov–Smirnov test[3]. The Shapiro–Wilk test is based on the correlation between the data and the corresponding normal scores and will have a value of 1.0 for perfect normality.

A distribution that passes these tests of normality provides extreme confidence that parametric tests can be used. However, variables that do not pass these tests may not be so non-normally distributed that parametric tests cannot be used, especially if the sample size is large. This is not to say that the results of these tests can be ignored but rather that a considered decision using the results of all the available tests of normality needs to be made.

For both the Shapiro–Wilk and Kolmogorov–Smirnov tests, a P value less than 0.05 indicates that the distribution is significantly different from normal. The P values are shown in the column labelled Sig. in the Tests of Normality table. Birth weight marginally fails the Shapiro–Wilk test but the P values for gestational age and length of stay show that they have potentially non-normal distributions. The Kolmogorov–Smirnov test shows that the distribution of birth weight is not significantly different from a normal distribution with a P value greater than 0.2. However, the Kolmogorov–Smirnov test indicates that the distributions of both gestational age and length of stay are significantly different from a normal distribution at $P < 0.0001$.

These tests of normality do not provide any information about why a variable is not normally distributed and therefore, it is always important to obtain skewness and kurtosis values using *Analyze → Descriptive Statistics → Explore* and to request plots in order to identify any reasons for non-normality.

Normality plots

Finally, from the commands in Box 2.2, descriptive and normality plots were requested for each variable. All of the plots should be inspected because each plot gives very different information.

The histograms show the frequency of measurements and the shape of the data and therefore provide a visual judgement of whether the distribution approximates to a bell shape. Histograms also show whether there are any gaps in the data, whether there are any outlying values and how far any outlying values are from the remainder of the data.

The normal Q–Q plot shows each data value plotted against the value that would be expected if the data came from a normal distribution. The values in the plot are the quantiles of the variable distribution plotted against the quantiles that would be expected if the distribution was normal. If the variable was normally distributed, the points would fall directly on the straight line. Any deviations from the straight line indicate some degree of non-normality.

The detrended normal Q–Q plots show the deviations of the points from the straight line of the normal Q–Q plot. If the distribution is normal, the points will cluster randomly around the horizontal line at zero with an equal spread of points above and below the line. If the distribution is non-normal, the points will be in a pattern such as J or an inverted U distribution and the horizontal line may not be in the centre of the data.

The box plot shows the median as the black horizontal line inside the box and the inter-quartile range as the length of the box. The inter-quartile range indicates the 25th to 75th percentiles, that is the range in which the central 25% to 75% of the data points lie. The whiskers are the lines extending from the top and bottom of the box. The whiskers represent the minimum and maximum values when they are within 1.5 times above or below the inter-quartile range. If values are outside this range, they are plotted as outlying or extreme values.

Any outlying values that are between 1.5 and 3 box lengths from the upper or lower edge of the box are shown as open circles, and are identified with the corresponding number of the data base row. Extreme values that are more than three box lengths from the upper or lower edge of the box are shown as asterisks. Extreme and/or outlying values should be checked to see whether they are univariate outliers (Chapter 3). If there are several extreme values at either end of the range of the data or the median is not in the centre of the box, the variable will not be normally distributed. If the median is closer to the bottom end of the box than to the top, the data are positively skewed. If the median is closer to the top end of the box, the data are negatively skewed.

In Figure 2.4 the histogram for birth weight shows that this distribution is not strictly bell shaped but the normal Q–Q plot follows an approximately normal distribution apart from the tails, and the box plot is symmetrical with no outlying or extreme values. These features indicate that the mean value will be an accurate estimate of the centre of the data and that the standard deviation will accurately describe the spread.

In Figure 2.5 the histogram for gestational age shows that this distribution has a small tail to the left and only deviates from normal at the lower end of the normal Q–Q plot. The box plot for this variable appears to be symmetrical but has a few outlying values and one extreme value at the lower end of the data values.

In contrast, in Figure 2.6 the histogram for length of stay has a marked tail to the right so that the distribution deviates markedly from a straight line on the normal Q–Q plot. On the detrended normal Q–Q plot, the pattern is similar to a U shape. The box plot shows many outlying values and multiple extreme values at the upper end of the distribution. Some of the outlying and extreme values overlap each other so that it is difficult to identify the cases. By double clicking on the box plot, the plot will be enlarged in the *Chart Editor* and the case numbers can be seen more clearly. By clicking on the case numbers, the display option can be altered so that the outliers and/or extreme values can be identified by their ID or case number.

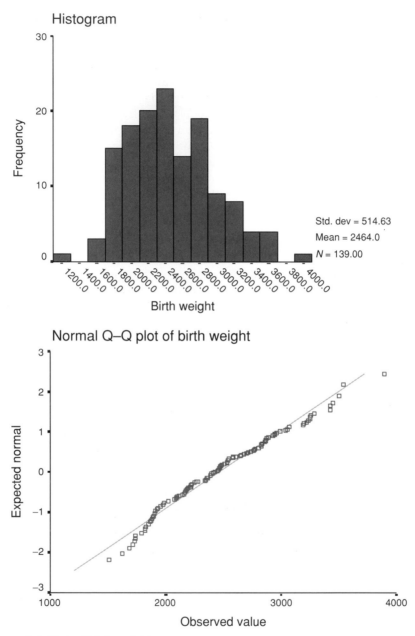

Figure 2.4 Plots of birth weight.

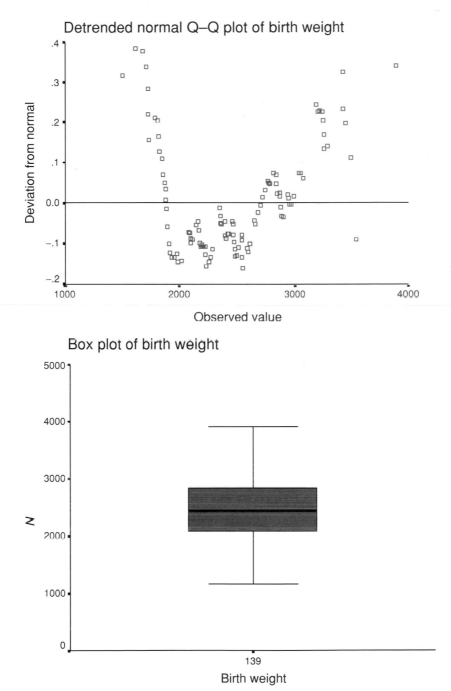

Figure 2.4 *Continued*

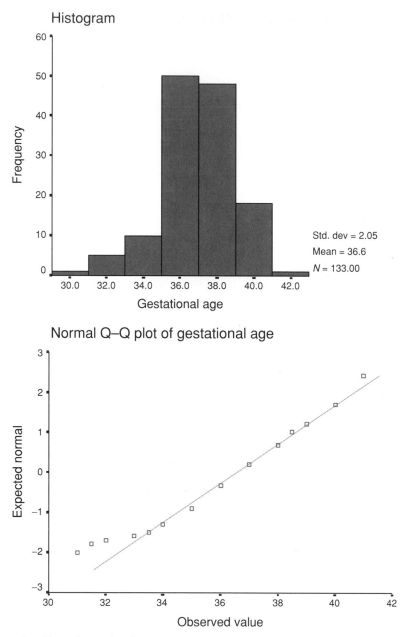

Figure 2.5 Plots of gestational age.

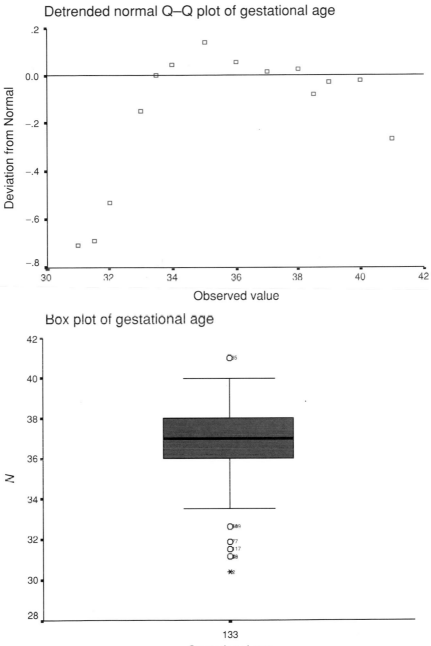

Figure 2.5 *Continued*

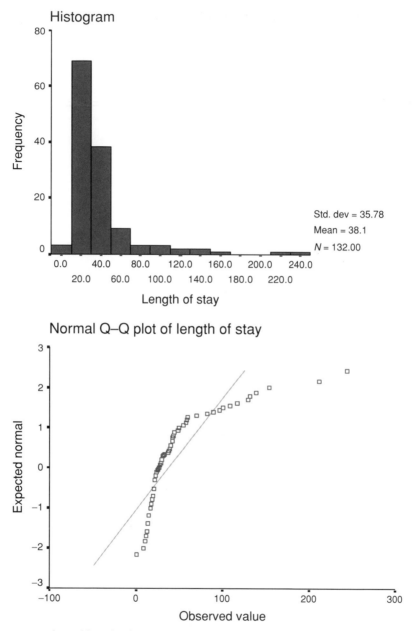

Figure 2.6 Plots of length of stay.

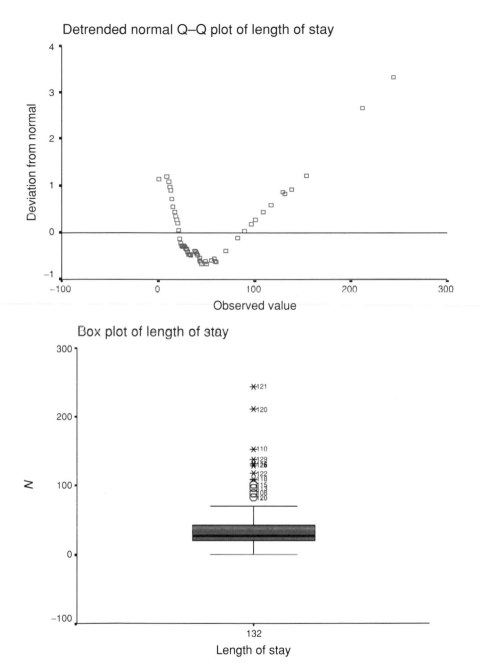

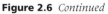

Figure 2.6 *Continued*

Kolmogorov–Smirnov test

In addition to the above tests of normality, a Kolmogorov–Smirnov test can be obtained as shown in Box 2.3.

Box 2.3 SPSS commands to conducting a one sample of normality

SPSS Commands
surgery – SPSS Data Editor
        Analyze → Non parametric Tests → 1-Sample K-S
One-Sample Kolmogorov-Smirnov Test
        Highlight Birth weight, Gestational age, Length of stay and click into Test
        Variable List
        Test Distribution - tick Normal (default)
        Click on Options
One-sample K-S: Options
        Missing Values – tick Exclude cases test-by-test (default)
        Click Continue
One-Sample Kolmogorov-Smirnov Test
        Click OK

NPar Tests

One-Sample Kolmogorov–Smirnov Test

		Birth weight	Gestational age	Length of stay
N		139	133	132
Normal parameters[a,b]	Mean	2463.99	36.564	38.05
	Std. deviation	514.632	2.0481	35.781
Most extreme	Absolute	0.067	0.151	0.241
Differences	Positive	0.067	0.105	0.241
	Negative	−0.043	−0.151	−0.202
Kolmogorov–Smirnov Z		0.792	1.741	2.771
Asymp. sig. (two-tailed)		0.557	0.005	0.000

[a] Test distribution is normal.
[b] Calculated from data.

The P values for the test of normality in the One-Sample Kolmogorov–Smirnov Test table are different from Kolmogorov–Smirnov P values obtained in *Analyze → Descriptive Statistics → Explore* because the one-sample test shown here is without the Lilliefors correction. Without the correction applied this test, which is based on slightly different assumptions about the mean and the variance of the normal distribution being tested for fit, is extremely conservative. Once again, the P values suggest that birth weight is normally distributed but gestational age and length of stay do not pass this test of normality with P values less than 0.05.

Table 2.4 Summary of whether descriptive statistics and plots indicate a normal distribution

	Mean– median	Mean ± 2 SD	Skewness and kurtosis	Critical values	K-S test	Plots	Overall decision
Birth weight	Probably	Yes	Yes	Yes	Yes	Probably	Yes
Gestational age	Yes	Yes	Yes	No	No	Probably	Yes
Length of stay	No	No	No	No	No	No	No

Deciding whether a variable is normally distributed

The information from the descriptive statistics and normality plots can be summarised as shown in Table 2.4. In the table, Yes indicates that the distribution is within normal range and No indicates that the distribution is outside the normal range.

Clearly, the results of tests of normality are not always in agreement. By considering all of the information together, a decision can be made about whether the distribution of each variable is normal enough to justify using parametric tests or whether the deviation from normal is so marked that non-parametric or categorical tests need to be used. These decisions, which sometimes involve subjective judgements, should be based on all processes of checking for normality.

Table 2.4 shows that parametric tests are appropriate for analysing birth weight because this variable is normally distributed. The variable gestational age is approximately normally distributed with some indications of a small deviation. However the mean value is a good estimate of the centre of the data. Parametric tests are robust to some deviations from normality if the sample size is large, say greater than 100 as is this sample. If the sample size had been small, say less than 30, then this variable would have to be perfectly normally distributed rather than approximately normally distributed before parametric tests could be used.

Length of stay is clearly not normally distributed and therefore this variable needs to be either transformed to normality to use parametric tests, analysed using non-parametric tests or transformed to a categorical variable. There are a number of factors to consider in deciding whether a variable should be transformed. Parametric tests generally provide more statistical power than non-parametric tests but if a parametric test does not have a non-parametric equivalent then transformation is essential. However, transformation can increase difficulties in interpreting the results because few people think naturally in transformed units. For example, if length of stay is transformed by calculating its square root, the results of parametric tests will be presented in units of the square root of length of stay and will be more difficult to interpret and to compare with results from other studies.

Transforming skewed distributions

Various mathematical formulae can be used to transform a skewed distribution to normality. When a distribution has a marked tail to the right hand side, a logarithmic transformation of scores is often effective[4]. The advantage of logarithmic transformations is that they give interpretable results after being back-transformed into original units[5]. Other common transformations include square roots and reciprocals[6]. When data are transformed and differences in transformed mean values between two or more groups are compared, the summary statistics will not apply to the means of the original data but will apply to the medians of the original data[6].

Length of stay can be transformed to logarithmic values using the commands shown in Box 2.4. The transformation LG10 can be clicked in from the Functions box and the variable can be clicked in from the variable list. Either base e or base 10 logarithms can be used but base 10 logarithms are a little more intuitive in that $0 = 1$ (10^0), $1 = 10$ (10^1), $2 = 100$ (10^2), etc. and are therefore a little easier to interpret and communicate. When using logarithms, any values that are zero will naturally be declared as invalid and registered as missing values in the transformed variable.

Box 2.4 SPSS commands for computing a new variable

SPSS Commands
surgery - SPSS Data Editor
        Transform → Compute
Compute Variable
        Target Variable = LOS2
        Scroll down Functions and highlight LG10 (numexpr) and click the arrow
            next to Functions
        Click Length of stay from the Variable list to obtain Numeric Expression =
            LG10 (lengthst)
        Click OK

On completion of the logarithmic transformation, an error message will appear in the output viewer of SPSS specifying any case numbers that have been set to system missing. In this data set, case 32 has a value of zero for length of stay and has been transformed to a system missing value for logarithmic length of stay. If there are only a few cases that cannot be log transformed, the number of system missing values may not be important. However if many cases have zero or negative values, a constant can be added to each value to ensure that the logarithmic transformation can be undertaken[7]. For example, if the minimum value is −2.2, then a constant of 3 can be added to all values. This value can be subtracted again when the summary statistics are transformed back to original units.

Whenever a new variable is created, it must be labelled and its format must be adjusted. The log-transformed length of stay can be re-assigned in Variable View by adding a label 'Log length of stay' to ensure that the output is self-documented. In addition, the number of decimal places can be adjusted to an appropriate number, in this case three. Once a newly transformed variable is obtained, its distribution must be checked again using the *Analyze →* *Descriptive Statistics → Explore* commands shown in Box 2.2, which will provide the following output.

Explore

Case Processing Summary

	Cases					
	Valid		Missing		Total	
	N	Per cent	N	Per cent	N	Per cent
Log length of stay	131	92.9%	10	7.1%	141	100.0%

The Case Processing Summary table shows that there are now 131 valid cases for log-transformed length of stay compared with 132 valid cases for length of stay because case 32, which had a zero value, could not be transformed and has been assigned a system missing value.

Descriptives

			Statistic	Std. error
Log length of stay	Mean		1.4725	0.02623
	95% confidence interval for mean	Lower bound	1.4206	
		Upper bound	1.5244	
	5% trimmed mean		1.4644	
	Median		1.4314	
	Variance		0.090	
	Std. deviation		0.30018	
	Minimum		0.00	
	Maximum		2.39	
	Range		2.39	
	Inter-quartile range		0.3010	
	Skewness		−0.110	0.212
	Kurtosis		4.474	0.420

The Descriptives table shows that mean log length of stay is 1.4725 and the median value is 1.4314. The two values are only 0.0411 units apart, which suggests that the distribution is now much closer to being normally distributed. Also, the skewness value is now closer to zero, indicating no significant skewness. The kurtosis value of 4.474 indicates that the distribution remains peaked, although not as markedly as before. The values for two standard deviations below and above the mean value, that is $1.4725 \pm (2 \times 0.3)$ or 0.87 and 2.07 respectively, are much closer to the minimum and maximum values of 0 and 2.39 for the variable.

Following transformation there is no need to request information of extreme values because the same data points are still the extreme points.

Dividing skewness by its standard error, that is $-0.110/0.212$, gives the critical value of -0.52, indicating a normal distribution. However, dividing the kurtosis by its standard error, that is $4.474/0.42$, gives the critical value of 10.65, confirming that the distribution remains too peaked to conform to normality. In practice, peakness is not as important as skewness for deciding when to use parametric tests because deviations in kurtosis do not bias mean values.

Tests of Normality

	Kolmogorov–Smirnov[a]			Shapiro-Wilk		
	Statistic	df	Sig.	Statistic	df	Sig.
Log length of stay	0.097	131	0.004	0.916	131	0.000

[a] Lilliefors Significance Correction.

In the Tests of Normality table, the results of the Kolmogorov–Smirnov and Shapiro–Wilk tests indicate that the distribution remains significantly different from a normal distribution at $P = 0.004$ and $P < 0.0001$ respectively.

The histogram for the log-transformed variable shown in Figure 2.7 conforms to a bell shape distribution better than the original variable except for some outlying values in both tails and a gap in the data on the left. Such gaps are a common feature of data distributions when the sample size is small but they need to be investigated when the sample size is large as in this case. The lowest extreme value for log length of stay is a univariate outlier. Although log length of stay is not perfectly normally distributed, it will provide less biased P values than the original variable if parametric tests are used.

Care must be taken when transforming summary statistics in log units back into their original units[5]. In general, it is best to carry out all statistical tests using the transformed scale and only transform summary statistics back into original units in the final presentation of the results. Thus, the interpretation of the statistics should be undertaken using summary statistics of the transformed variable. When a logarithmic mean is anti-logged it is called a geometric mean. The standard deviation (spread) cannot be back transformed to have the usual interpretation although the 95% confidence interval can be back transformed and will have the usual interpretation.

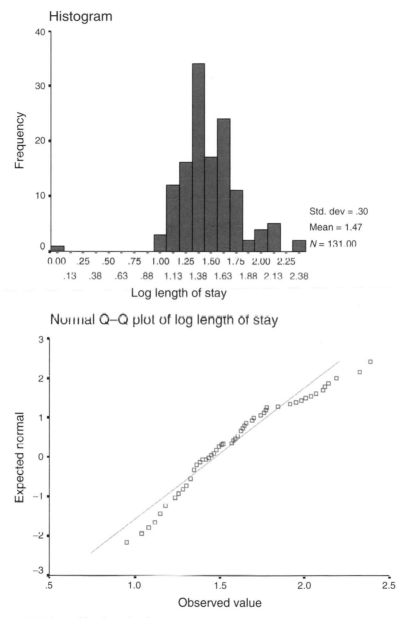

Figure 2.7 Plots of log length of stay.

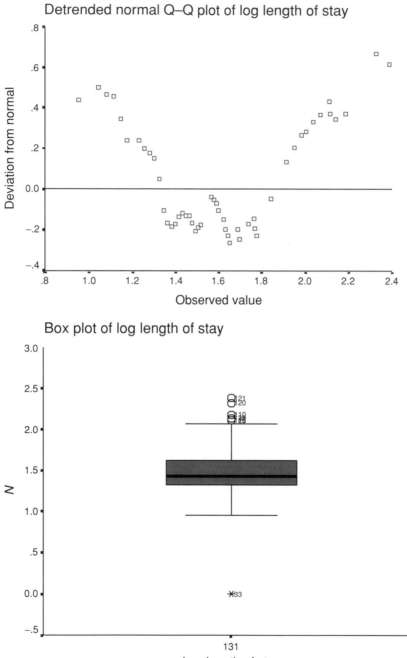

Figure 2.7 *Continued*

Summarising descriptive statistics

In all research studies, it is important to report details of the characteristics of the study sample or study groups to describe the generalisability of the results. For this, statistics that describe the centre of the data and its spread are appropriate. Therefore, for variables that are normally distributed, the mean and the standard deviation are reported. For variables that are non-normally distributed, the median and the inter-quartile range are reported.

Statistics of normally distributed variables that describe precision, that is the standard error and 95% confidence interval, are more useful for comparing groups or making inferences about differences between groups. Table 2.5 shows how to present the characteristics of the babies in the **surgery.sav** data set. In presenting descriptive statistics, no more than one decimal point greater than in the units of the original measurement should be used[8].

Table 2.5 Baseline characteristics of the study sample

Characteristic	N	**Distribution in sample** **Mean (SD) or median (IQ range)**
Birth weight	139	2464.0 g (SD 514.6)
Gestational age	133	36.6 weeks (SD 2.0)
Length of stay	132	27.0 days (IQ range 21.8 days)

Testing for normality in published results

When critically appraising journal articles, it may be necessary to transform a measure of spread to a measure of precision, or vice versa, for comparing with results from other studies. Computing a standard deviation from a standard error, or vice versa, is simple because the formula is

Standard error (SE) = Standard deviation (SD)$/\sqrt{n}$

where n is the sample size.

Also, by adding and subtracting two standard deviations from the mean, it is possible to roughly estimate whether the distribution of the data conforms to a bell shaped distribution. For example, Table 2.6 shows summary statistics of lung function shown as the mean and standard deviation in a sample of children with severe asthma. In this table, FEV_1 is forced expiratory volume in one second and it is rare that this value would be below 30%, even in a child with severe lung disease.

Table 2.6 Mean lung function values of two study groups

%predicted normal value	Active group	Control group	P value
FEV_1 (mean ± SD)	37.5 ± 16.0	36.0 ± 15.0	0.80

In the active group, the lower value of the 95% range of per cent predicted FEV_1 is 37.5% − (2 × 16.0)%, which is 5.5%. Similarly the lower value of

95% range for the control group is 6.0%. Both of these values for predicted FEV_1 are implausible and are a clear indication that the data are skewed, that the standard deviation is not an appropriate statistic to describe the spread of the data and that parametric tests cannot be used to compare the groups.

If the lower estimate of the 95% range is too low, as in Table 2.6, the mean will be an overestimate of the median value. If the lower estimate is too high, the mean value will be an underestimate of the median value. In Table 2.6, the variables are significantly skewed with a tail to the right hand side. In this case, the median and inter-quartile range would provide more accurate estimates of the centre, of the differences between the groups and spread of the data and non-parametric tests would be needed to compare the groups.

Notes for critical appraisal

Questions to ask when assessing descriptive statistics published in the literature are shown in Box 2.5.

Box 2.5 Questions for critical appraisal

The following questions should be asked when appraising published results:
- Have several tests of normality been considered and reported?
- Are appropriate statistics used to describe the centre and spread of the data?
- Do the values of the mean ±2 SD represent a reasonable 95% range?
- If a distribution is skewed, has the mean of either group been underestimated or overestimated?
- If the data are skewed, have the median and inter-quartile range been reported?

References

1. Healy MJR. Statistics from the inside. 11. Data transformations. Arch Dis Child 1993; 68: 260–264.
2. Lang TA, Secic M. How to report statistics in medicine. Philadelphia, PA: American College of Physicians, 1997; p. 48.
3. Stevens J. Applied multivariate statistics for the social sciences (3rd edition). Mahwah, NJ: Lawrence Erlbaum Associates, 1996; pp 237–260.
4. Chinn S. Scale, parametric methods, and transformations. Thorax 1991; 46: 536–538.
5. Bland JM, Altman DG. Transforming data. BMJ 1996; 312: 770.
6. Tabachnick BG, Fidell LS. Using multivariate statistics (4th edition). Boston: Allyn and Bacon, 2001; pp 82–88.
7. Peat JK, Unger WR, Combe D. Measuring changes in logarithmic data, with special reference to bronchial responsiveness. J Clin Epidemiol 1994; 47: 1099–1108.
8. Altman DG, Bland JM. Presentation of numerical data. BMJ 1996; 312: 572.

CHAPTER 3

Continuous variables: comparing two independent samples

Do not put faith in what statistics say until you have carefully considered what they do not say.
WILLIAM W. WATT

Objectives

The objectives of this chapter are to explain how to:
- conduct an independent two sample parametric or non-parametric test
- assess for homogeneity of variances
- interpret effect sizes and 95% confidence intervals
- report the results in a table or a graph
- critically appraise the analysis of data from two independent groups in the literature

---

Comparing the means of two independent samples

A two-sample t-test is a parametric test used to estimate whether the mean value of a normally distributed outcome variable is significantly different between two groups of participants. This test is also known as a Student's t-test or an independent samples t-test. Two-sample t-tests are classically used when the outcome is a continuous variable and when the explanatory variable is binary. For example, this test would be used to assess whether mean height is significantly different between a group of males and a group of females.

A two-sample t-test is used to assess whether two mean values are similar enough to have come from the same population or whether their difference is large enough for the two groups to have come from different populations. Rejecting the null hypothesis of a two-sample t-test indicates that the difference in the means of the two groups is large and is not due to either chance or sampling variation.

The assumptions that must be met to use a two-sample t-test are shown in Box 3.1.

> **Box 3.1** Assumptions for using a two-sample t-test
>
> The assumptions that must be satisfied to conduct a two-sample t-test are:
> - the groups must be independent, that is each participant must be in one group only
> - the measurements must be independent, that is a participant's measurement can be included in their group once only
> - the outcome variable must be on a continuous scale
> - the outcome variable must be normally distributed in each group

The first two assumptions in Box 3.1 are determined by the study design. To conduct a two-sample t-test, each participant must be on a separate row of the spreadsheet and each participant must be included in the spreadsheet once only. In addition, one of the variables must indicate the group to which the participant belongs.

The fourth assumption that the outcome variable must be normally distributed in each group must also be met. If the outcome variable is not normally distributed in each group, a non-parametric test or a transformation of the outcome variable will be needed. However, two-sample t-tests are fairly robust to some degree of non-normality if the sample size is large and if there are no influential outliers. The definition of a 'large' sample size varies but there is common consensus that t-tests can be used when the sample size of each group contains at least 30 to 50 participants. If the sample size is less than 30, if outliers significantly influence one of the distributions or if the distribution is non-normal, then a two-sample t-test should not be used.

One- and two-tailed tests

When a hypothesis is tested, it is possible to conduct a one-tailed (sided) or a two-tailed (sided) test. A one-tailed test is used to test an effect in one direction only (i.e. $mean_1 > mean_2$) whereas a two-tailed test is used to decide whether one mean value is smaller or larger than another mean value (i.e. $mean_1 \neq mean_2$). In the majority of studies, it is important to always use a two-tailed test. If a one-tailed test is used, the direction should be specified in the study design prior to data collection. As shown in Figure 3.1, a two-tailed test halves the level of significance (i.e. 0.05) in each tail of the distribution.

Assuming that the null hypothesis of no difference between population means is true and pairs of samples were repeatedly compared to each other, in 95% of the cases the observed t values would fall within the critical t value range and differences would be due to sampling error. Observed t values that fall outside this critical range, which occurs in 5% of the cases, represent an unlikely t value to occur when the null hypothesis is true, therefore the null hypothesis is rejected.

For a two-tailed test, 2.5% of the rejection region is placed in the positive tail of the distribution (i.e. $mean_1 > mean_2$) and 2.5% is placed in the negative tail (i.e. $mean_1 < mean_2$). When a one-tailed test is used, the 5% rejection region

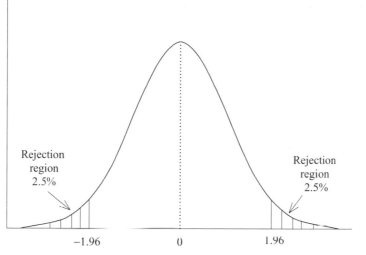

Figure 3.1 Statistical model and rejection regions for a two-tailed *t*-test with $P = 0.05$.

is placed only in one tail of the distribution. For example, if the hypothesis $mean_1 > mean_2$ was being tested, the 5% rejection region would be in the positive end of the tail. This means that for one-tailed tests, P values on the margins of significance are reduced and that the difference is more likely to be significant. For this reason, one-tailed tests are rarely used in health research.

Homogeneity of variance

In addition to testing for normality, it is also important to inspect whether the variance (the square of the standard deviation) in each group is similar, that is whether there is homogeneity of variances between groups. If the variance is different between the two groups, that is there is heterogeneity of variances, then the degrees of freedom and t value associated with a two-sample t-test are calculated differently. In this situation, a fractional value for degrees of freedom is used and the t-test statistics is calculated using individual group variances. In SPSS, Levene's test for equality of variances is an automatic part of the two-sample t-test routine and the information is printed in the SPSS output.

Effect size

Effect size is a term used to describe the size of the difference in mean values between two groups relative to the standard deviation. Effect sizes are important because they can be used to describe the magnitude of the difference between two groups in either experimental or observational study designs. The effect size between two independent groups is calculated as follows:

Effect size = $(Mean_2 - Mean_1)/SD$

where SD denotes the standard deviation.

Effect sizes are measured in units of the standard deviation. The standard deviation around each group's mean value indicates the spread of the measurements in each group and is therefore useful for describing the distance between the two mean values. If the variances of the two groups are homogeneous then the standard deviation of either group can be used in calculating the effect size[1]. If there is an experimental group (i.e. a group in which a treatment is being tested) and a control group, the standard deviation of the control group should be used. If the sample size of the control group is large, the standard deviation will be an unbiased estimate of the population who have not been given the treatment. When the sample size is small or when there is no control group, the pooled standard deviation, which is the average of the standard deviations of the two groups, is used. The pooled standard deviation is the root mean square of the two standard deviations and is calculated as:

$$\text{Pooled standard deviation} = \sqrt{\left[\frac{(SD_1{}^2 + SD_2{}^2)}{2}\right]}$$

where SD_1 = standard deviation of group 1 and SD_2 = standard deviation of group 2.

An effect size of 0.2 is considered small, 0.5 is considered medium and 0.8 is considered large[2]. Effect size is generally interpreted assuming that the two groups have a normal distribution and can be considered as the average percentile ranking of the experimental group relative to the control group. Therefore, an effect size of 1 indicates that the mean of the experimental group is at the 84th percentile of the control group[1].

Figure 3.2 shows the distribution of a variable in two groups that have mean values that are one standard deviation apart, that is an effect size of 1 SD.

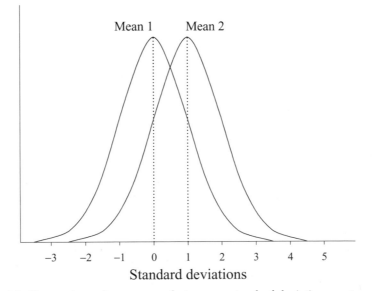

Figure 3.2 Mean values of two groups that are one standard deviation apart.

Study design

Two-sample t-tests can be used to analyse data from any type of study design where the explanatory variable falls into two groups, e.g. males and females, cases and controls, and intervention and non-intervention groups. For a two-sample t-test, there must be no relation or dependence between the participants in each of the two groups. Therefore, two-sample t-tests cannot be used to analyse scores from follow-up studies where data from a participant are obtained on repeated occasions for the same measure or for matched case-control studies in which participants are treated as pairs in the analyses. In these types of studies, a paired t-test should be used.

It is important to interpret significant P values in the context of the size of the difference between the groups and the sample size. The size of the study sample is an important determinant of whether a difference in means between two groups is statistically significant. Ideally, studies should be designed and conducted with a sample size that is sufficient for a clinically important difference between two groups to become statistically significant.

If a small effect size and/or a lower level of significance is used, then a large sample size will be needed to detect the effect with sufficient power[2]. When designing a study, a power analysis should be conducted to calculate the sample size that is needed to detect a pre-determined effect size with sufficient statistical power. If the sample size is too small, then type II errors may occur, that is a clinically important difference between groups will not be statistically significant. The influence of sample size can make the results of statistical tests difficult to interpret. In addition to specialised computer programs, there are a number of resources that can be used to calculate sample size and assess the power of a study (see Useful Web sites).

In many studies, the two groups will have unequal sample sizes. In this situation, a two-sample t-test can still be used but in practice leads to a loss of statistical power, which may be important when the sample size is small. For example, a study with three times as many cases as controls and a total sample size of 100 participants (75 cases and 25 controls) has roughly the same statistical power as a balanced study with 76 participants (38 cases and 38 controls)[3]. Thus, the unbalanced study requires the recruitment of an extra 24 participants to achieve the same statistical power.

Research question

The data file **babies.sav** contains the information of birth length, birth weight and head circumference measured at 1 month of age in 256 babies. The babies were recruited during a population study in which one of the inclusion criteria was that the babies had to have been a term birth. The research question and null hypothesis are shown below. Unlike the null hypothesis, the research question usually specifies the direction of effect that is expected. Nevertheless, a two-tailed test should be used because the direction of effect could be in either direction and if the effect is in a direction that is not expected, it is usually important to know this especially in experimental studies. In this example, all three outcome measurements (birth length, birth weight and head circumference) are continuous and the explanatory measurement (gender) is a binary group variable.

Questions:	Are males longer than females?
	Are males heavier than females?
	Do males have a larger head circumference than females?
Null hypothesis:	There is no difference between males and females in length.
	There is no difference between males and females in weight.
	There is no difference between males and females in head circumference.
Variables:	Outcome variables = birth length, birth weight and head circumference (continuous)
	Explanatory variable = gender (categorical, binary)

The appropriate statistic that is used to test differences between groups is the *t* value. If the *t* value obtained from the two-sample *t*-test falls outside the *t* critical range and is therefore in the rejection region, the *P* value will be small and the null hypothesis will be rejected. In SPSS, the *P* value is calculated so it is not necessary to check statistical tables to obtain *t* critical values. When the null hypothesis is rejected, the conclusion is made that the difference between groups is statistically significant and did not occur by chance. It is important to remember that statistical significance does not only reflect the size of the difference between groups but also reflects the sample size. Thus, small unimportant differences between groups can be statistically significant when the sample size is large.

Statistical analyses

Before differences in outcome variables between groups can be tested, it is important that all of the assumptions specified in Box 3.1 are checked. In the data file **babies.sav**, the first assumption is satisfied because all the males are in one group (coded 1) and all the females are in a separate group (coded 2). In addition, each participant appears only once in their group, therefore the groups and the measurements are independent. All three outcome variables are on a continuous scale for each group, so the fourth assumption of the outcome variable being normally distributed must be tested. Descriptive statistics need to be obtained for the distribution of each outcome variable in each group rather than for the entire sample. It is also important to check for univariate outliers, calculate the effect size and test for homogeneity of variances. It is essential to identify outliers that tend to bias mean values of groups and make them more different or more alike than median values show they are.

Box 3.2 shows how to obtain the descriptive information for each group in SPSS.

Box 3.2 SPSS commands to obtain descriptive statistics

SPSS Commands
babies – SPSS Data Editor
 Analyze→ Descriptive Statistics→ Explore
Explore
 Highlight Birth weight, Birth length, and Head circumference and click
  into Dependent List
 Highlight Gender and click into Factor List
 Click on Plots
Explore: Plots
 Boxplots – Factor levels together (default setting)
 Descriptive – untick Stem and leaf (default setting), tick Histogram and
  tick Normality plots with tests
 Click Continue
Explore
 Click on Options
Explore: Options
 Missing Values – tick Exclude cases pairwise
 Click Continue
Explore
 Click OK

The Case Processing Summary table indicates that there are 119 males and 137 females in the sample and that none of the babies have missing values for any of the variables.

Explore

Case Processing Summary

		Cases					
		Valid		Missing		Total	
	Gender	N	Percent	N	Percent	N	Percent
Birth weight (kg)	Male	119	100.0%	0	.0%	119	100.0%
	Female	137	100.0%	0	.0%	137	100.0%
Birth length (cms)	Male	119	100.0%	0	.0%	119	100.0%
	Female	137	100.0%	0	.0%	137	100.0%
Head circumference (cms)	Male	119	100.0%	0	.0%	119	100.0%
	Female	137	100.0%	0	.0%	137	100.0%

Descriptives

	Gender			Statistic	Std. error
Birth weight (kg)	Male	Mean		3.4430	0.03030
		95% confidence	Lower bound	3.3830	
		interval for mean	Upper bound	3.5030	
		5% trimmed mean		3.4383	
		Median		3.4300	
		Variance		0.109	
		Std. deviation		0.33057	
		Minimum		2.70	
		Maximum		4.62	
		Range		1.92	
		Inter-quartile range		0.4700	
		Skewness		0.370	0.222
		Kurtosis		0.553	0.440
	Female	Mean		3.5316	0.03661
		95% confidence	Lower bound	3.4592	
		interval for mean	Upper bound	3.6040	
		5% trimmed mean		3.5215	
		Median		3.5000	
		Variance		0.184	
		Std. deviation		0.42849	
		Minimum		2.71	
		Maximum		4.72	
		Range		2.01	
		Inter-quartile range		0.5550	
		Skewness		0.367	0.207
		Kurtosis		−0.128	0.411
Birth length (cm)	Male	Mean		50.333	0.0718
		95% confidence	Lower bound	50.191	
		interval for mean	Upper bound	50.475	
		5% trimmed mean		50.342	
		Median		50.500	
		Variance		0.614	
		Std. deviation		0.7833	
		Minimum		49.0	
		Maximum		51.5	
		Range		2.5	
		Inter-quartile range		1.000	
		Skewness		−0.354	0.222
		Kurtosis		−0.971	0.440
	Female	Mean		50.277	0.0729
		95% confidence	Lower bound	50.133	
		interval for mean	Upper bound	50.422	

Continued

	Gender			Statistic	Std. error
			5% trimmed mean	50.264	
			Median	50.000	
			Variance	0.728	
			Std. deviation	0.8534	
			Minimum	49.0	
			Maximum	52.0	
			Range	3.0	
			Inter-quartile range	1.500	
			Skewness	−0.117	0.207
			Kurtosis	−1.084	0.411
Head circumference (cm)	Male		Mean	34.942	0.1197
		95% confidence interval for mean	Lower bound	34.705	
			Upper bound	35.179	
			5% trimmed mean	34.967	
			Median	35.000	
			Variance	1.706	
			Std. deviation	1.3061	
			Minimum	31.5	
			Maximum	38.0	
			Range	6.5	
			Inter-quartile range	2.000	
			Skewness	−0.208	0.222
			Kurtosis	0.017	0.440
	Female		Mean	34.253	0.1182
		95% confidence interval for mean	Lower bound	34.019	
			Upper bound	34.486	
			5% trimmed mean	34.301	
			Median	34.000	
			Variance	1.914	
			Std. deviation	1.3834	
			Minimum	29.5	
			Maximum	38.0	
			Range	8.5	
			Inter-quartile range	1.500	
			Skewness	−0.537	0.207
			Kurtosis	0.850	0.411

The first check of normality is to compare the mean and median values provided by the Descriptives table and summarised in Table 3.1. The differences between the mean and median values are small for birth weight and relatively small for birth length and for head circumference.

Information from the Descriptives table indicates that the skewness and kurtosis values are all less than or close to ±1, suggesting that the data are

Table 3.1 Testing for a normal distribution

	Gender	Mean – median	Skewness (SE)	Skewness/SE (critical value)	Kurtosis (SE)	Kurtosis/SE (critical value)
Birth weight	Male	0.013	0.370 (0.222)	1.67	0.553 (0.440)	1.26
	Female	0.032	0.367 (0.207)	1.77	−0.128 (0.411)	−0.31
Birth length	Male	−0.167	−0.354 (0.222)	−1.59	−0.971 (0.440)	−2.21
	Female	0.277	−0.117 (0.207)	−0.57	−1.084 (0.411)	−2.64
Head	Male	−0.058	−0.208 (0.222)	−0.94	0.017 (0.440)	0.04
circumference	Female	0.253	−0.537 (0.207)	−2.59	0.850 (0.411)	2.07

approximately normally distributed. Calculations of normality statistics for skewness and kurtosis in Table 3.1 show that the critical values of kurtosis/SE for birth length for both males and females are less than −1.96 and outside the normal range, indicating that the distributions of birth length are relatively flat. The head circumference of females is negatively skewed because the critical value of skewness/SE is less than −1.96 and outside the normal range. Also, the distribution of head circumference for females is slightly peaked because the critical value of kurtosis/SE for this variable is outside the normal range of +1.96.

From the Descriptives table, it is possible to also compute effect sizes and estimate homogeneity of variances as shown in Table 3.2. The effect sizes using the pooled standard deviation are small for birth weight, very small for birth length and medium for head circumference. The variance of birth weight for females compared to males is 0.109:0.184 or 1:1.7. This indicates that females have a wider spread of birth weight scores, which is shown by similar minimum values for males and females (2.70 vs 2.71 kg) but a higher maximum value for females (4.62 vs 4.72 kg). For birth length and head circumference, males and females have similar variances with ratios of 1:1.12 and 1:1.1 respectively.

Table 3.2 Effect sizes and homogeneity of variances

	Difference in means and SD	Effect size (SD)	Maximum and minimum variance	Variance ratio
Birth weight	3.443 − 3.532/0.38	−0.23	0.184, 0.109	1:1.7
Birth length	50.33 − 50.28/0.82	0.06	0.728, 0.614	1:1.2
Head circumference	34.94 − 34.25/1.35	0.51	1.914, 1.706	1:1.1

Tests of Normality

	Gender	Kolmogorov–Smirnov[a]			Shapiro–Wilk		
		Statistic	df	Sig.	Statistic	df	Sig.
Birth weight (kg)	Male	0.044	119	0.200*	0.987	119	0.313
	Female	0.063	137	0.200*	0.983	137	0.094
Birth length (cm)	Male	0.206	119	0.000	0.895	119	0.000
	Female	0.232	137	0.000	0.889	137	0.000
Head circumference (cm)	Male	0.094	119	0.012	0.977	119	0.037
	Female	0.136	137	0.000	0.965	137	0.001

*This is a lower bound of the true significance.
[a] Lilliefors significance correction.

The Tests of Normality table shows that the distribution of birth weight for males and females is not significantly different from a normal distribution and therefore passes the test of normality. However, both the Kolmogorov–Smirnov and Shapiro–Wilk tests of normality indicate that birth length and head circumference for males and females are significantly different from a normal distribution.

The histograms shown in Figure 3.3 indicate that the data for birth weight of males and females follow an approximately normal distribution with one or two outlying values to the right hand side. The box plots shown in Figure 3.3 indicate that there is one outlying value for males and two outlying values for females that are 1.5 to 3 box lengths from the upper edge of the box. Both groups have outlying values at the high end of the data range that would tend to increase the mean value of each group. To check whether these outlying values are univariate outliers, the mean of the group is subtracted from the outlying value and then divided by the standard deviation of the group. This calculation converts the outlying value to a z score. If the absolute value of the z score is greater than 3, then the value is a univariate outlier[4]. If the sample size is very small, then an absolute z score greater than 2 should be considered to be a univariate outlier[4].

For the birth weight of males, the outlying value is the maximum value of 4.62 and is case 249. By subtracting the mean from this value and dividing by the standard deviation that is $((4.62 - 3.44)/0.33)$, a z value of 3.58 is obtained indicating that case 249 is a univariate outlier. This score is an extreme value compared to the rest of the data points and should be checked to ensure that it is not a transcribing or data entry error. Checking shows that the score was entered correctly and came from a minority ethnic group. There is only one univariate outlier and the sample size is large and therefore it is unlikely that this outlier will have a significant influence on the summary statistics. If the sample size is large, say at least 100 cases, then a few cases with z scores greater than the absolute value of 3 would be expected by chance[4].

If there were more than a few univariate outliers, a technique that can be used to reduce the influence of outliers is to transform the scores so that the shape of the distribution is changed. The outliers will still be present on the tails of the transformed distribution, but their influence will be reduced[5]. If there are only a few outliers, another technique that can be used is to change the score for the outlier so it is not so extreme, for example by changing the score to one point larger or smaller than the next extreme value in the distribution[5].

For illustrative purposes, the case that is a univariate outlier for birth weight of males will be changed so that it is less extreme. Using the *Analyze* → *Descriptive Statistics* → *Explore* commands and requesting outliers as shown in Box 2.2 the next extreme value is obtained, which is case 149 with a value of 4.31. If a value of 1 were added to the next extreme value this would give a value of 5.31, which would be the changed value for the univariate outlier, case 249. However, this value is higher than the actual value of case 249, therefore this technique is not suitable. An alternative is that the univariate outlier is changed to a value that is within three z scores of the mean. For birth weight

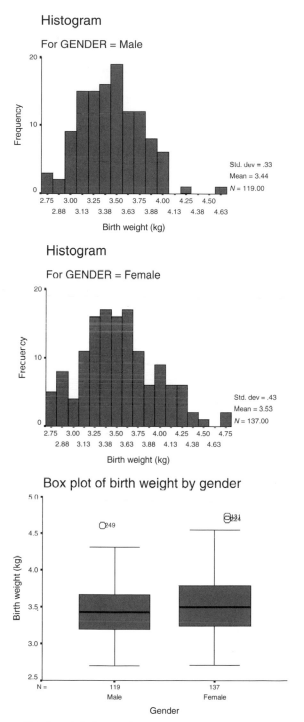

Figure 3.3 Plots of birth weight by gender.

of males, this value would be 4.43 that is $(0.33 \times 3) + 3.44$. This value is lower than the present value of case 249 and slightly higher than the next extreme value, case 149. Therefore, the value of case 249 is changed from 4.62 to 4.43. This information should be recorded in the study handbook and the method recorded in any publications.

After the case has been changed, the Descriptives table for birth weight of males should be obtained with new summary statistics. This table shows that the new maximum value for birth weight is 4.43. The mean of 3.4414 is almost the same as the previous mean of 3.4430, and the standard deviation, skewness and kurtosis values of the group have slightly decreased, indicating a slightly closer approximation to a normal distribution.

Descriptives

	Gender			Statistic	Std. error
Birth weight (kg)	Male	Mean		3.4414	0.02982
		95% confidence	Lower bound	3.3824	
		interval for mean	Upper bound	3.5005	
		5% trimmed mean		3.4383	
		Median		3.4300	
		Variance		0.106	
		Std. deviation		0.32525	
		Minimum		2.70	
		Maximum		4.43	
		Range		1.73	
		Inter-quartile range		0.4700	
		Skewness		.235	0.222
		Kurtosis		.028	0.440
	Female	Mean		3.5316	0.03661
		95% confidence	Lower bound	3.4592	
		interval for mean	Upper bound	3.6040	
		5% trimmed mean		3.5215	
		Median		3.5000	
		Variance		0.184	
		Std. deviation		0.42849	
		Minimum		2.71	
		Maximum		4.72	
		Range		2.01	
		Inter-quartile range		0.5550	
		Skewness		0.367	0.207
		Kurtosis		−0.128	0.411

For the birth weight of females, cases 131 and 224 are outlying values and are also from the same minority ethic group as case 249. Case 131 is the higher of the two values and is the maximum value of the group with a value of 4.72, which is 2.77 standard deviations above the group mean and is not a univariate outlier. Therefore, case 224 is not a univariate outlier and the values of both cases 131 and 224 are retained.

Another alternative to transforming data or changing the values of univariate outliers is to omit the outliers from the analysis. If there were more univariate outliers from the same minority ethnic group, the data points could be included so that the results could be generalised to all ethnic groups in the recruitment area. Alternatively, all data points from the minority group could be omitted regardless of outlier status although this would limit the generalisability of the results.

The decision of whether to omit or include outlying values is always difficult. If the sample was selected as a random sample of the population, omission of some participants from the analyses should not be considered.

The histograms shown in Figure 3.4 indicate that birth length of males and females does not follow a classic normal distribution and explains the kurtosis statistics for males and females in the Descriptives table. The birth length of both males and females has a narrow range of only 49 to 52 cm as shown in the Descriptives table. The histograms show that birth length is usually recorded to the nearest centimetre and rarely to 0.5 cm (Figure 3.4). This rounding of birth length may be satisfactory for obstetric records but it would be important to ensure that observers measure length to an exact standard in a research study. Since birth length has only been recorded to the nearest centimetre, summary statistics for this variable should be reported using no more than one decimal place.

The box plots shown in Figure 3.4 confirm that females have a lower median birth length than males but have a wider absolute range of birth length values as indicated by the length of the box. This suggests that the variances of each group may not be homogeneous.

The histograms for head circumference shown in Figure 3.5 indicate that the data are approximately normally distributed although there is a slight tail to the left for females. This is confirmed by the box plot in Figure 3.5 that shows a few outlying values at the lower end of the distribution, indicating that a few female babies have a head circumference that is smaller than most other babies in the group. The smallest value is case 184 with a head circumference of 29.5, which has a z score of 3.44 and is a univariate outlier. The next smallest value is case 247 with a value of 30.2, which has a z score of 2.93. There is only one univariate outlier, which is expected in this large sample as part of normal variation. It is unlikely that this one outlier will have a significant impact on summary statistics, so it is not adjusted and is included in the data analyses. The maximum value for head circumference of females is case 108 with a value of 38, which has a z value of 2.71 and is not a univariate outlier.

Finally, after the presence of outliers has been assessed and all tests of normality have been conducted, the tests of normality can be summarised as shown in Table 3.3. In the table, 'yes' indicates that the distribution is within the normal range and 'no' indicates that the distribution is outside the normal range.

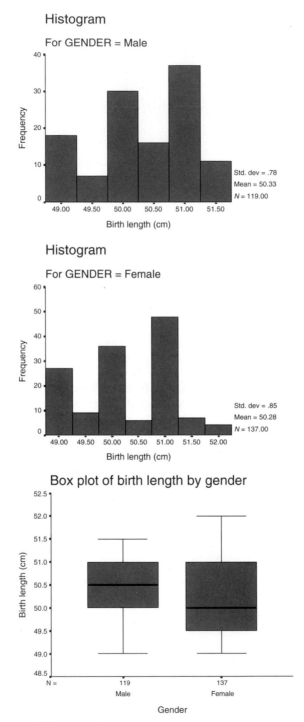

Figure 3.4 Plots of birth length by gender.

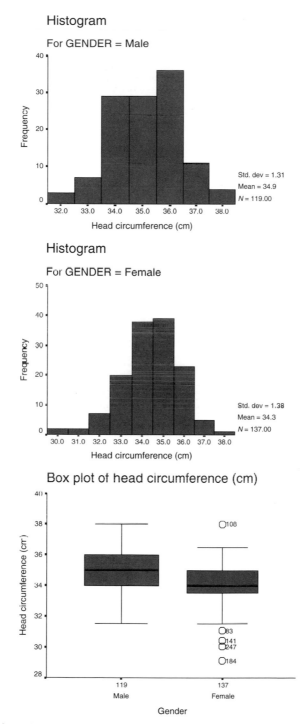

Figure 3.5 Plots of head circumference by gender.

Table 3.3 Summary of whether descriptive statistics indicates a normal distribution in each group

		Mean – median	Skewness	Kurtosis	K-S test	Plots	Overall decision
Birth weight	Males	Yes	Yes	Yes	Yes	Yes	Yes
	Females	Yes	Yes	Yes	Yes	Yes	Yes
Birth length	Males	Yes	Yes	No	No	No	Yes
	Females	Probably	Yes	No	No	No	Yes
Head circumference	Males	Yes	Yes	Yes	No	Yes	Yes
	Females	Probably	No	No	No	Yes	Yes

Based on all checks of normality, the birth weight of males and females is normally distributed so a two-sample t-test can be used. The distribution of birth length of males and females has a flat shape but does not have any outliers. While birth length of both males and females has some kurtosis, this has less impact on summary statistics than if the data were skewed. The variable head circumference is normally distributed for males but for females has some slight skewness caused by a few outlying values. However, the mean and median values for females are not largely different. Also, in the female group there is only one outlier and the number of outlying values is small and the sample size is large, and a t-test will be robust to these small deviations from normality. Therefore, the distribution of each outcome variable is approximately normally distributed for both males and females, and a two-sample t-test can be used to test between group differences.

Two-sample t-test

A two-sample t-test is basically a test of how different two group means are in terms of their variance. Clearly, if there was no difference between the groups, the difference to variance ratio would be close to zero. The t value becomes larger as the difference between the groups increases in respect to their variances. An approximate formula for calculating a t value, when variances are equal is:

$$t = (x_1 - x_2)/\sqrt{(s_p^2/n_1 + s_p^2/n_2)}$$

where x is the mean, s_p^2 is the pooled variance and n is the sample size of each group. Thus, t is the difference between the mean values for the two groups divided by the standard error of the difference. When variances of the two groups are not equal, that is Levene's test for equality of variances is significant, individual group variances and not the pooled variance are used in calculating the t value. Box 3.3 shows the SPSS commands to obtain a two-sample t-test in which the numbered coding for each group has to be entered.

Box 3.3 SPSS commands to obtain a two-sample *t*-test

SPSS Commands
babies – SPSS Data Editor
       Analyze → Compare Means → Independent Samples T Test
Independent-Samples T-Test
       Highlight Birth weight, Birth length and Head circumference and click into
              Test Variable(s)
       Highlight Gender and click into Group Variable
       Click on Define Groups
Define Groups
       Enter coding: 1 for Group 1 and 2 for Group 2
       Click Continue
Independent-Samples T-Test
       Click OK

T-Test

Group Statistics

	Gender	*N*	Mean	Std. deviation	Std. error mean
Birth weight (kg)	Male	119	3.4414	0.32525	0.02982
	Female	137	3.5316	0.42849	0.03661
Birth length (cm)	Male	119	50.333	0.7833	0.0718
	Female	137	50.277	0.8534	0.0729
Head circumference (cm)	Male	119	34.942	1.3061	0.1197
	Female	137	34.253	1.3834	0.1182

The first Group Statistics table shows summary statistics, which are identical to the statistics obtained in *Analyze → Descriptive Statistics → Explore*. However, there is no information in this table that would allow the normality of the distributions in each group or the presence of influential outliers to be assessed. Thus, it is important to always obtain full descriptive statistics to check for normality prior to conducting a two-sample *t*-test.

In the Independent Samples Test table (p. 70), the first test is Levene's test of equal variances. A *P* value for this test that is less than 0.05 indicates that the variances of the two groups are significantly different and therefore that the *t* statistics calculated assuming variances are not equal should be used. The variable birth weight does not pass the test for equal variances with a *P* value of 0.007 but this was expected because the statistics in the Descriptives table showed a 1:1.7, or almost two-fold, difference in variance (Table 3.2). For this variable, the statistics calculated assuming variances are not equal is appropriate. However, both birth length and head circumference pass the test

Independent Samples Test

		Levene's test for equality of variances		t-test for equality of means				95% confidence interval of the difference	
		F	Sig.	t	df	Sig. (Two-tailed)	Mean difference	Std. error difference	Lower	Upper
Birth weight (kg)	Equal variances assumed	7.377	0.007	−1.875	254	0.062	−0.0902	0.04812	−0.18498	0.00455
	Equal variances not assumed			−1.911	249.659	0.057	−0.0902	0.04721	−0.18320	0.00277
Birth length (cm)	Equal variances assumed	2.266	0.133	0.538	254	0.591	0.055	0.1030	−0.1473	0.2581
	Equal variances not assumed			0.541	253.212	0.589	0.055	0.1023	−0.1461	0.2569
Head circumference (cm)	Equal variances assumed	0.257	0.613	4.082	254	0.000	0.689	0.1689	0.3568	1.0221
	Equal variances not assumed			4.098	252.221	0.000	0.689	0.1682	0.3581	1.0208

of equal variances and the differences between genders can be reported using the *t* statistics that have been calculated assuming equal variances.

For birth weight, the appropriate *t* statistic can be read from the line *Equal variances not assumed*. The *t* statistic for birth length and head circumference can be read from the line *Equal variances assumed*. The *t*-test *P* value indicates the likelihood that the differences in mean values occurred by chance. If the likelihood is small, that is less than 0.05, the null hypothesis can be rejected. For birth weight, the *P* value for the difference between the genders does not reach statistical significance with a *P* value of 0.057. This *P* value indicates that there is a 5.7%, or 57 in 1000, chance of finding this difference if the two groups in the population have equal means.

For birth length, there is clearly no difference between the genders with a *P* value of 0.591. For head circumference, there is a highly significant difference between the genders with a *P* value of <0.0001. The head circumference of female babies is significantly lower than the head circumference of male babies. This *P* value indicates that there is less than a 1 in 1000 chance of this difference being found by chance if the null hypothesis is true.

Confidence intervals

Confidence intervals are invaluable statistics for estimating the precision around a summary statistic such as a mean value and for estimating the magnitude of the difference between two groups. For mean values, the 95% confidence interval is calculated as follows:

Confidence interval (CI) = Mean ± (1.96 × SE)

where SE = standard error.

Thus, using the data from the Group Statistics table provided in the SPSS output for a *t*-test, the confidence interval for birth weight for males would be calculated as follows:

95% confidence interval = 3.441 + (1.96 × 0.0298) = 3.383, 3.499

These values correspond to the 95% confidence interval lower and upper bounds shown in the Descriptives table. To calculate the 99% confidence interval, the critical value of 2.57 instead of 1.96 would be used in the calculation. This would give a wider confidence interval that would indicate the range in which the true population mean lies with more certainty.

The confidence intervals of two groups can be used to assess whether there is a significant difference between the two groups. If the 95% confidence interval of one group does not overlap with the confidence interval of another, there will be a statistically significant difference between the two groups. The interpretation of the overlapping of confidence intervals when two groups are compared is shown in Table 3.4.

Table 3.4 Interpretation of 95% confidence intervals

Relative position of confidence intervals	Statistical significance between groups
Do not overlap	Highly significant difference
Overlap, but one summary statistic is not within the confidence interval for the other	Possibly significant, but not highly
Overlap to a large extent	Definitely not significant

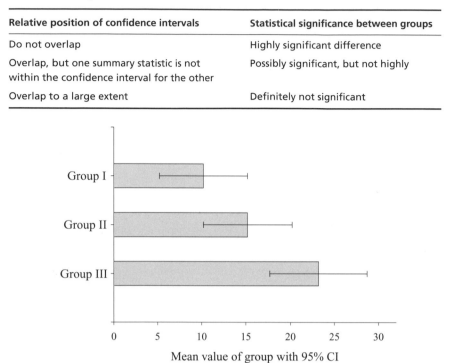

Mean value of group with 95% CI

Figure 3.6 Interpretation of the overlap between 95% confidence intervals.

Figure 3.6 shows the mean values of an outcome measurement, say per cent change from baseline, in three independent groups. The degree of overlap of the confidence intervals reflects the P values. For the comparison of group I vs III the confidence intervals do not overlap and the group means are significantly different at $P < 0.0001$. For the comparison of group I vs II, the confidence intervals overlap to a large extent and the group means are not significantly different at $P = 0.52$. For the comparison of group II vs III, where one summary statistic is not within the confidence interval of the other group, the difference between group means is marginally significant at $P = 0.049$.

In the data set, **babies.sav** the means and confidence intervals of the outcome variable for each group can be summarised as shown in Table 3.5. The overlap of the 95% confidence intervals confirms the between group P values.

Finally, in the Independent Samples Test table, the mean difference and its 95% confidence interval were also reported. The mean difference is the absolute difference between the mean values for males and females. The direction of the mean difference is determined by the coding used for gender. With males coded as 1 and females as 2, the differences are represented as males – females. Therefore, this section of the table indicates that males have a mean

Table 3.5 Summary of mean values and interpretation of 95% confidence intervals

	Mean (95% CI) Males	Mean (95% CI) Females	Overlap of CI	Significance
Birth weight	3.44 (3.38, 3.50)	3.53 (3.46, 3.60)	Slight	$P = 0.06$
Birth length	50.3 (50.1, 50.5)	50.3 (50.1, 50.4)	Large	$P = 0.59$
Head circumference	34.9 (34.7, 35.2)	34.3 (34.0, 34.5)	None	$P < 0.0001$

birth weight that is 0.0902 kg lower than females but a mean birth length that is 0.055 cm longer and a mean head circumference that is 0.689 cm larger than females.

Obviously, a zero value for mean difference would indicate no difference between groups. Thus, a 95% confidence interval around the mean difference that contains the value of zero, as it does for birth length, suggests that the two groups are not significantly different. A confidence interval that is shifted away from the value of zero, as it is for head circumference, indicates with 95% certainty that the two groups are different. The slight overlap with zero for the 95% confidence interval of the difference for birth weight reflects the marginal P value.

Reporting the results in a table

The results from two-sample t-tests can be reported as shown in Table 3.6. In addition to reporting the P value for the difference between genders, it is important to report the characteristics of the groups in terms of their mean values and standard deviations, the effect size and the mean between group difference and 95% confidence interval. Except for effect size, these statistics are all provided on the SPSS t-test output.

Table 3.6 Summary of birth details by gender

	Males Mean (SD)	Females Mean (SD)	Effect size (SD)	Mean difference and 95% CI	P value
Birth weight (kg)	3.44 (0.33)	3.53 (0.43)	−0.23	−0.09 (−0.18, −0.003)	0.06
Birth length (cm)	50.3 (0.78)	50.3 (0.85)	0.06	0.06 (−0.15, 0.26)	0.59
Head circumference (cm)	34.9 (1.31)	34.3 (1.38)	0.51	0.69 (0.36, 1.02)	<0.0001

The P values show the significance of the differences, but the effect size and mean difference give an indication of the magnitude of the differences between the groups. As such, these statistics give a meaningful interpretation to the P values.

Reporting results in a graph

Graphs are important tools for conveying the results of research studies. The most informative figures are clear and self-explanatory. For mean values from continuous data, dot plots are the most appropriate graph to use. In summarising data from continuous variables, it is important that bar charts are only used when the distance from zero has a meaning and therefore when the zero value is shown on the axis.

Box 3.4 shows how to draw a dot plot with error bars in SPSS.

Box 3.4 SPSS commands to draw a dot plot

SPSS Commands
babies – SPSS Data Editor
        Graphs → Error Bar
Error Bar
        Click Simple
        Click Define
Define Simple Error Bar: Summaries for Groups of Cases
        Highlight Birth weight and click into Variable
        Highlight Gender and click into Category Axis
        Click OK

The commands in Box 3.4 can then be repeated for birth length and head circumference to produce the graphs shown in Figure 3.7. Note that the scales on the y-axis of the three graphs shown in Figure 3.7 are different and therefore it is not possible to compare the graphs with one another or combine them.

However, in each graph shown in Figure 3.7, the degree of overlap of the confidence intervals provides an immediate visual image of the differences between genders. The graphs show that female babies are slightly heavier with a small overlap of 95% confidence intervals and that they are not significantly shorter because there is a large overlap of the 95% confidence intervals. However, males have a significantly larger head circumference because there is no overlap of confidence intervals. The extent to which the confidence intervals overlap in each of the three graphs provides a visual explanation of the P values obtained from the two-sample t-tests.

Drawing a figure in SigmaPlot

For publication quality, the differences between groups can be presented in a graph using SigmaPlot. In the example below, only the data for head circumference are plotted but the same procedure could be used for birth weight and length. First, the width of confidence interval has to be calculated using the Descriptives table obtained from *Analyze → Descriptive Statistics → Explore*.

Width of 95% CI = Mean − Lower bound of 95% CI

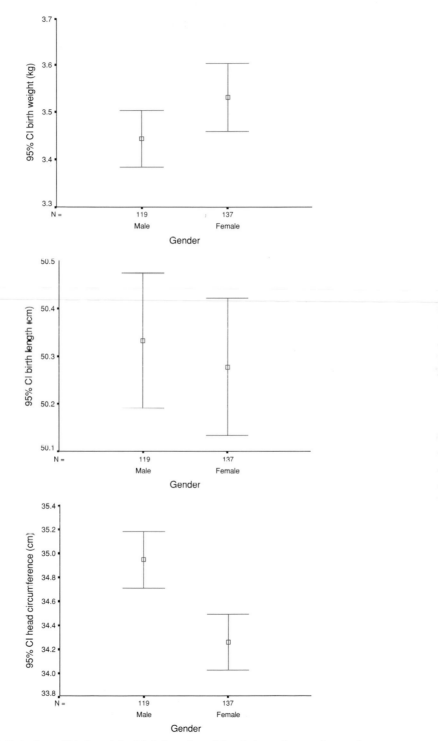

Figure 3.7 Dot plots of birth weight, birth length and head circumference by gender.

Thus, the width of the confidence interval for head circumference is as follows:

Width of 95% CI = 34.94 − 34.71 = 0.23 (males)

= 34.25 − 34.02 = 0.23 (females)

The numerical values of the mean and the width of the 95% confidence interval are then entered into the SigmaPlot spreadsheet as follows and the commands in Box 3.5 can be used to draw a dot plot as shown in Figure 3.8.

Column 1	Column 2
34.94	0.23
34.25	0.23

Box 3.5 SigmaPlot commands for drawing a dot plot

SigmaPlot Commands
SigmaPlot – [Data 1*]
Graph → Create Graph
Create Graph – Type
       Highlight Scatter Plot, click Next
Create Graph –Style
       Highlight Simple Error Bars, click Next
Create Graph – Error Bars
       Symbol Values = Worksheet Columns (default), click Next
Create Graph – Data Format
       Highlight Single Y, click Next
Create Graph – Select Data
       Data for Y = use drop box and select Column 1
       Data for Error = use drop box and select Column 2,
       Click Finish

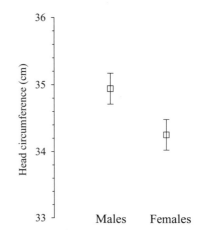

Figure 3.8 Mean head circumference at 1 month by gender.

Once the plot is obtained, the graph can be customised by changing the axes, axis labels, graph colours, etc. using options under the menu *Graph → Graph Properties*.

Alternatively, the absolute mean differences between males and females could be presented in a graph. Birth length and head circumference were measured in the same scale (cm) and therefore can be plotted on the same figure. Birth weight is in different units (kg) and would need to be presented in a different figure.

The width of the confidence intervals is calculated from the mean difference and lower 95% confidence interval of the difference, as follows:

$$\text{Width of 95\% CI for birth length} = 0.055 - (-0.147) = 0.202$$

$$\text{Width of 95\% CI for head circumference} = 0.689 - 0.357 = 0.332$$

These values are then entered into the SigmaPlot spreadsheet as follows:

Column 1	Column 2
0.055	0.202
0.689	0.332

Box 3.6 shows how a horizontal scatter plot can be drawn in SigmaPlot to produce Figure 3.9. The decision whether to draw horizontal or vertical dot plots is one of personal choice; however, horizontal plots have the advantage that longer descriptive labels can be included in a way that they can be easily read.

Box 3.6 SigmaPlot commands for horizontal dot plot

SigmaPlot Commands
SigmaPlot – [Data 1]*
Graph → Create Graph
Create Graph – Type
　　　Highlight Scatter Plot, click Next
Create Graph – Style
　　　Highlight Horizontal Error Bars, click Next
Create Graph – Error Bars
　　　Symbol Values = Worksheet Columns (default), click Next
Create Graph – Data Format
　　　Highlight Many X, click Next
Create Graph – Select Data
　　　Data for X1 = use drop box and select Column 1
　　　Data for Error 1 = use drop box and select Column 2
Click Finish

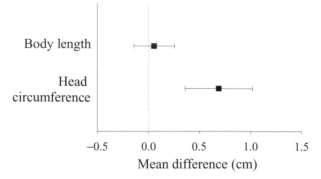

Figure 3.9 Mean difference in body length and head circumference between males and females at 1 month of age.

Rank based non-parametric tests

Rank based non-parametric tests are used when the data do not conform to a normal distribution. If the data are clearly skewed, if outliers have an important effect on the mean value or if the sample size in one or more of the groups is small, say between 20 and 30 cases, then a rank based non-parametric test should probably be used. These tests rely on ranking and summing the scores in each group and may lack sufficient power to detect a significant difference between two groups when the sample size is very small.

The non-parametric test that is equivalent to a two-sample *t*-test is the Mann–Whitney U test, which the Wilcoxon rank sum produces the same result as W test. The Mann–Whitney U test is based on the ranking of measurements from two samples to estimate whether the samples are from the same population. In this test, no assumptions are made about the distribution of the measurements in either group.

The assumptions for the Mann–Whitney U test are shown in Box 3.7.

Box 3.7 Assumptions for Mann–Whitney U test to compare two independent samples

The assumptions for the Mann–Whitney U test are:
• the data are randomly sampled from the population
• the groups are independent, that is each participant is in one group only

Research question

The spreadsheet **surgery.sav**, which was used in Chapter 2, contains the data for 141 babies who attended hospital for surgery, their length of stay and whether they had an infection during their stay.

Question: Do babies who have an infection have a longer stay in hospital?

Null hypothesis:	That there is no difference in length of stay between babies who have an infection and babies who do not have an infection
Variables:	Outcome variable = length of stay (continuous)
	Explanatory variable = infection (categorical, binary)

Statistical analyses

Descriptive statistics and the distribution of the outcome variable length of stay in each group can be inspected using the commands shown in Box 3.2 with length of stay as the dependent variable and infection as the factor.

Infection

Descriptives

	Infection			Statistic	Std. error
Length of stay	No	Mean		33.20	3.706
		95% confidence interval for mean	Lower bound	25.82	
			Upper bound	40.58	
		5% trimmed mean		28.25	
		Median		22.50	
		Variance		1098.694	
		Std. deviation		33.147	
		Minimum		0	
		Maximum		244	
		Range		244	
		Inter-quartile range		19.75	
		Skewness		4.082	0.269
		Kurtosis		21.457	0.532
	Yes	Mean		45.52	5.358
		95% confidence interval for mean	Lower bound	34.76	
			Upper bound	56.28	
		5% trimmed mean		40.36	
		Median		37.00	
		Variance		1492.804	
		Std. deviation		38.637	
		Minimum		11	
		Maximum		211	
		Range		200	
		Inter-quartile range		28.50	
		Skewness		2.502	0.330
		Kurtosis		7.012	0.650

Continued

Tests of Normality

	Infection	Kolmogorov–Smirnov[a]			Shapiro–Wilk		
		Statistic	df	Sig.	Statistic	df	Sig.
Length of stay	No	0.252	80	0.000	0.576	80	0.000
	Yes	0.262	52	0.000	0.707	52	0.000

[a] Lilliefors significance correction.

The Descriptives table shows that the mean and median values for length of stay for babies with no infection are 33.20 – 22.50, or 10.70 units apart and 45.52 – 37.00, or 8.52 units apart for babies with an infection. The variances are unequal at 1098.694 for no infection and 1492.804 for infection, that is a ratio of 1:1.4. The skewness statistics are all above 2 and the kurtosis statistics are also high, indicating that the data are peaked and are not normally distributed. The P values for the Kolmogorov–Smirnov and the Shapiro–Wilk tests are shown in the column labelled Sig. and are less than 0.05 for both groups, indicating that the data do not pass the tests of normality in either group.

The histograms and plots shown in Figure 3.10 confirm the results of the tests of normality. The histograms show that both distributions are positively skewed with tails to the right. The Q–Q plot for each group does not follow the line of normality and is significantly curved. The box plots show a number of extreme and outlying values. The maximum value for length of stay of babies with no infection is 6.36 z scores above the mean, while for babies with an infection the maximum value is 4.28 z scores above the mean.

The normality statistics for babies with an infection and babies without an infection are summarised in Table 3.7, with 'no' indicating that the distribution is outside the normal range.

For both groups, the data are positively skewed and could possibly be transformed to normality using a logarithmic transformation. Without transformation, the most appropriate test for analysing length of stay is a rank based non-parametric test, which can be obtained using the commands shown in Box 3.8.

The Mann–Whitney U test is based on ranking the data values as if they were from a single sample. For illustrative purposes, a subset of the data, that is the first 20 cases in the data set with valid length of stay are shown in Table 3.8. Firstly, the data are sorted in order of magnitude and ranked. Data points that are equal share tied ranks. Thus, the two data points of 13 share the ranks of 7 and 8 and are rated at 7.5 each. Similarly, the four data points of 17 share the ranks from 17 to 20 and are ranked at 18.5 each, which is the mean of the four rankings. Once the ranks are assigned, they are then summed for each of the groups.

In SPSS, the mean rank and the sum of the ranks are calculated for each group. In the Ranks table all cases are included. The sum of ranks and mean ranks gives a direction of effect but because the data are ranked, the dimension is different from the original measurement and is therefore difficult to communicate. The Mann–Whitney U and the Wilcoxon W that are obtained from SPSS are two derivations of the same test and are best reported as the Mann–Whitney U test. The Test Statistics table shows that the P value for the difference between groups is $P = 0.004$ which is statistically significant. The asymptotic significance value is reported when the sample size is large, say more than 30 cases, otherwise the *Exact* button at the bottom of the command screen can be used to calculate P values for a small sample.

The difference between the groups could be reported in a table as shown in Table 3.9.

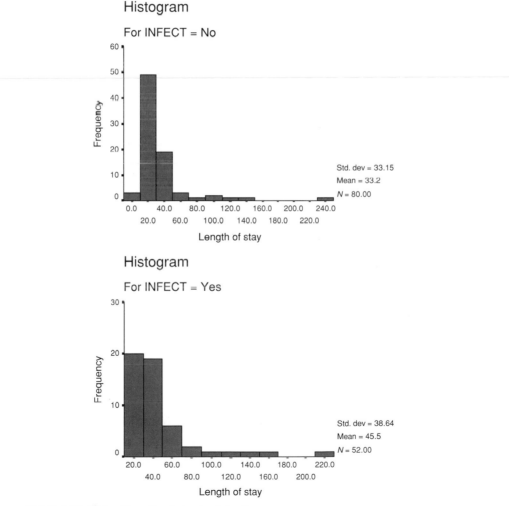

Figure 3.10 Plots of length of stay by infection.

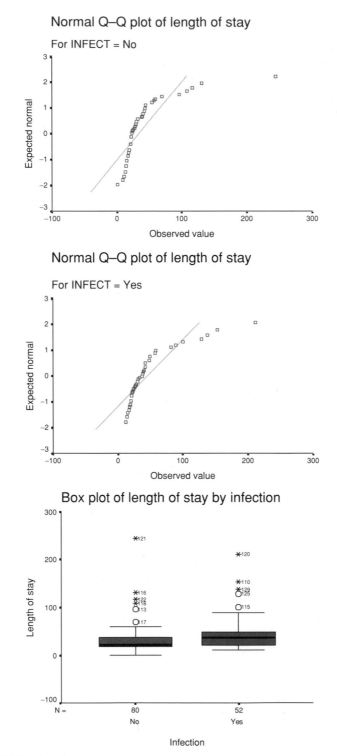

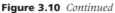

Figure 3.10 *Continued*

Table 3.7 Summary of statistics to assess whether data are within normal limits or outside normal range

Group	Mean – median	Skewness	Kurtosis	Shapiro–Wilk test	K-S test	Plots	Overall decision
No	No	No	No	No	No	No	No
Yes	No	No	No	No	No	No	No

Box 3.8 SPSS commands to obtain a non-parametric test for two independent groups

SPSS Commands
surgery – SPSS Data Editor
  Analyze → Nonparametric Tests → 2 Independent Samples
Two-Independent-Samples Test
  Highlight Length of stay into Test Variable List
  Highlight Infection into Grouping Variable
  Test Type tick Mann-Whitney U (default setting)
  Click on Define Groups
Two Independent Samples: Define Groups
  Group1 = 1
  Group 2 = 2
  Click Continue
Two-Independent-Samples Test
  Click OK

NPar Tests
Mann–Whitney Test

Ranks

	Infection	N	Mean rank	Sum of ranks
Length of stay	No	80	58.88	4710.00
	Yes	52	78.23	4068.00
	Total	132		

Test Statistics[a]

	Length of stay
Mann–Whitney U	1470.000
Wilcoxon W	4710.000
Z	−2.843
Asymp. sig. (two-tailed)	0.004

[a] Grouping variable: infection.

Table 3.8 Ranking data to compute non-parametric statistics

ID	Length of stay	Infection group	Rank Group 1	Rank Group 2
32	0	1	1	
33	1	1	2	
12	9	1	3	
16	11	1	4.5	
22	11	2		4.5
28	12	2		6
20	13	1	7.5	
27	13	1	7.5	
10	14	1	10.5	
11	14	1	10.5	
24	14	1	10.5	
25	14	2		10.5
14	15	1	14.5	
19	15	1	14.5	
23	15	2		14.5
30	15	1	14.5	
13	17	1	18.5	
15	17	1	18.5	
17	17	1	18.5	
21	17	2		18.5
		Sum of ranks	156	54
		N	15	5
		Mean	10.5	10.8

Another approach to non-normal data is to divide the outcome variable into categorical centile groups as discussed in Chapter 7. Decision about whether to use non-parametric tests, to transform the variable or to categorise the values requires careful consideration. The decision should be based on the size of the sample, the effectiveness of the transformation in normalising the data and the ways in which the relationship between the explanatory and outcome variables is best presented.

Notes for critical appraisal

Questions to ask when assessing descriptive statistics published in the literature are shown in Box 3.9.

Table 3.9 Length of stay for babies with infection and without infection

	Infection absent	Infection present	P value
Number			
Length of stay	80	52	
Median and IQ range	22.50 (19.75)	45.52 (37.00)	0.004

Box 3.9 Questions for critical appraisal

The following questions should be asked when appraising published results:

- are any cases included in a group more than once, for example are any follow-up data treated as independent data?
- is there evidence that the outcome variable is normally distributed in each group?
- if the variance of the two groups is unequal, has the correct P value, that is the P value with equal variances not assumed, been reported?
- are the summary statistics appropriate for the distributions?
- are there any influential outliers that could have increased the difference in mean values between the groups?
- Are mean values presented appropriately in figures as dot plots or are histograms used inappropriately?
- are mean values and the differences between groups presented with 95% confidence intervals?

References

1. Cohen J. Statistical power analysis for the behavioural sciences (2nd edition). Hillsdale, NJ: Lawrence Erlbaum Associates, 1988; p. 44.
2. Cohen J. A power primer. Psychol Bull 1992; 1:155–159.
3. Peat JK, Mellis CM, Williams K, Xuan W. Health science research. In: A handbook of quantitative methods. Crows Nest, Australia: Allen and Unwin, 2002; pp 128–147.
4. Stevens J. Applied multivariate statistics for the social sciences (3rd edition). Mahwah, NJ: Lawrence Erlbaum Associates, 1996; p. 17.
5. Tabachnick BG, Fidell LS. Using multivariate statistics (4th edition). Boston, USA: Allyn and Bacon, 2001; pp 66–71.

CHAPTER 4

Continuous variables: paired and one-sample t-tests

A statistician is a person who likes to prove you wrong, 5% of the time.
TAKEN FROM AN INTERNET BULLETIN BOARD

Objectives

The objectives of this chapter are to explain how to:
- analyse paired or matched data
- use paired t-tests and one-sample t-tests
- interpret results from non-parametric paired tests
- report changes or differences in paired data in appropriate units

In addition to two-sample (independent) t-tests, there are also two other t-tests that can be used to analyse continuous data, that is paired t-tests and one-sample (single sample) t-tests. All three types of t-test can be one-tailed or two-tailed tests but one-tailed t-tests are rarely used.

A paired t-test is used to estimate whether the means of two related measurements are significantly different from one another. This test is used when two continuous variables are related because they are collected from the same participant at different times, from different sites on the same person at the same time or from cases and their matched controls[1]. Examples of paired study designs are:

- data from a longitudinal study
- measurements collected before and after an intervention in an experimental study
- differences between related sites in the same person, for example limbs, eyes or kidneys
- matched cases and controls

For a paired t-test, there is no explanatory (group) variable. The outcome of interest is the difference in the outcome measurements between each pair or between each case and its matched control, that is the within-pair differences. When using a paired t-test, the variation between the pairs of measurements is the most important statistic and the variation between the participants, as when using a two-sample t-test, is of little interest. In effect, a paired t-test is used to assess whether the mean of the differences between the two related measurements is significantly different from zero.

For related measurements, the data for each pair of values must be entered on the same row of the spreadsheet. Thus, the number of rows in the data sheet is the same as the number of participants when the outcome variable is measured twice for each participant or is the number of participant-pairs when cases and controls are matched. When each participant is measured on two occasions, the effective sample size is the number of participants. In a matched case-control study, the number of case-control pairs is the effective sample size and not the total number of participants. For this reason, withdrawals, loss of follow-up data and inability to recruit matched controls reduce both power and the generalisability of the paired t-test because participants with missing paired values have to be excluded from the analyses.

Assumptions for a paired t-test

Independent two-sample t-tests cannot be used for analysing paired or matched data because the assumption that the two groups are independent, that is data are collected from different or non-matched participants, would be violated. Treating paired or matched measurements as independent samples will artificially inflate the sample size and lead to inaccurate analyses.

The assumptions for using paired t tests are shown in Box 4.1.

> **Box 4.1** Assumptions for a paired t-test
>
> For a paired t-test the following assumptions must be met:
> • the outcome variable has a continuous scale
> • the differences between the pairs of measurements are normally distributed

The data file **growth.sav** contains the body measurements of 277 babies measured at 1 month and at 3 months of age.

Questions:	Does the weight of babies increase significantly in a 2-month growth period?
	Does the length of babies increase significantly in a 2-month growth period?
	Does the head circumference of babies increase significantly in a 2-month growth period?
Null hypotheses:	The weight of babies is not different between the two time periods.
	The length of babies is not different between the two time periods.
	The head circumference of babies is not different between the two time periods.
Variables:	Outcome variables = weight, length and head circumference measured at 1 month of age and 3 months of age (continuous)

The decision of whether to use a one- or two-tailed test must be made when the study is designed. If a one-tailed t-test is used, the null hypothesis is more likely to be rejected than if a two-tailed test is used (Chapter 3). In general, two-tailed tests should always be used unless there is a good reason for not doing so and a one-tailed test should only be used when the direction of effect is specified in advance[2]. In this example, it makes sense to test for a significant increase in body measurements because there is certainty that a decrease will not occur and there is only one biologically plausible direction of effect. Therefore a one-tailed test is appropriate for the alternate hypothesis.

To test the assumption that the differences between the two outcome variables is normally distributed, the differences between measurements taken at 1 month and at 3 months must first be computed as shown in Box 4.2.

Box 4.2 SPSS commands to transform variables

SPSS Commands
growth – SPSS Data Editor
        Transform → Compute
Compute Variable
        Target Variable = diffwt
        Numeric Expression = Weight at 3mo – Weight at 1mo
        Click OK

By clicking on the *Reset* button in *Compute Variable* all fields will be reset to empty and the command sequence shown in Box 4.2 can be used to compute the following variables:

diffleng = Length at 3mo – Length at 1mo, and

diffhead = Head circumference at 3mo – Head circumference at 1mo

Once the new variables are created, they should be labelled and have the number of decimal places adjusted to be appropriate. The distribution of these differences between the paired measurements can then be examined using the commands shown in Box 4.3 to obtain histograms. While only histograms have been obtained in this example, in practice a thorough investigation of all tests of normality should be undertaken using *Analyze → Descriptive Statistics → Explore* and other options discussed in Chapter 2.

Box 4.3 SPSS commands to obtain frequency histograms

SPSS Commands
        Graphs → Histogram
Histogram
        Variable = Weight 3mo-1mo
        Tick box 'Display normal curve'
        Click OK

The command sequence in Box 4.3 can then be repeated with the variables Length 3m-1mo and Head 3mo-1mo to produce the histograms shown in Figure 4.1. The histograms indicate that all three difference variables are fairly normally distributed with only a slight skew to the right hand side. A paired *t*-test will be robust to these small departures from normality because with 277 babies the sample size is large.

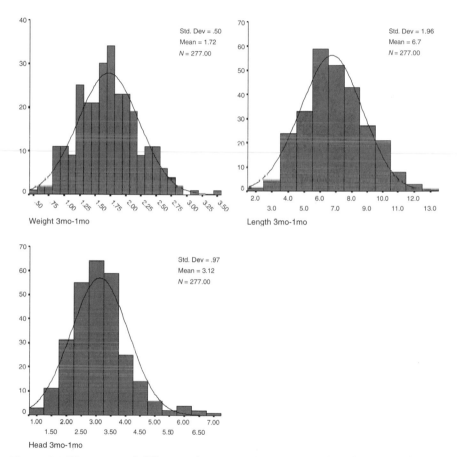

Figure 4.1 Histograms of differences between babies at 1 month and 3 months for weight, length and head circumference.

The SPSS commands to conduct a paired samples *t*-test to examine whether there has been a significant increase in weight, length and head circumference are shown in Box 4.4. By holding down the Ctrl key, two variables can be highlighted and clicked over simultaneously into the Paired Variables box.

Box 4.4 SPSS commands to obtain a paired samples *t*-test

SPSS Commands
growth – SPSS Data Editor
    Analyze → Compare Means → Paired-Samples T Test
Paired-Samples T-Test
    Highlight Weight at 1mo (Variable 1) and Weight at 3mo (Variable 2) and
        click over into the Paired Variables box (weight1m – weight3m)
    Highlight Length at 1mo (Variable 1) and Length at 3mo (Variable 2) and
        click over into the Paired Variables box (length1m – length3m)
    Highlight Head circumference at 1m (Variable 1) and Head circumference
        at 3mo (Variable 2) and click over into the Paired Variables box (head1m
        – head3m)
    Click OK

t-test

Paired Samples Statistics

		Mean	N	Std. deviation	Std. error mean
Pair 1	Weight at 1 mo (kg)	4.415	277	0.6145	0.0369
	Weight at 3 mo (kg)	6.131	277	0.7741	0.0465
Pair 2	Length at 1 mo (cm)	54.799	277	2.3081	0.1387
	Length at 3 mo (cm)	61.510	277	2.7005	0.1623
Pair 3	Head circumference at 1 mo (cm)	37.918	277	1.3685	0.0822
	Head circumference at 3 mo (cm)	41.039	277	1.3504	0.0811

Paired Samples Correlations

		N	Correlation	Sig.
Pair 1	Weight at 1 mo (kg) & Weight at 3 mo (kg)	277	0.768	0.000
Pair 2	Length at 1 mo (cm) & Length at 3 mo (cm)	277	0.703	0.000
Pair 3	Head circumference at 1 mo (cm) & Head circumference at 3 mo (cm)	277	0.746	0.000

The Paired Samples Statistics table provides summary statistics for each variable but does not give any information that is relevant to the paired *t*-test. The

Paired Samples Correlations table shows the correlations between each of the paired measurements. This table should be ignored because it does not make sense to test the hypothesis that two related measurements are associated with one another.

Paired Samples Test

		Paired differences							
		Mean	Std. deviation	Std. error Mean	95% confidence interval of the difference		t	df	Sig. (Two-tailed)
					Lower	Upper			
Pair 1	Weight at 1 mo (kg) − weight at 3 mo (kg)	−1.717	0.4961	0.0298	−1.775	−1.658	−57.591	276	0.000
Pair 2	Length at 1mo (cm) − length at 3 mo (cm)	−6.710	1.9635	0.1180	−6.943	−6.478	−56.881	276	0.000
Pair 3	Head circumference at 1 mo (cm) − head circumference at 3 mo (cm)	−3.121	0.9697	0.0583	−3.236	−3.006	−53.565	276	0.000

The Paired Samples Test table provides important information about the *t*-test results. The second column, which is labelled Mean, gives the main outcome statistic, that is the mean within-pair difference. When conducting a paired *t*-test, the means of the differences between the pairs of variables are computed as part of the test. The only way to control the direction of the mean differences is by organising the order of variables in the spreadsheet. In the data set, weight at 1 month occurs before weight at 3 months, so it is not possible to obtain a paired samples *t*-test with weight at 3mo as Variable 1 and weight at 1mo as Variable 2 unless the data set is re-organised.

The mean paired differences column in the table indicates that at 1 month, babies were on average 1.717 kg lower in weight, 6.71 cm smaller in length and 3.121 cm smaller in head circumference than at 3 months of age. These mean values do not answer the research question of whether babies increased significantly in measurements over a 2-month period but rather answer the question of whether the babies were smaller at a younger age.

The 95% confidence intervals of the differences, which are calculated as the mean paired differences ± (1.96 * SE of mean paired differences), do not contain the value of zero for any variable which also indicates that the difference in body size between 1 and 3 months is statistically significant. The *t* value is calculated as the mean differences divided by their standard error. Because the standard error becomes smaller as the sample size becomes larger, the *t* value increases as the sample size increases for the same mean difference. Thus, in this example with a large sample size of 277 babies, relatively small mean differences are highly statistically significant.

The *P* values provided in the Paired Samples Test table are for a two-tailed test, so they have to be adjusted for a one-sample test by halving the *P* value. In this example, the *P* values are <0.0001 so that halving them will also render a highly significant P value. The P values (one tailed) from the paired t-tests for all three variables indicate that each null hypothesis should be rejected and that there is a significant increase in body measurements between the two time periods. By multiplying the mean difference values by -1, to obtain the mean difference in the correct direction (i.e. weight at 3 months − weight at 1 month), babies over a 2-month period were significantly heavier ($+1.72$ kg, $P < 0.0001$), longer ($+6.71$ cm, $P < 0.0001$) and had a larger head circumference ($+3.12$ cm, $P < 0.0001$). As with any statistical test, it is important to decide whether the size of mean difference between measurements would be considered clinically important in addition to considering statistical significance.

Non-parametric test for paired data

A non-parametric equivalent of the paired t-test is the Wilcoxon signed rank test, which is also called the Wilcoxon matched pairs test and is used when lack of normality in the differences is a concern or when the sample size is small. The Wilcoxon signed rank test is used to test whether the median of the differences is equal to zero.

An assumption of the Wilcoxon signed rank test is that the paired differences are independent and come from the same continuous and symmetric population distribution. This test is relatively resistant to outliers. However, the number of outliers should not be large relative to the sample size and the amount of skewness should be equal in both groups. When the sample size is small, symmetry may be difficult to assess.

In this test, the absolute differences between paired scores are ranked and difference scores that are equal to zero, that is indicate no difference between pairs, are excluded from the analysis. Thus, this test is not suitable when a large proportion of paired differences are equal to zero because this effectively reduces the sample size.

If the difference values in the **growth.sav** data set did not have a normal distribution, the Wilcoxon signed rank test could be obtained using the SPSS commands in Box 4.5.

Box 4.5 SPSS commands to conduct a non-parametric paired test

SPSS Commands

growth – SPSS Data Editor
   Analyze → Nonparametric Tests → 2 Related Samples
Two Related Samples
   Click on Weight at 1mo (Variable 1) and click on Weight at 3mo
      (Variable 2)
   Click on the arrow to place variables under Test Pair(s) List (weight1m –
      weight3m)
   Click on Length at 1mo (Variable 1) and click on Length at 3mo
      (Variable 2)

> Click on the arrow to place variables under Test Pair(s) List
> (length1m – length3m)
> Click on Head circumference at 1mo (Variable 1) and click on Head
> circumference at 3mo (Variable 2)
> Click on the arrow to place variables under Test Pair(s) List (head1m –
> head3m)
> Test Type = tick Wilcoxon (default setting)
> Click Options
> Two-Related-Samples: Options
> Tick Quartiles
> Click Continue
> Two Related Samples
> Click OK

NPar tests

Descriptive Statistics

	N	25th	50th (median)	75th
			Percentiles	
Weight at 1 mo (kg)	277	4.000	4.350	4.815
Length at 1 mo (cm)	277	53.000	54.500	56.500
Head circumference at 1 mo (cm)	277	37.000	38.000	39.000
Weight at 3 mo (kg)	277	5.550	6.040	6.680
Length at 3 mo (cm)	277	59.500	61.500	63.500
Head circumference at 3 mo (cm)	277	40.000	41.000	42.000

Instead of providing information about mean values, this non-parametric test provides the median and the 25th and 75th percentile values as summary statistics. These are the summary statistics that would be used in box plots or reported in tables of results.

Wilcoxon Signed Rank Test

Ranks

		N	Mean Rank	Sum of Ranks
Weight at 3 mo (kg) – weight at 1 mo (kg)	Negative ranks	0[a]	0.00	0.00
	Positive ranks	277[b]	139.00	38503.00
	Ties	0[c]		
	Total	277		

Continued

Ranks *continued*

		N	Mean Rank	Sum of Ranks
Length at 3 mo (cm) − length at 1 mo (cm)	Negative ranks	0[d]	0.00	0.00
	Positive ranks	277[e]	139.00	38503.00
	Ties	0[f]		
	Total	277		
Head circumference at 3 mo (cm) − Head circumference at 1 mo (cm)	Negative ranks	0[g]	0.00	0.00
	Positive ranks	277[h]	139.00	38503.00
	Ties	0[i]		
	Total	277		

[a] Weight at 3 months (kg) < Weight at 1 month (kg)
[b] Weight at 3 months (kg) > Weight at 1 month (kg)
[c] Weight at 1 month (kg) = Weight at 3 months (kg)
[d] Length at 3 months (cm) < Length at 1 month (cm)
[e] Length at 3 months (cm) > Length at 1 month (cm)
[f] Length at 1 month (cm) = Length at 3 months (cm)
[g] Head circumference at 3 months (cm) < Head circumference at 1 month (cm)
[h] Head circumference at 3 months (cm) > Head circumference at 1 month (cm)
[i] Head circumference at 1 month (cm) = Head circumference at 3 months (cm)

Test Statistics[b]

	Weight at 3 months (kg) − weight at 1 month (kg)	Length at 3 months (cm) − length at 1 month (cm)	Head circumference at 3 months (cm) − head circumference at 1 month (cm)
Z	−14.427[a]	−14.438[a]	−14.470[a]
Asymp. sig. (two-tailed)	0.000	0.000	0.000

[a] Based on negative ranks.
[b] Wilcoxon signed ranks test.

The P values that are computed are based on the ranks of the absolute values of the differences between time 1 (1 month) and time 2 (3 months). The number of negative ranks where time 1 is lower than time 2 is compared to the number of positive ranks where time 1 is higher than time 2 with the zero ranks omitted. In this test the summary statistics are given the opposite direction of effect to the paired t-test and, in this case, give the correct direction of effect.

The Ranks table indicates that, as expected, no babies have a negative rank that is a lower measurement at 1 month than at 3 months. The table also shows that there are no ties, that is no babies with the same difference scores. Although this table does not provide any useful information for communicating the size of effect, it does indicate the correct direction of effect. The test statistics with a P value of <0.0001 for all variables show that there has been a significant increase in all measurements from 1 month (baseline) to 3 months. Because the data are fairly normally distributed, both the parametric test and the non-parametric test give the same P values.

The results of this non-parametric test would be reported as for a paired t-test except that the median differences rather than the mean differences would be reported and, if required, the inter-quartile range and the z score would be reported rather than the standard deviation and the paired t value.

Standardising for differences in baseline measurements

With paired data, the differences between the pairs are sometimes not an appropriate outcome of interest. It is often important that the differences are standardised for between-subject differences in baseline values. One method is to compute a per cent change from baseline. Another method is to calculate the ratio between the follow-up and baseline measurements. It is important to choose a method that is appropriate for the type of data collected and that is easily communicated.

For babies' growth, per cent change is a simple method to standardise for differences in body size at baseline, that is at 1 month of age. The syntax shown in Box 4.6 can be used to compute per cent growth in weight, length and head circumference.

Box 4.6 SPSS commands to compute per cent changes

SPSS Commands
growth – SPSS Data Editor
> *Transform → Compute*
Compute Variable
> *Target Variable = perwt*
> *Numeric Expression = (Weight at 3mo – Weight at 1mo) * 100/*
> > *Weight at 1mo*
> *Click Paste*
Syntax1 – SPSS Syntax Editor
> *Run → All*

The syntax can then be repeated to compute:

Perleng = (Length at 3mo - Length at 1mo)*100/Length at 1mo, and

Perhead = (Head circumference at 3mo - Head circumference at 1mo)*100/
> *Head circumference at 1mo*

The paste and run commands list the transformations in the syntax window as shown below. This information can then be printed and stored for documentation. Once the computations are complete, the new variables need to be labelled in the Variable View window.

COMPUTE perwt = (weight3m − weight1m)*100/weight1m.
EXECUTE.

COMPUTE perlen = (length3m − length1m)*100/length1m.
EXECUTE.

COMPUTE perhead = (head3m − head1m)*100/head1m.
EXECUTE.

An assumption of paired *t*-tests is that the differences between the pairs of measurements are normally distributed, therefore the distributions of the per cent changes need to be examined. Again, the distributions should be fully checked for normality using *Analyze → Descriptive Statistics → Explore* as discussed in Chapter 2. The histograms shown in Figure 4.2 can be obtained

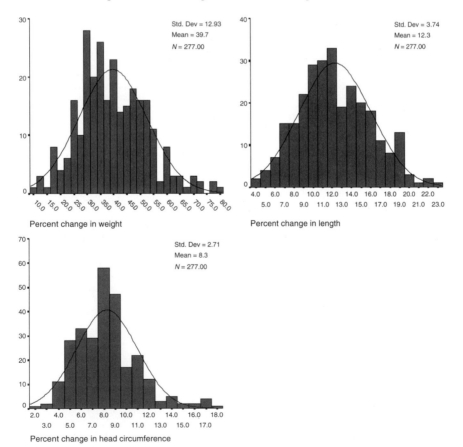

Figure 4.2 Histograms of per cent change in weight, length and head circumference.

using the commands shown in Box 4.3. The histograms for per cent change in weight and head circumference have a small tail to the right, but the sample size is large and the tails are not so marked that the assumptions for using a paired t-test would be violated.

Single-sample *t*-test

The research question has now changed slightly because rather than considering absolute differences between time points, the null hypothesis being tested is whether the mean per cent changes over time are significantly different from zero. With differences converted to a per cent change, there is now a single continuous outcome variable and no group variable. Thus, a one-sample t-test, which is also called a single-sample t-test, can be used to test whether there is a statistically significant difference between the mean per cent change and a fixed value such as zero.

A one-sample test is more flexible than a paired t-test, which is limited to testing whether the mean difference is significantly different from zero. One-sample t-tests can be used, for example, to test if the sample has a different mean from 100 points if the outcome being measured is IQ or from 40 hours if the outcome measured is the average working week. A one-sample t-test is a parametric test and the only assumption is that the data, in this case per cent increases, are normally distributed.

Computing per cent changes provides control over the units that the changes are expressed in and their direction of effect. However, if the differences computed in Box 4.2 were used as the outcome and a one-sample t-test was used to test for a difference from zero, the one-sample t-test would give exactly the same P values as the paired t-test although the direction of effect would be correctly reversed.

For the research question, the command sequence shown in Box 4.7 can be used to compute a one-sample t-test to test whether the per cent changes in weight, length and head circumference are significantly different from zero.

Box 4.7 SPSS commands to conduct a one-sample *t*-test

SPSS Commands
Growth – SPSS Data Editor
> *Analyze → Compare Means → One-Sample T Test*
One-Sample T Test
> *Highlight the variables Percent change in weight, Percent change in length and Percent change in head circumference and click into the Test Variable(s) box*
> *Test Value = 0 (default setting)*
> *Click OK*

t-test

One-Sample Statistics

	N	Mean	Std. deviation	Std. error mean
Per cent change in weight	277	39.7264	12.9322	0.7770
Per cent change in length	277	12.2980	3.7413	0.2248
Per cent change in head circumference	277	8.2767	2.7115	0.1629

The One-Sample Statistics table gives more relevant statistics with which to answer the research question because the mean within-participant per cent changes and their standard deviations are provided. The means in this table show that the per cent increase in weight over 2 months is larger than the per cent increase in length and head circumference.

One-Sample Test

					95% confidence interval of the difference	
	t	df	Sig. (two-tailed)	Mean difference	Lower	Upper
Per cent change in weight	51.126	276	0.000	39.7264	38.1968	41.2561
Per cent change in length	54.708	276	0.000	12.2980	11.8555	12.7406
Per cent change in head circumference	50.803	276	0.000	8.2767	7.9559	8.5974

Test value = 0

In the One-Sample Test table, the *t* values are again computed as mean difference divided by the standard error and, in this table, are highly significant for all measurements. The highly significant *P* values are reflected in the 95% confidence intervals, none of which contain the zero value. The outcomes are now all in the same units, that is per cent change, and therefore growth rates between the three variables can be directly compared. This was not possible before when the variables were in their original units of measurement. This summary information could be reported as shown in Table 4.1. In some disciplines, the *t* value is also reported with its degrees of freedom, for example as $t(276) = 51.13$ but because the only interpretation of the *t* value and its degrees of freedom is the *P* value, it is often excluded from summary tables.

Table 4.1 Mean body measurements and per cent change between 1 and 3 months in 277 babies

	1 month Mean (SD)	3 months Mean (SD)	Per cent increase and 95% CI	P value
Weight (kg)	4.42 (0.62)	6.13 (0.77)	39.7 (38.2, 41.3)	<0.0001
Length (cm)	54.8 (2.3)	61.5 (2.7)	12.3 (11.9, 12.7)	<0.0001
Head circumference (cm)	37.9 (1.4)	41.0 (1.4)	8.3 (7.9, 8.6)	<0.0001

Research question

The research question can now be extended to ask if certain groups, such as males and females, have different patterns or rates of growth.

Questions:	Over a 2-month period: - do males increase in weight significantly more than females? - do males increase in length significantly more than females? do males increase in head circumference significantly more than females?
Null hypothesis:	Over a 2-month period: - there is no difference between males and females in weight growth. - there is no difference between males and females in length growth. - there is no difference between males and females in head circumference growth.
Variables:	Outcome variables = per cent increase in length, weight and head circumference (continuous) Explanatory variable = gender (categorical, binary)

The research question then becomes a two-sample *t*-test again because there is a continuously distributed variable (per cent change) and a binary group variable with two levels that are independent (male, female). The SPSS commands shown in Box 3.3 in Chapter 3 can be used to obtain the following output.

t-test

Group Statistics

	Gender	N	Mean	Std. deviation	Std. error mean
Per cent change in weight	Male	148	42.0051	13.2656	1.0904
	Female	129	37.1121	12.0676	1.0625

Continued

Group Statistics *continued*

	Gender	N	Mean	Std. deviation	Std. error mean
Per cent change in length	Male	148	12.6818	3.3079	0.2719
	Female	129	11.8577	4.1533	0.3657
Per cent change in head	Male	148	8.2435	2.5066	0.2060
circumference	Female	129	8.3147	2.9385	0.2587

The means in the Group Statistics table show that males have a higher increase in weight and length than females but a slightly lower increase in head circumference. These statistics are useful for summarising the magnitude of the differences in each gender.

In the Independent Samples Test table (opposite), Levene's test of equality of variances shows that the variances are not significantly different between genders for weight ($P = 0.374$) and head circumference ($P = 0.111$). For these two variables, the *Equal variances assumed* rows in the table are used. However, the variance in per cent change for length is significantly different between the genders ($P = 0.034$) and therefore the appropriate t value, degrees of freedom and P value for this variable are shown in the *Equal variances not assumed* row. An indication that the variances are unequal could be seen in the previous Group Statistics table, which shows that the standard deviation for per cent change in length is 3.3079 for males and 4.1533 for females. An estimate of the variances can be obtained by squaring the standard deviations to give 10.94 for males and 17.25 for females, which is a variance ratio of 1:1.6.

Thus, the Independent Samples Test table shows that per cent increase in weight is significantly different between the genders at $P = 0.002$, per cent increase in length does not reach significance between the genders at $P = 0.072$ and per cent increase in head circumference is not clearly not different between the genders at $P = 0.828$. This is reflected in the 95% confidence intervals, which do not cross zero for weight, cross zero marginally for length and encompass zero for head circumference.

Presenting the results

The growth patterns for weight are different between genders and therefore it is important to present the one-sample *t*-test results for each gender separately. If no between-gender differences were found, the summary statistics for the entire sample could be presented. In this case, one-sample *t*-tests are used to test whether the mean per cent increase is significantly different from zero for each gender. This can be achieved using the *Split File* option shown in Box 4.8. After the commands have been completed, the message *Split File On* will appear in the bottom right hand side of the Data Editor screen. The advantage of using *Split File* rather than *Select Cases* is that the output will be automatically documented with group status.

Independent Samples Test

		Levene's test for equality of variances		t-test for equality of means						95% confidence interval of the difference	
		F	Sig.	t	df	Sig. (Two-tailed)	Mean difference	Std. error difference		Lower	Upper
Per cent change in weight	Equal variances assumed	0.792	0.374	3.193	275	0.002	4.8930	1.53240		1.87633	7.90976
	Equal variances not assumed			3.214	274.486	0.001	4.8930	1.52247		1.89583	7.89025
¶ Per cent change in length	Equal variances assumed	4.518	0.034	1.837	275	0.067	0.8241	0.44873		−0.05928	1.70748
	Equal variances not assumed			1.808	243.779	0.072	0.8241	0.45569		−0.07350	1.72170
¶ Per cent change in head circumference	Equal variances assumed	2.561	0.111	−0.217	275	0.828	−0.0711	0.32717		−0.71521	0.57294
	Equal variances not assumed			−0.215	253.173	0.830	−0.0711	0.33074		−0.72248	0.58021

> **Box 4.8** SPSS commands to compare gender means
>
> **SPSS Commands**
> *growth – SPSS Data Editor*
>   *Data → Split File*
> *Split File*
>   *Click Compare groups*
>   *Highlight Gender and click over into 'Groups Based on'*
>   *Click OK*

The one-sample *t*-test for each gender can then be obtained using the commands shown in Box 4.7 to produce the following output.

t-test

One-Sample Statistics

Gender		N	Mean	Std. deviation	Std. error mean
Male	Per cent change in weight	148	42.0051	13.2656	1.0904
	Per cent change in length	148	12.6818	3.3079	0.2719
	Per cent change in head circumference	148	8.2435	2.5066	0.2060
Female	Per cent change in weight	129	37.1121	12.0676	1.0625
	Per cent change in length	129	11.8577	4.1533	0.3657
	Per cent change in head circumference	129	8.3147	2.9385	0.2587

One-Sample Test

Gender		t	df	Sig. (Two-tailed)	Mean difference	95% confidence interval of the difference	
						Lower	Upper
Male	Per cent change in weight	38.522	147	0.000	42.0051	39.8502	44.1601
	Per cent change in length	46.640	147	0.000	12.6818	12.1445	13.2192
	Per cent change in head circumference	40.010	147	0.000	8.2435	7.8363	8.6507

Continued

						95% confidence interval of the difference	
Gender		t	df	Sig. (Two-tailed)	Mean difference	Lower	Upper
Female	Per cent change in weight	34.929	128	0.000	37.1121	35.0098	39.2144
	Per cent change in length	32.426	128	0.000	11.8577	11.1342	12.5813
	Per cent change in head cir-cumference	32.138	128	0.000	8.3147	7.8027	8.8266

The One-Sample Statistics table gives the same summary statistics as obtained in the two-sample *t*-test but gives a *P* value for the significance of the per cent change from baseline for each gender and also gives the 95% confidence intervals around the mean changes. Another alternative to obtaining summary means for each gender is to use the commands shown in Box 4.9, but with the *Split File* option removed.

Box 4.9 SPSS commands to obtain summary mean values

SPSS Commands
growth – SPSS Data Editor
        Data → Split File
Split File
        Click Analyze all cases, do not create groups
        Click OK
growth – SPSS Data Editor
        Analyze → Compare Means → Means
Means
        Click variables for weight, length, head circumference at 1 month (weight1m, length1m, head1m) and at 3 months (weight3m, length3m, head3m) and all three percent changes (perwt, perlen, perhead) into the Dependent List box
        Click Gender over into the Independent List box
        Click OK

Means
Report

Gender		Weight at 1 mo (kg)	Length at 1 mo (cm)	Head circumference at 1 mo (cm)	Weight at 3 mo (kg)	Length at 3 mo (cm)	Head circumference at 3 mo (cm)	Per cent change in weight	Per cent change in length	Per cent change in head circumference
Male	Mean	4.534	55.249	38.259	6.389	62.218	41.393	42.0051	12.6818	8.2435
	N	148	148	148	148	148	148	148	148	148
	Std. deviation	0.6608	2.5636	1.3252	0.7829	2.6185	1.1411	13.26558	3.30790	2.50656
Female	Mean	4.278	54.283	37.526	5.836	60.698	40.632	37.1121	11.8577	8.3147
	N	129	129	129	129	129	129	129	129	129
	Std. deviation	0.5269	1.8539	1.3160	0.6507	2.5704	1.4575	12.06764	4.15334	2.93850
Total	Mean	4.415	54.799	37.918	6.131	61.510	41.039	39.7264	12.2980	8.2767
	N	277	277	277	277	277	277	277	277	277
	Std. deviation	0.6145	2.3081	1.3685	0.7741	2.7005	1.3504	12.93223	3.74134	2.71147

The Report table completes the information needed to report the results as shown in Table 4.2. Although a one-tailed P value is used for the significance of increases in body size, a two-tailed P value is used for between-gender comparisons.

Table 4.2 Mean body measurements and per cent change between 1 and 3 months in 148 male and 129 female babies

		1 month Mean (SD)	3 months Mean (SD)	Per cent change and 95% CI	P value for change from baseline	P value for difference between genders
Weight (kg)	Male	4.53 (0.66)	6.39 (0.78)	42.0 (39.9, 44.2)	<0.0001	0.002
	Female	4.28 (0.53)	5.84 (0.65)	37.1 (35.0, 39.2)	<0.0001	
Length (cm)	Male	55.2 (2.6)	62.2 (2.6)	12.7 (12.1, 13.2)	<0.0001	0.072
	Female	54.3 (1.9)	60.7 (2.6)	11.9 (11.1, 12.6)	<0.0001	
Head circumference (cm)	Male	38.3 (1.3)	41.4 (1.1)	8.2 (7.8, 8.7)	<0.0001	0.828
	Female	37.5 (1.3)	40.6 (1.5)	8.3 (7.8, 8.8)	<0.0001	

When plotting summary statistics of continuous variables, the choice of whether to use bar charts or dot points is critical. Bar charts should always begin at zero so that their lengths can be meaningfully compared. When the distance from zero has no meaning, mean values are best plotted as dot points. For example, mean length would not be plotted using a bar chart because no baby has a zero length. However, bar charts are ideal for plotting per cent changes where a zero value is plausible. The results can be plotted as bar charts in SigmaPlot by entering the data as follows and using the commands shown in Box 4.10. The means for males are entered in column 1 and the 95% confidence interval width in column 2. The values for females are entered in columns 3 and 4. The column titles should not be entered in the spreadsheet cells.

Column 1	Column 2	Column 3	Column 4
42.0	2.1	37.1	2.1
12.7	0.6	11.9	0.6
8.2	0.4	8.3	0.4

Box 4.10 SigmaPlot commands for graphing per cent change results

SigmaPlot Commands
SigmaPlot – [Data 1]
Graph → Create Graph

> *Create Graph – Type*
>   *Highlight Horizontal Bar Chart, click Next*
> *Create Graph –Style*
>   *Highlight Grouped Error Bars, click Next*
> *Create Graph – Error Bars*
>   *Symbol Values = Worksheet Columns (default), click Next*
> *Create Graph – Data Format*
>   *Highlight Many X, click Next*
> *Create Graph – Select Data*
>   *Data for Set 1 = use drop box and select Column 1*
>   *Data for Error 1 = use drop box and select Column 2*
>   *Data for Set 2 = use drop box and select Column 3*
>   *Data for Error 2 = use drop box and select Column 4*
>   *Click Finish*

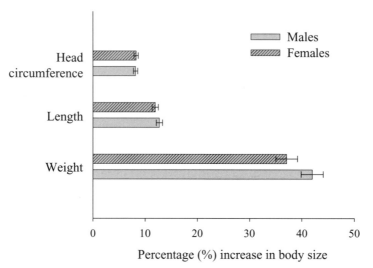

Figure 4.3 Per cent increase in growth from age 1 to 3 months.

The plot can then be customised by changing the axes, fills, labels etc in *Graph → Graph Properties* menus.

Notes for critical appraisal

Questions to ask when assessing statistics from paired or matched data are shown in Box 4.11.

Box 4.11 Questions for critical appraisal

The following questions should be asked when appraising published results from paired or matched data:
- Has an appropriate paired t-test or single sample test been used?
- Do the within-pair differences need to be standardised for baseline differences, that is presented as per cent changes or ratios?
- Are the within-pair differences normally distributed?
- If summary statistics are reported, are they in the same units of change so that they can be directly compared if necessary?
- Have rank based non-parametric tests been used for non-normally distributed differences?
- Have descriptive data been reported for each of the pair of variables in addition to information of mean changes?

References

1. Bland JM, Altman DG. Matching. BMJ 1994; 309: 1128.
2. Bland JM, Altman DG. One and two sided tests of significance. BMJ 1994; 309: 248.

CHAPTER 5

Continuous variables: analysis of variance

I discovered, though unconsciously and insensibly, that the pleasure of observing and reasoning was a much higher one that that of skill and sports.
CHARLES DARWIN.

Objectives

The objectives of this chapter are to explain how to:
- decide when to use an ANOVA test
- run and interpret the output from a one-way or a factorial ANOVA
- understand between-group and within-group differences
- classify factors into fixed, interactive or random effects
- test for a trend across the groups within a factor
- perform post-hoc tests
- build a multivariate ANCOVA model
- report the findings from an ANOVA model
- test the ANOVA assumptions

A two-sample t-test can only be used to assess the significance of the difference between the mean values of two independent groups. To compare differences in the mean values of three or more independent groups, analysis of variance (ANOVA) is used. Thus, ANOVA is suitable when the outcome measurement is a continuous variable and when the explanatory variable is categorical with three or more groups. An ANOVA model can also be used for comparing the effects of several categorical explanatory variables at one time or for comparing differences in the mean values of one or more groups after adjusting for a continuous variable, that is a covariate.

A one-way ANOVA is used when the effect of only one categorical variable (explanatory variable) on a single continuous variable (outcome) is explored, for example when the effect of socioeconomic status, which has three groups (low, medium and high), on weight is examined. The concept of ANOVA can be thought of as an extension of a two-sample t-test but the terminology used is quite different. A factorial ANOVA is used when the effects of two or more categorical variables (explanatory variables) on a single continuous variable (outcome) are explored, for example when the effects of gender and socioeconomic status on weight are examined.

An analysis of covariance (ANCOVA) is used when the effects of one or more categorical factors (explanatory variables) on a single continuous variable (outcome) are explored after adjusting for the effects of one or more continuous variables (covariates). A covariate is any variable that correlates with the outcome variable. For example, ANCOVA would be used to test for the effects of gender and socioeconomic status on weight after adjusting for height.

For both ANOVA and ANCOVA, the theory behind the model must be reliable in that there must be biological plausibility or scientific reason for the effects of the factors being tested. In this, it is important that the factors are independent and not related to one another. For example, it would not make sense to test for differences in mean values of an outcome between groups defined according to education and socioeconomic status when these two variables are related. Once the results of an analysis of variance are obtained, they can only be generalised to the population if the data were collected from a random sample, and a significant P value cannot be taken as evidence of causality.

Building an ANOVA model

When building an ANOVA or ANCOVA model, it is important to build the model in a logical and considered way. The process of model building is as much an art as a science. Descriptive and summary statistics should always be obtained first to provide a good working knowledge of the data before beginning the bivariate analyses or multivariate modelling. In this way, the model can be built up in a systematic way, which is preferable to including all variables in the model and then deciding which variables to remove from the model, that is, using a backward elimination process. Table 5.1 shows the steps in the model building process.

Table 5.1 Steps in building an ANOVA model

Type of analysis	SPSS procedure	Purpose
Univariate analyses	Explore	Examine cell sizes Obtain univariate means Test for normality
Bivariate analyses	Crosstabulations One-way ANOVA	Ensure adequate cell sizes Estimate differences in means and homogeneity of variances Examine trends across groups within a factor
Multivariate analyses	Factorial ANOVA ANCOVA	Test several explanatory factors or adjust for covariates Test normality of residuals Test influence of multivariate outliers

Assumptions for ANOVA models

The assumptions for ANOVA, which must be met in all types of ANOVA models, are shown in Box 5.1.

Box 5.1 Assumptions for using ANOVA

The assumptions that must be met when using one-way or factorial ANOVA are as follows:
- the participants must be independent, that is each participant appears only once in their group
- the groups must be independent, that is each participant must be in one group only
- the outcome variable is normally distributed
- all cells have an adequate sample size
- the cell size ratio is no larger than 1:4
- the variances are similar between groups
- the residuals are normally distributed
- there are no influential outliers

The first two assumptions are similar to the assumptions for two-sample t-tests and any violation will invalidate the analysis. In practice, this means that each participant should appear on one data row of the spreadsheet only and thus will be included in the analysis once only. When cases appear in the spreadsheet on more than one occasion then repeated ANOVA should be used in which case the ID numbers are included as a factor.

When an ANOVA is conducted, the data are divided into cells according to the number of groups in the explanatory variable. Small cell sizes, that is cell sizes less than 10, are always problematic because of the lack of precision in calculating the mean value for the cell. The minimum cell size in theory is 10 but in practice 30 is preferred. In addition to creating imprecision, low cell counts lead to a loss of statistical power. The assumption of a low cell size ratio is also important. A cell size imbalance of more than 1:4 across the model would be a concern, for example when one cell has 10 cases and another cell has 60 cases and the ratio is then 1:6.

It may be difficult to avoid small cell sizes because it is not possible to predict the number of cases in each cell prior to data collection. Even in experimental studies in which equal numbers can be achieved in some groups, drop-outs and missing data can lead to unequal cell sizes. If small cells are present, they can be re-coded into larger cells but only if it is possible to meaningfully interpret the re-coding.

Both the assumptions of a normal distribution and equality of the variance of the outcome variable between cells should be tested before ANOVA is conducted. However, as with a t-test, ANOVA is robust to some deviations from normality of distributions and some imbalance of variances. The assumption that the outcome variable is normally distributed is of most importance when the sample size is small and/or when univariate outliers increase or decrease mean values between cells by an important amount and therefore influence perceived differences between groups. The main effects of non-normality and unequal variances, especially if there are outliers, are to bias the P values. However, the direction of the bias may not be clear.

When variances are not significantly different between cells, the model is said to be homoscedastic. The assumption of equal variances is of most importance when there are small cells, say cells with less than 30 cases, when the cell size ratio is larger than 1:4 or when there are large differences in variance between cells, say larger than 1:10. The main effect of unequal variance is to reduce statistical power and thus lead to type II errors. Equality of variances should be tested in bivariate analyses before running an ANOVA model and then re-affirmed in the final model.

One-way ANOVA

A one-way ANOVA test is very similar to a two-sample t-test but in ANOVA the explanatory variable, which is called a factor, has more than two groups. For example, a factor could be participants' residential area with three groups: inner city, outer suburbs and rural. A one-way ANOVA is used to test the null hypothesis that each group within the factor has the same mean value.

The ANOVA test is called an analysis of variance and not an analysis of means because this test is used to assess whether the mean values of different groups are far enough apart in terms of their spread (variance) to be considered significantly different. Figure 5.1 shows how a one-way ANOVA model in which the factor has three groups can be conceptualised.

If a factor has four groups, it is possible to conduct three independent two-sample t-tests, that is to test the mean values of group 1 vs 2, group 3 vs 4

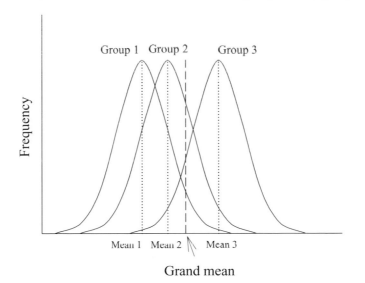

Figure 5.1 Concept of an ANOVA model.

and group 1 vs 4. However, this approach of conducting multiple two-sample *t*-tests increases the probability of obtaining a significant result merely by chance (a type I error). The probability of a type I error not occurring for each *t*-test is 0.95 (i.e. $1 - 0.05$). The three tests are independent, therefore the probability of a type I error not occurring over all three tests is $0.95 \times 0.95 \times 0.95$, or 0.86. Therefore, the probability of at least one type I error occurring over the three two-sample *t*-tests is 0.14 (i.e. $1 - 0.86$), which is higher than the *P* level set at 0.05.[1] A one-way ANOVA is therefore used to investigate the differences between several groups within a factor in one model and to reduce the number of pairwise comparisons that are made.

Within- and between-group variance

To interpret the output from an ANOVA model, it is important to have a concept of the mathematics used in conducting the test. In one-way ANOVA, the data are divided into their groups as shown in Figure 5.1 and a mean for each group is computed. Each mean value is considered to be the predicted value for that particular group of participants. In addition, a grand mean is calculated as shown in Table 5.2. The grand mean which is also shown in Figure 5.1, is the mean for all of the data and will only be the average of the three group means when the sample size in each group is equal.

Table 5.2 Means computed in one-way ANOVA

Group$_1$	Group$_2$	Group$_3$	Total sample
Group mean$_1$	Group mean$_2$	Group mean$_3$	Grand mean

The ANOVA analysis is then based on calculating the difference of each participant's observed value from their group mean, which is regarded as their predicted value, and also the difference from the grand mean. Thus, the following calculations are made for each participant:

Within-group difference = group mean − observed measurement

Between-group difference = grand mean − observed measurement

The within-group difference is the variation of each participant's measurement from their own group mean and is thought of as the explained variation. The between-group difference is the variation of each participant's measurement from the grand mean and is thought of as the unexplained variation. An important concept in ANOVA is that the within-group differences, which are also called residual or error values, are normally distributed.

In calculating ANOVA statistics, the within-group differences are squared and then summed to compute the within-group variance. The between-group differences are also squared and then summed to compute the between-group variance. The effect of squaring the values is to remove the effects of negative values, which would balance out the positive values.

The F value is calculated as the mean between-group variance divided by the mean within-group variance, that is the unexplained variance divided by the explained variance. Thus, the F value indicates whether the between-group variation is greater than would be expected by chance. The higher the F value, the more significant the ANOVA test because the groups (factors) are accounting for a higher proportion of the variance. Obviously, if more of the participants are closer to their group mean than to the grand mean, then the within-group variance will be lower than the between-group variance and F will be large. If the within-group variance is equal to the between-group variance, then F will be equal to 1 indicating that there is no significant difference in means between the groups of the factor.

If there are only two groups in a factor and only one factor, then a one-way ANOVA is equivalent to a two-sample t-test and F is equal to t^2. This relationship holds because t is calculated from the mean divided by the standard error (SE) in the same units as the original measurements whereas F is calculated from the variance, which is in squared units.

Research question

The spreadsheet **weights.sav** contains the data from a population sample of 550 term babies who had their weight recorded at 1 month of age. The babies also had their parity recorded, that is their birth order in their family.

Question: Are the weights of babies related to their parity?
Null hypothesis: That there is no difference in mean weight between groups defined by parity.
Variables: Outcome variable = weight (continuous)
                   Explanatory variable = parity (categorical, four groups)

The first statistics to obtain are the cell means and cell sizes. The number of children in each parity group can be obtained using the *Analyze → Descriptive Statistics → Frequencies* command sequences shown in Box 1.9.

Frequency table

Parity

		Frequency	Per cent	Valid per cent	Cumulative per cent
Valid	Singleton	180	32.7	32.7	32.7
	One sibling	192	34.9	34.9	67.6
	two siblings	116	21.1	21.1	88.7
	three or more siblings	62	11.3	11.3	100.0
	Total	550	100.0	100.0	

The Frequency table shows that the sample size of each group is large in that all cells have more than 30 participants. The cell size ratio is 62:192 or 1:3 and does not violate the ANOVA assumptions. Thus, the ANOVA model will be robust to some degrees of non-normality, outliers and unequal variances. However, it is still important to validate the ANOVA assumptions of normality and equal variances between groups. An awareness of any violations of these assumptions before running the model may influence how the results are interpreted, especially if any P values are of marginal significance. A small cell with a small variance compared to the other groups has the effect of inflating the F value, that is of increasing the chance of a type I error. On the other hand, a small cell with large variance compared to the other groups reduces the F value and increases the chance of a type II error.

Summary statistics and checks for normality can be obtained using the *Analyze → Descriptive Statistics → Explore* command sequence shown in Box 2.2 in Chapter 2. In this example, the dependent variable is weight and the factor list is parity. The plots that are most useful to request are the box plots, histograms and normality plots.

Descriptives

	Parity			Statistic	Std. error
Weight (kg)	Singleton	Mean		4.2589	0.04617
		95% confidence	Lower bound	4.1678	
		interval for mean	Upper bound	4.3501	
		5% trimmed mean		4.2588	
		Median		4.2500	
		Variance		0.384	
		Std. deviation		0.61950	
		Minimum		2.92	
		Maximum		5.75	
		Range		2.83	
		Inter-quartile range		0.9475	
		Skewness		0.046	0.181
		Kurtosis		−0.542	0.360
	One sibling	Mean		4.3887	0.04277
		95% confidence	Lower bound	4.3043	
		interval for mean	Upper bound	4.4731	
		5% trimmed mean		4.3709	
		Median		4.3250	
		Variance		0.351	
		Std. deviation		0.59258	
		Minimum		3.17	
		Maximum		6.33	
		Range		3.16	
		Inter-quartile range		0.8350	
		Skewness		0.467	0.175
		Kurtosis		0.039	0.349
	Two siblings	Mean		4.4601	0.05619
		95% confidence	Lower bound	4.3488	

Continued

Parity				Statistic	Std. error
		interval for mean	Upper bound	4.5714	
		5% trimmed mean		4.4525	
		Median		4.4700	
		Variance		0.366	
		Std. deviation		0.60520	
		Minimum		3.09	
		Maximum		6.49	
		Range		3.40	
		Inter-quartile range		0.8225	
		Skewness		0.251	0.225
		Kurtosis		0.139	0.446
Weight (kg)	Three or more siblings	Mean		4.4342	0.06798
		95% confidence	Lower bound	4.2983	
		interval for mean	Upper bound	4.5701	
		5% trimmed mean		4.4389	
		Median		4.4450	
		Variance		0.287	
		Std. deviation		0.53526	
		Minimum		3.20	
		Maximum		5.48	
		Range		2.28	
		Inter-quartile range		0.7100	
		Skewness		−0.029	0.304
		Kurtosis		−0.478	0.599

The Descriptives table shows that means and medians for weight in each group are approximately equal and the values for skewness and kurtosis are all between +1 and −1 suggesting that the data are close to normally distributed. The variances in each group are 0.384, 0.331, 0.366 and 0.287 respectively. The variance ratio between the lowest and highest values is 0.287:0.384 which is 1:1.3.

Tests of Normality

		Kolmogorov–Smirnova[a]			Shapiro–Wilk		
	Parity	Statistic	df	Sig.	Statistic	df	Sig.
Weight (kg)	Singleton	0.038	180	0.200*	0.992	180	0.381
	One sibling	0.065	192	0.049	0.983	192	0.018
	Two siblings	0.059	116	0.200*	0.990	116	0.579
	Three or more siblings	0.070	62	0.200*	0.985	62	0.672

* This is a lower bound of the true significance.
[a] Lilliefors significance correction.

The Kolmogorov–Smirnov statistics in the Tests of Normality table suggest that the data for singletons, babies with two siblings, and babies with three or more siblings conform to normality with P values above 0.05. However, the data for babies with one sibling do not conform to a normal distribution because the P value of 0.049 is less than 0.05. Again, this is a conservative test of normality and failure to pass it does not always mean that ANOVA cannot be used unless other tests also indicate non-normality.

The histograms shown in Figure 5.2 confirm the tests of normality and show that the distribution for babies with one sibling has slightly spread tails so that

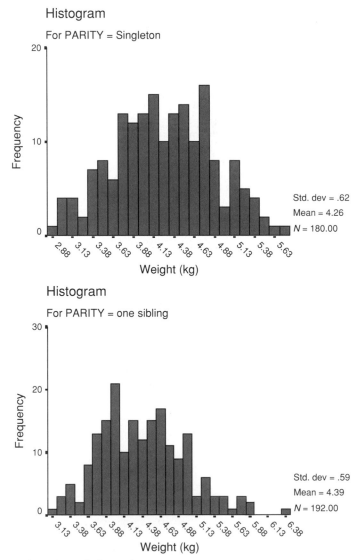

Figure 5.2 Plots of weight by parity.

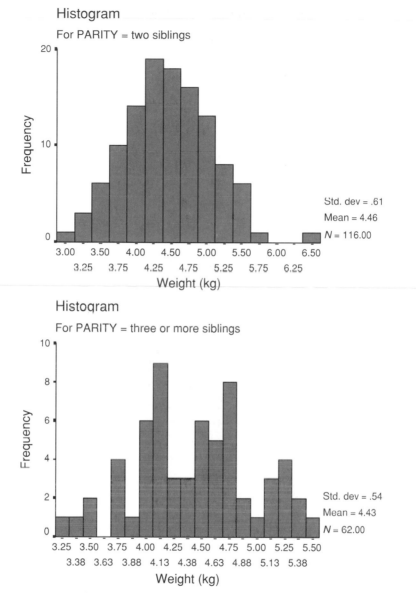

Figure 5.2 *Continued*

it does not conform absolutely to a bell shaped curve. The normal Q–Q plots shown in Figure 5.2 have small deviations at the extremities. The normal Q–Q plot for babies with one sibling deviates slightly from normality at both extremities. Although the histogram for babies with three or more siblings is not classically bell shaped, the normal Q–Q plot suggests that this distribution conforms to normality.

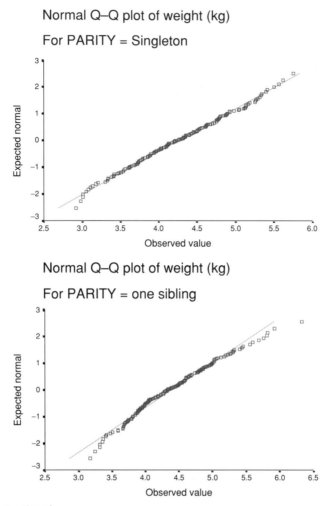

Figure 5.2 *Continued*

The box plots in Figure 5.2 indicate that there are two outlying values, one in the group of babies with one sibling and one in the group of babies with two siblings. It is unlikely that these outlying values, which are also univariate outliers, will have a large influence on the summary statistics and ANOVA result because the sample size of each group is large. However, the outliers should be confirmed as correct values and not data entry or data recording errors. Once they are verified as correctly recorded data points, the decision to include or omit outliers from the analyses is the same as for any other statistical tests. In a study with a large sample size, it is expected that there

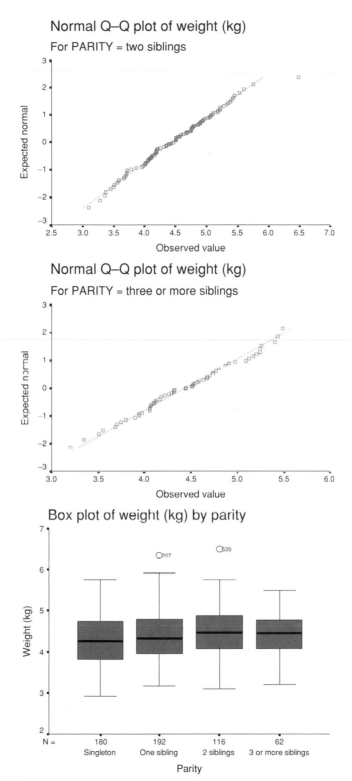

Figure 5.2 *Continued*

will be a few outliers (Chapter 3). In this data set, the outliers will be retained in the analyses and the extreme residuals will be examined to ensure that these values do not have undue influence on the results. The characteristics of the sample that need to be considered before conducting an ANOVA test and the features of the data set are summarised in Table 5.3.

Table 5.3 Characteristics of the data set

Characteristic	
Independence	Yes
Smallest cell size	62
Cell ratio	1:3
Variance ratio	1:1.3
Approximately normal distribution in each group	Yes
Number of outlying values	2
Number of univariate outliers	2

Running the one-way ANOVA

After the assumptions for using ANOVA have been checked and are validated, a one-way ANOVA can be obtained using the SPSS commands shown in Box 5.2.

Box 5.2 SPSS commands to obtain a one-way ANOVA

SPSS Commands
weights – SPSS Data Editor
       Analyze → Compare Means → One-Way ANOVA
One-Way ANOVA
       Highlight Weight and click over into Dependent List
       Highlight Parity and click over into Factor
       Click on Post-hoc
One-Way ANOVA: Post Hoc Multiple Comparisons
       Tick LSD, Bonferroni and Duncan, click Continue
One-Way ANOVA
       Click on Options
One-Way ANOVA: Options
       Tick Descriptive, Homogeneity of variance test, Means Plot, click Continue
One-Way ANOVA
       Click OK

One way

Descriptives
Weight (kg)

	N	Mean	Std. deviation	Std. error	95% confidence interval for mean Lower bound	Upper bound	Minimum	Maximum
Singleton	180	4.2589	0.61950	0.04617	4.1678	4.3501	2.92	5.75
One sibling	192	4.3887	0.59258	0.04277	4.3043	4.4731	3.17	6.33
Two siblings	116	4.4601	0.60520	0.05619	4.3488	4.5714	3.09	6.49
Three or more siblings	62	4.4342	0.53526	0.06798	4.2983	4.5701	3.20	5.48
Total	550	4.3664	0.60182	0.02566	4.3160	4.4168	2.92	6.49

The summary statistics in the Descriptives table produced in a one-way ANOVA are identical to the statistics obtained using the command sequence *Analyze → Descriptive Statistics → Explore*. The descriptive statistics provided by the ANOVA commands show useful summary information but do not give enough details to check the normality of the distributions of weight in each group.

Test of Homogeneity of Variances
Weight (kg)

Levene statistic	df1	df2	Sig.
0.639	3	546	0.590

Homogeneity of variances is a term that is used to indicate that groups have the same or similar variances (Chapter 3). Thus, in the Test of Homogeneity of Variances table, the *P* value of 0.590 in the significance column, which is larger than the critical value of 0.05, indicates that the variance of each group is not significantly different from one another.

ANOVA
Weight (kg)

	Sum of squares	df	Mean square	F	Sig.
Between groups	3.477	3	1.159	3.239	0.022
Within groups	195.365	546	0.358		
Total	198.842	549			

The ANOVA table shows how the sum of squares is partitioned into between-group and within-group effects. The average of each sum of squares is needed to calculate the F value. Therefore, each sum of squares is divided by its respective degree of freedom (df) to compute the mean variance, which is called the mean square. The degrees of freedom for the between-group sum of squares is the number of groups minus 1, that is $4 - 1 = 3$, and for the within-group sum of squares is the number of cases in the total sample minus the number of groups, that is $550 - 4 = 546$.

In this model, the F value, which is the between-group mean square divided by the within-group mean square, is large at 3.239 and is significant at $P = 0.022$. This indicates that there is a significant difference in the mean values of the four parity groups.

The amount of variation in weight that is explained by parity can be calculated as the between-group sum of squares divided by the total sum of squares to provide a statistic that is called eta squared as follows:

$$Eta^2 = \text{Between-group sum of squares/Total sum of squares}$$
$$= 3.477/198.842$$
$$= 0.017$$

This statistic indicates that only 1.7% of the variation in weight is explained by parity. Alternatively, eta^2 can be obtained using the commands *Analyze→ Compare Means→Means*, clicking on Options and requesting *ANOVA table and eta*. This will produce the same ANOVA table as above and include eta^2 but does not include a test of homogeneity or allow for post-hoc testing.

Post-hoc tests

Although the ANOVA statistics show that there is a significant difference in mean weights between parity groups, they do not indicate which groups are significantly different from one another. Specific group differences can be assessed using planned contrasts, which are decided before the ANOVA is run and which strictly limit the number of comparisons conducted[2]. Alternatively, post-hoc tests, which involve all possible comparisons between groups, can be used. Post-hoc tests are often considered to be data dredging and therefore inferior to the thoughtfulness of planned or *a priori* comparisons[3]. Some post-hoc tests preserve the overall type I error rate, but for other post-hoc tests the chance of a type I error increases with the number of comparisons made.

It is always better to run a small number of planned comparisons rather than a large number of unplanned post-hoc tests. Strictly speaking, the between-group differences that are of interest and the specific between-group comparisons that are made should be decided prior to conducting the ANOVA. In addition, planned and post-hoc tests should only be requested after the main ANOVA has shown that there is a statistically significant difference between groups. When the F test is not significant, it is unwise to explore whether there are any between-group differences[2].

A post-hoc test may consist of pairwise comparisons, group-wise comparisons or a combination of both. Pairwise comparisons are used to compare the differences between each pair of means. Group-wise comparisons are used to identify subsets of means that differ significantly from each other. Post-hoc tests also vary from being exceedingly conservative to simply conducting to multiple t-tests with no adjustment for multiple comparisons. A conservative test is one in which the actual significance is smaller than the stated significance level. Thus, conservative tests may incorrectly fail to reject the null hypothesis because a larger effect size between means is required for significance. Table 5.4 shows some commonly used post-hoc tests, their assumptions and the type of comparisons made.

Table 5.4 Types of comparisons produced by post-hoc tests

Post-hoc test	Requires equal group sizes	Group-wise subsets	Pairwise comparisons with a 95% CI
Equal variance assumed			
Conservative tests			
Scheffe	No	Yes	Yes
Tukey's honestly significant difference (HSD)	Yes	Yes	Yes
Bonferroni	No	No	Yes
Liberal tests			
Student–Newman–Keuls (SNK)	Yes	Yes	No
Duncan	Yes	Yes	No
Least significance difference (LSD)	Yes	No	Yes
Equal variance not assumed			
Games Howell	No	No	Yes
Dunnett's C	No	No	Yes

The choice of post-hoc test should be determined by equality of the variances, equality of group sizes and by the acceptability of the test in a particular research discipline. For example, Scheffe is often used in psychological medicine, Bonferroni in clinical applications and Duncan in epidemiological studies. The advantages of using a conservative post-hoc test have to be balanced against the probability of type II errors, that is missing real differences[4,5]. In the ANOVA test for the **weights.sav** data, the following post-hoc comparisons were requested:

Post-hoc tests

Multiple Comparisons
Dependent Variable: Weight (kg)

	(I) Parity	(J) Parity	Mean difference (I−J)	Std. error	Sig.	95% confidence interval Lower bound	Upper bound
LSD	Singleton	One sibling	−0.1298*	0.06206	0.037	−0.2517	−0.0078
		Two siblings	−0.2011*	0.07122	0.005	−0.3410	−0.0612
		Three or more siblings	−0.1752*	0.08809	0.047	−0.3483	−0.0022
	One sibling	Singleton	0.1298*	0.06206	0.037	0.0078	0.2517
		Two siblings	−0.0714	0.07034	0.311	−0.2096	0.0668
		Three or more siblings	−0.0455	0.08738	0.603	−0.2171	0.1261
	Two siblings	Singleton	0.2011*	0.07122	0.005	0.0612	0.3410
		One sibling	0.0714	0.07034	0.311	−0.0668	0.2096
		Three or more siblings	0.0259	0.09410	0.783	−0.1590	0.2107
	Three or more siblings	Singleton	0.1752*	0.08809	0.047	0.0022	0.3483
		One sibling	0.0455	0.08738	0.603	−0.1261	0.2171
		Two siblings	−0.0259	0.09410	0.783	−0.2107	0.1590
Bonferroni	Singleton	One sibling	−0.1298	0.06206	0.222	−0.2941	0.0346
		Two siblings	−0.2011*	0.07122	0.029	−0.3897	−0.0126
		Three or more siblings	−0.1752	0.08809	0.283	−0.4085	0.0580
	One sibling	Singleton	0.1298	0.06206	0.222	−0.0346	0.2941
		Two siblings	−0.0714	0.07034	1.000	−0.2577	0.1149
		Three or more siblings	−0.0455	0.08738	1.000	−0.2769	0.1859
	Two siblings	Singleton	0.2011*	0.07122	0.029	0.0126	0.3897
		One sibling	0.0714	0.07034	1.000	−0.1149	0.2577
		Three or more siblings	0.0259	0.09410	1.000	−0.2233	0.2751
	Three or more siblings	Singleton	0.1752	0.08809	0.283	−0.0580	0.4085
		One sibling	0.0455	0.08738	1.000	−0.1859	0.2769
		Two siblings	−0.0259	0.09410	1.000	−0.2751	0.2233

*The mean difference is significant at the 0.05 level.

The Multiple Comparisons table shows pairwise comparisons generated using the least significance difference (LSD) and Bonferroni post-hoc tests. The LSD test is the most liberal post-hoc test because it performs all possible tests between means. This test is not normally recommended when more than three groups are being compared or when there are unequal variances or cell sizes. With no adjustments made for multiple tests or comparisons, the results of the LSD test amount to multiple t-testing and has been included here only for comparison with the Bonferroni test.

The Multiple Comparisons table shows the mean difference between each pair of groups, the significance and the confidence intervals around the difference in means between groups. SigmaPlot can be used to plot the LSD mean differences and 95% confidence intervals as a scatter plot with horizontal error bars using the commands shown in Box 3.6 to obtain Figure 5.3. This figure shows that three of the comparisons have error bars that cross the zero line of no difference, and the differences are not statistically significant using the LSD test. The remaining three comparisons do not cross the zero line of no difference and are statistically significant as indicated by the P values in the Multiple Comparisons table.

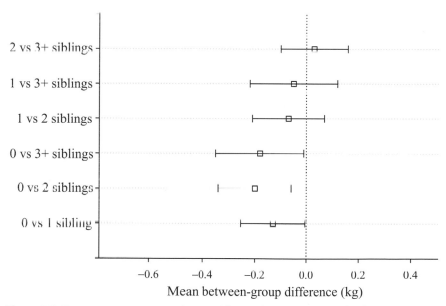

Figure 5.3 Between-group comparisons with no adjustment for multiple testing.

The Bonferroni post-hoc comparison is a conservative test in which the critical P value of 0.05 is divided by the number of comparisons made. Thus, if five comparisons are made, the critical value of 0.05 is divided by 5 and the adjusted new critical value is $P = 0.01$. In SPSS the P levels in the Multiple Comparisons table have already been adjusted for the number of multiple comparisons. Therefore, each *P* level obtained from a Bonferroni test in the Multiple Comparisons table should be evaluated at the critical level of 0.05.

By using the Bonferroni test, which is a conservative test, the significant differences between some groups identified by the LSD test are now non-significant. The mean values are identical but the confidence intervals are adjusted so that they are wider as shown in Figure 5.4. The 95% error bars show that only one comparison does not cross the zero line of difference compared to three comparisons using the LSD test.

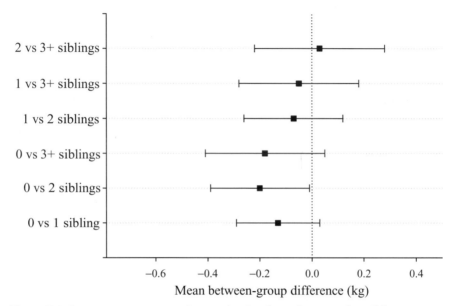

Figure 5.4 Between-group comparisons using Bonferroni corrected confidence intervals.

Homogeneous subsets

Weight (kg)

| | Parity | N | Subset for alpha = 0.05 | |
			1	2
Duncan[a,b]	Singleton	180	4.2589	
	One sibling	192	4.3887	4.3887
	Three or more siblings	62		4.4342
	Two siblings	116		4.4601
	Sig.		0.104	0.403

Means for groups in homogeneous subsets are displayed.
[a] Uses harmonic mean sample size = 112.633.
[b] The group sizes are unequal. The harmonic mean of the group sizes is used. Type I error levels are not guaranteed.

The Duncan test shown in the Homogeneous Subsets table is one of the more liberal post-hoc tests. Under this test, there is a progressive comparison between the largest and smallest mean values until a difference that is not significant at the $P < 0.05$ level is found and the comparisons are stopped. In this way, the number of comparisons is limited. The output from this test is presented as subsets of groups that are not significantly different from one another. The between-group P value (0.05) is shown in the top row of the Homogenous subtests table and the within-group P values at the foot of the columns. Thus in the table, the mean values for groups of singletons and babies with one sibling are not significantly different from one another with a P value of 0.104. Similarly, the mean values of groups with one sibling, two siblings, or three or more siblings are not significantly different from one another with a P value of 0.403. Singletons do not appear in the same subset as babies with two siblings or with three or more siblings which indicates that the mean weight of singletons is significantly different from these two groups at the $P < 0.05$ level.

The means plot provides a visual presentation of the mean value for each group. The means plot shown in Figure 5.5 indicates that there is a trend for weight to increase with increasing parity and helps in the interpretation of the post-hoc tests. It also shows why the group with one sibling is not significantly

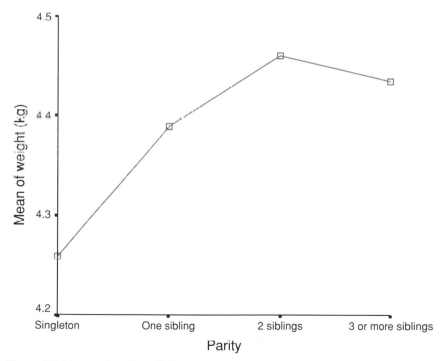

Figure 5.5 Means plot of weight by parity.

different from singletons or babies with two siblings or with three or more siblings, and why singletons are significantly different from the groups with two siblings or with three or more siblings.

If the means plot shown in Figure 5.5 was to be published, it would be best plotted in SigmaPlot with 95% confidence intervals around each mean value included to help interpret the between-group differences. Also, the line connecting the mean value of each group should be removed because the four groups are independent of one another.

Trend test

The increase in weight with increasing parity suggests that it is appropriate to test whether there is a significant linear trend for weight to increase across the groups within this factor. A trend test can be performed by re-running the one-way ANOVA and ticking the Polynomial option in the Contrasts box with the Degree: Linear (default) option used. As the polynomial term implies, an equation is calculated across the model.

One way

ANOVA
Weight (kg)

			Sum of squares	df	Mean square	F	Sig.
Between groups	(Combined)		3.477	3	1.159	3.239	0.022
	Linear term	Unweighted	1.706	1	1.706	4.768	0.029
		Weighted	2.774	1	2.774	7.754	0.006
		Deviation	0.703	2	0.351	0.982	0.375
Within groups			195.365	546	0.358		
Total			198.842	549			

If each of the parity cells had the same number of cases then the unweighted linear term would be used to assess the significance of the trend. However, the cell sizes are unequal and therefore the weighted linear term is used. The table shows that the weighted linear term sum of squares is significant at the $P = 0.006$ level indicating that there is a significant trend for mean weight to increase as parity or the number of siblings increases.

Reporting the results

In addition to presenting the between-group comparisons shown in Figure 5.3, the results from the one-way ANOVA can be summarised as shown in Table 5.5. When describing the table it is important to include details stating that weight was approximately normally distributed in each group and that the group sizes were all large (minimum 62) with a cell size ratio of 1:3 and a variance ratio of 1:1.3. The significant difference in weight at 1 month between children with different parities can be described as $F = 3.24$, $df = 3$, 546, $P = 0.022$ with a significant linear trend for weight to increase with increasing parity ($P = 0.006$). The degrees of freedom are conventionally shown as the between-group and within-group degrees of freedom separated with a comma. Although the inclusion of the F value and degrees of freedom is optional since their only interpretation is the P value, some journals request that they are reported.

Table 5.5 Reporting results from a one-way ANOVA

Parity	N	Mean (SD)	F (df)	P value	P value trend
Singletons	180	4.26 (0.62)	3.24 (3, 546)	0.022	0.006
One sibling	192	4.39 (0.59)			
Two siblings	116	4.46 (0.61)			
Three or more siblings	62	4.43 (0.54)			

When designing the study, only one post-hoc test should be planned and conducted if the ANOVA was significant. If the Bonferroni post-hoc test had been conducted, it could be reported that the only significant difference in mean weights was between singletons and babies with two siblings ($P = 0.029$) with no significant differences between any other groups.

If Duncan's post-hoc test had been conducted, it could be reported that babies with two siblings and babies with three or more siblings were significantly heavier than singletons ($P < 0.05$). However, babies with one sibling did not have a mean weight that was significantly different from either singletons ($P = 0.104$) or from babies with two siblings, or with three or more siblings ($P = 0.403$).

Factorial ANOVA models

A factorial ANOVA is used to test for differences in mean values between groups when there are two or more factors, or explanatory variables, with two or more groups each included in a single multivariate analysis. In SPSS, factorial ANOVA is accessed through the *Analyze → General Linear Models → Univariate* command sequence. The term univariate may seem confusing in this context but in this case refers to there being only one outcome variable rather than only one explanatory factor.

In a factorial ANOVA, the data are divided into cells according to the number of participants in each group of each factor stratified by the other factors. The more explanatory variables that are included in a model, the greater the likelihood of creating small or empty cells. The cells can be conceptualised as shown in Table 5.6. The number of cells in a model is calculated by multiplying the number of groups in each factor. For a model with three factors that have three, two and four groups respectively as shown in Table 5.6, the number of cells is $3 \times 2 \times 4$, or 24 cells in total.

Table 5.6 Cells in the analysis of a model with three factors (three-way ANOVA)

FACTOR 1	Group 1		Group 2		Group 3	
FACTOR 2	Group 1	Group 2	Group 1	Group 2	Group 1	Group 2
FACTOR 3						
Group 1	$m_{1,1,1}$	$m_{2,1,1}$	$m_{1,2,1}$	$m_{2,2,1}$	$m_{1,3,1}$	$m_{2,3,1}$
2	$m_{1,1,2}$	$m_{2,1,2}$	$m_{1,2,2}$	$m_{2,2,2}$	$m_{1,3,2}$	$m_{2,3,2}$
3	$m_{1,1,3}$	$m_{2,1,3}$	$m_{1,2,3}$	$m_{2,2,3}$	$m_{1,3,3}$	$m_{2,3,3}$
4	$m_{1,1,4}$	$m_{2,1,4}$	$m_{1,2,4}$	$m_{2,2,4}$	$m_{1,3,4}$	$m_{2,3,4}$

In factorial ANOVA, the within-group differences are calculated as the distance of each participant from its cell mean rather than from the group mean as in one-way ANOVA. However, the between-group differences are again calculated as the difference of each participant from the grand mean, that is the mean of the entire data set. As with one-way ANOVA, all of the differences are squared and summed, and then the mean square is calculated.

Fixed factors, interactions and random factors

Both fixed and random effects can be incorporated in factorial ANOVA models. Factorial ANOVA is mostly used to examine the effects of fixed factors which are factors in which all possible groups are included, for example males and females or number of siblings. When using fixed factors, the differences between the specified groups are the statistics of interest.

Sometimes the effect of one fixed factor is modified by another fixed factor, that is it interacts with it. The presence of a significant interaction between two or more factors or between a factor and a covariate can be tested in a factorial ANOVA model. The interaction term is computed as a new variable by multiplying the factors together and then included in the model or can be requested on an SPSS option.

Factors are considered to be random when only a sample of a wider range of groups is included. For example, factors may be classified as having random effects when only three or four ethnic groups are represented in the sample but the results will be generalised to all ethnic groups in the community. In this case, only general differences between the groups are of interest because the results will be used to make inferences to all possible ethnic groups rather than to only the groups in the sample.

It is important to classify groups as random factors if the study sample was selected by recruiting, for example, specific sports teams, schools or doctors' practices and the results will be generalised to all sports teams, schools or doctors' practices or if different sports teams, schools or doctors' practices would be selected in the future. In these types of study designs, there is a cluster sampling effect and the group is entered into the model as a random factor.

The classification of factors as fixed or random effects has implications for interpreting the results of the ANOVA. In random effect models, any unequal variance between cells is less important when the numbers in each cell are equal. However, when there is increasing inequality between the numbers in each cell, then differences in variance become more problematic. The use of fixed or random effects can give very different P values because the F statistic is computed differently. For fixed effects, the F value is calculated as the between-group mean square divided by the error mean square whereas for random effects, the F value is calculated as the between-group mean square divided by the interaction mean square.

Research question

Differences in weights between genders can be tested using a two-sample t-test and differences between different parities were tested in the previous example using a one-way ANOVA. However, maternal education status (Year 10 school, Year 12 school or university) in addition to gender and parity can be tested together as explanatory factors in a three-way ANOVA model. These factors are all fixed factors.

Question:	Are the weights of babies related to their gender, parity or maternal level of education?
Null hypothesis:	That there is no difference in mean weight between groups defined according to gender, parity and level of education
Variables:	Outcome variable = weight (continuous)
	Explanatory variables = gender (categorical, two groups), parity (categorical, four groups) and maternal education (categorical, three groups)

The number of cells in the ANOVA model will be 2 (gender) $\times$ 3 (maternal education) $\times$ 4 (parity), or 24 cells. First, the summary statistics need to be obtained to verify that there are an adequate number of babies in each cell. This can be achieved by splitting the file by gender which has the smallest number of groups and then generating two tables of parity by maternal education as shown in Box 5.3.

Box 5.3 SPSS commands to obtain cell sizes

SPSS Commands
weights – SPSS Data Editor
   Data → Split File
Split File
   Tick 'Organise output by groups'
   Highlight Gender and click into 'Groups Based on' box
   Click OK
weights – SPSS Data Editor
   Analyze → Descriptive Statistics → Crosstabs
Crosstabs
   Highlight Maternal education and click into Rows
   Highlight Parity and click into Columns
   Click OK

Gender = male

Maternal Education * Parity Crosstabulation
Count

			Parity			
		Singleton	One sibling	Two siblings	Three or more siblings	Total
Maternal	year 10	15	40	26	17	98
education	year 12	22	16	8	4	50
	Tertiary	55	42	22	8	127
Total		92	98	56	29	275

[a] Gender = male.

Gender = female

Maternal Education * Parity Crosstabulation
Count

			Parity			
		Singleton	One sibling	Two siblings	Three or more siblings	Total
Maternal	year 10	24	36	21	19	100
education	year 12	19	15	13	2	49
	Tertiary	45	43	26	12	126
Total		88	94	60	33	275

[a] Gender = Female.

The Crosstabulations tables show that even with a large sample size of 550 babies, including three factors in the model will create some small cells with less than 10 cases and that there is a large cell imbalance. For males, the cell size ratio is 4:55, or 1:14, and for females the cell size ratio is 2:45, or 1:23. Without maternal education included, all cell sizes as indicated by the Total row and Total column totals are quite large. To increase the small cell sizes, it would make sense to combine the groups of two siblings and three or more siblings. This combining of cells is possible because the theory is valid and because the one-way ANOVA showed that the means of these two groups are not significantly different from one another. By combining these groups, the smallest cells will be larger at $8 + 4$ or 12 for males and $13 + 2$ or 15 for females. The cell ratios will then be 12:55, or 1:4.6 for males and 15:45, or 1:3 for females. The ratio for males is close to the assumption of 1:4 and within this assumption for females.

To combine the parity groups, the re-code commands shown in Box 1.10 can be used after removing the Split file option as shown in Box 5.4.

Box 5.4 SPSS commands to remove split file

SPSS Commands
weights – SPSS Data Editor
> *Data → Split File*
> *Tick 'Analyse all cases, do not create groups'*
> *Click OK*

The SPSS commands to obtain summary means for parity and maternal education in males and females separately are shown in Box 5.5.

Box 5.5 SPSS commands to obtain summary means

SPSS Commands
weights – SPSS Data Editor
> *Analyze → Compare Means → Means*
Means
> *Highlight Weight and click into Dependent List*
> *Highlight Gender, Maternal education and Parity recoded (3 levels),*
>   *click into Independent List*
> *Click OK*

Means
Weight (kg) * Gender
Weight (kg)

Gender	Mean	*N*	Std. deviation
Male	4.5923	275	0.62593
Female	4.1405	275	0.48111
Total	4.3664	550	0.60182

Weight (kg) * Maternal Education
Weight (kg)

Maternal education	Mean	N	Std. deviation
Year10	4.3529	198	0.55993
Year12	4.4109	99	0.69464
Tertiary	4.3596	253	0.59611
Total	4.3664	550	0.60182

Weight (kg) * Parity Recoded (Three Levels)
Weight (kg)

Parity re-coded (Three levels)	Mean	N	Std. deviation
Singleton	4.2589	180	0.61950
One sibling	4.3887	192	0.59258
Two or more siblings	4.4511	178	0.58040
Total	4.3664	550	0.60182

The Means tables show mean values in each group for each factor. There is a difference of 4.59 – 4.14, i.e. 0.45 kg between genders, a difference of 4.41 – 4.35, i.e. 0.06 kg between the highest and lowest maternal education groups and a difference of 4.45 – 4.26, i.e. 0.19 kg between the highest and lowest parity groups. These are not effect sizes in units of the standard deviations so the differences cannot be directly compared. In ANOVA, effect sizes can be calculated but the number of groups and the pattern of dispersion of the mean values across the groups need to be taken into account[6]. However, the absolute differences show that the largest difference is for gender followed by parity and that there is an almost negligible difference for maternal education. The effect of maternal education is so small that it is unlikely to be a significant predictor in a multivariate model.

The summary statistics can also be used to verify the cell size and variance ratios. A summary of this information validates the model and helps to interpret the output from the three-way ANOVA. The cell size ratio when parity is re-coded into three cells has been found to be adequate. The variance ratio for each factor, for example for parity, can be calculated by squaring the standard deviations from the Means table. For parity, the variance ratio is $(0.58)^2:(0.62)^2$ or 1:1.14.

Next, the distributions of the variables should be checked for normality using the methods described in Chapter 2 and for one-way ANOVA. The largest difference between mean values is between genders, therefore it is important to examine the distribution for each gender to identify any outlying values or outliers. In fact, the distribution of each group for each factor should be checked for the presence of any outlying values or univariate outliers. The output is not included here but the analyses should proceed in the knowledge that there are no influential outliers and no significant deviations from normality for any variable in the model.

The commands for running a three-way ANOVA to test for the effects of gender (two groups), parity (three groups) and maternal education (three groups) on weight and to test for a trend for weight to increase with increasing parity are shown in Box 5.6.

Box 5.6 SPSS commands to obtain a three-way ANOVA

SPSS Commands

weights – SPSS Data Editor

        Analyze → General Linear Model → Univariate

Univariate

        Highlight Weight and click into Dependent Variable

        Highlight Gender, Maternal education and Parity recoded (3 levels) and
            click into Fixed Factor(s)

        Click on Model

Univariate: Model

        Click on Custom

        Under Build Term(s) pull down menu and click on Main effects

        Highlight gender, education and parity1 and click over into Model

        Sum of squares: Type III on pull down menu (default)

        Tick Include intercept in model (default), click Continue

Univariate

        Click on Contrasts

Univariate Contrasts

        Factors: Highlight parity1

        Change Contrasts: pull down menu, highlight Polynomial, click Change,
        click Continue

Univariate

        Click on Plots

Univariate: Profile Plots

        Highlight gender, click into Horizontal Axis

        Highlight parity1, click in Separate Lines, click Add, click Continue

Univariate

        Click on Options

Univariate: Options

        Highlight gender, education and parity1 and click into 'Display
        Means for'

        Tick 'Compare main effects'

> *Confidence interval adjustment: LSD (none)(default)*
> *Click Continue*
> *Univariate*
> *   Click OK*

Univariate analysis of variance

Tests of Between-Subject Effects
Dependent Variable: Weight (kg)

Source	Type III Sum of Squares	df	Mean square	F	Sig.
Corrected model	32.613[a]	5	6.523	21.346	0.000
Intercept	9012.463	1	9012.463	29494.120	0.000
GENDER	28.528	1	28.528	93.361	0.000
EDUCATIO	0.604	2	0.302	0.989	0.373
PARITY1	4.327	2	2.164	7.080	0.001
Error	166.229	544	0.306		
Total	10684.926	550			
Corrected total	198.842	549			

[a] R squared = 0.164 (adjusted R squared = 0.156).

A three-way ANOVA shown in the Tests of Between-Subject Effects table is similar to a regression model. In the table, the first two rows show the Corrected Model and Intercept and indicate that the factors are significant predictors of weight. The corrected model sum of squares divided by the corrected total sum of squares, that is 32.613/198.842 or 0.164, is the variation that can be explained by the model and is the R squared value shown in the footnote. This value indicates that gender, maternal education and parity together explain 0.164 or 16.4% of the variation in weight. This is considerably higher than the 1.7% explained by parity only in a previous model.

The F values are the within-group mean square divided by the error mean square. The F values for the three factors show that both gender and parity are significant predictors of weight at 1 month with $P < 0.0001$ and $P = 0.001$ respectively, but that maternal educational status is not a significant predictor with $P = 0.373$. After combining two of the parity groups and adjusting for gender differences in the parity groups, the significance of parity in predicting weight has increased to $P = 0.001$ compared with $P = 0.022$ obtained from the one-way ANOVA previously conducted.

The sums of squares for the model, intercept, factors and the error term when added up manually equal 9244.764. This is less than the total sum of squares of 10 684.926 shown in the table, which also includes the sum of squares for all possible interactions between factors in the model, even though the inclusion of interactions was not requested.

Custom Hypothesis Tests

Contrast Results (K matrix)

Parity recoded (three levels) Polynomial contrast[a]		Dependent variable Weight (kg)
Linear	Contrast estimate	0.157
	Hypothesised value	0
	Difference (estimate − hypothesised)	0.157
	Std. error	0.042
	Sig.	0.000
	95% confidence interval for difference Lower bound	0.074
	Upper bound	0.240
Quadratic	Contrast estimate	−0.025
	Hypothesised value	0
	Difference (estimate − hypothesised)	−0.025
	Std. error	0.040
	Sig.	0.542
	95% confidence interval for difference Lower bound	−0.104
	Upper bound	0.055

[a] Metric = 1.000, 2.000, 3.000.

The polynomial linear contrast in the Contrast Results table shows that there is again a significant trend for weight to increase with parity at the $P < 0.0001$ level. The subscript to this table indicates that the outcome is being assessed over the three parity groups, that is the groups labelled 1, 2 and 3. The quadratic term is not relevant because there is no evidence to suggest that the relationship between weight and parity is curved rather than linear, and consistent with this, the quadratic contrast is not significant.

Estimated Marginal Means

Estimates
Dependent Variable: Weight (kg)

Gender	Mean	Std. error	95% confidence interval	
			Lower bound	Upper bound
Male	4.603	0.035	4.535	4.672
Female	4.148	0.035	4.079	4.216

The Estimated Marginal Means table shows mean values adjusted for the other factors in the model, that is the predicted mean values. Marginal means

Pairwise Comparisions
Dependent Variable: Weight (kg)

(I) gender	(J) gender	Mean difference (I−J)	Std. error	Sig.[a]	95% Confidence Interval for Difference[a]	
					Lower bound	Upper bound
Male	Female	0.456*	0.047	0.000	0.363	0.548
Female	Male	−0.456*	0.047	0.000	−0.548	−0.363

Based on estimated marginal means.
*The mean difference is significant at the 0.05 level.
[a] Adjustment for multiple comparisions: least significant difference (equivalent to no adjustments).

Univariate Tests
Dependent Variable: Weight (kg)

	Sum of squares	df	Mean square	F	Sig.
Contrast	28.528	1	28.528	93.361	0.000
Error	166.229	544	0.306		

The F tests the effect of gender. This test is based on the linearly independent pairwise comparisions among the estimated marginal means.

that are similar to the unadjusted mean values provide evidence that the model is robust. If the marginal means change by a considerable amount after adding an additional factor to the model, then the added factor is an important confounder or covariate. The significance of the comparisons in the Pairwise Comparisons table is based on a t value, that is the mean difference/SE, for the difference in marginal means without any adjustment for multiple comparisons.

In this model, the marginal means are adjusted for differences in the distribution of parity and maternal education in the two gender groups. The standard errors are identical in the two groups because the pooled data for all cases are used to compute a single estimate of the standard error. For this reason, it is important that the assumptions of equal variance and similar cell sizes in all groups are met. The marginal mean for males is 4.603 kg compared to a mean of 4.592 kg in the unadjusted analysis, and for females is 4.148 kg compared to 4.141 kg in the unadjusted analysis. Thus, the difference between genders in the adjusted ANOVA analysis is 0.456 kg compared with a difference of 0.452 kg that can be calculated from the previous Means table.

Pairwise comparisons for maternal education and parity were also requested although they have not been included here.

The Profile plot shown in Figure 5.6 indicates that the relative values in mean weights between groups defined according to parity are the same for both genders. In the plot, if the lines cross one another this would indicate an interaction between factors. However, in Figure 5.6, the lines are parallel which indicates that there is no interaction between gender and parity. Interactions are discussed in more detail in Chapter 6.

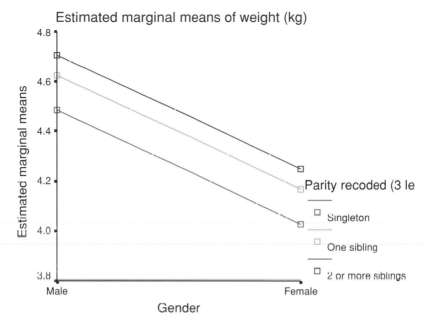

Figure 5.6 Profile plot of marginal means of weight by gender and parity.

Reporting the results

The results from the three-way ANOVA can be presented as shown in Table 5.7.

Table 5.7 Mean weights of babies at 1 month of age by gender, parity and maternal education

	N	Weight (kg) Mean (SD)	F (df)	P value	P value trend
Gender					
Males	275	4.59 (0.63)	93.36 (1, 544)	<0.0001	–
Females	275	4.14 (0.48)			
Parity					
Singletons	180	4.26 (0.62)	7.08 (2, 544)	0.001	<0.0001
One sibling	192	4.39 (0.59)			
Two or more siblings	178	4.45 (0.58)			
Maternal education					
Year 10 school	198	4.35 (0.56)	0.99 (2, 544)	0.373	–
Year 12 school	99	4.41 (0.69)			
Tertiary education	253	4.36 (0.60)			

The results could be described as follows: 'Table 5.7 shows the unadjusted mean weights of babies at 1 month of age by group. The F and P values were derived from a three-way ANOVA. The cell size was within the assumption of 1:4 for females and close to this assumption for males and the variance ratio was less than 1:2. There was a significant difference in weight between males and females and between groups defined according to parity, but not between groups defined according to maternal education status. A polynomial contrast indicated that the linear trend for weight to increase with parity was significant at $P < 0.0001$. Pairwise contrasts showed that the difference in marginal means between males and females was 0.46 kg (95% CI 0.36, 0.55). In addition, the difference in marginal means between singletons and babies with one sibling was statistically significant at -0.14 kg (95% CI -0.25, -0.03, $P = 0.015$) and the difference between singletons and babies with two or more siblings were statistically significant at -0.22 kg (95% CI -0.34, -0.11, $P < 0.0001$). Profile plots indicated that there was no interaction between gender and parity'.

Analysis of covariance

Analysis of covariance (ANCOVA) is used when it is important to examine group differences after adjusting the outcome variable for a continuously distributed explanatory variable (covariate). The ANCOVA analysis first produces a regression of the outcome on the covariate and then adjusts the cell means for the effect of the covariate. Adjusting for a covariate has the effect of reducing the residual (error) term by reducing the amount of noise in the model. As in regression, it is important that the association between the outcome and the covariate is linear. In ANCOVA, the residual terms are the distances of each individual from the regression line and not from the cell mean, thus the residual distances are smaller than in ANOVA.

The assumptions for ANCOVA are identical to the assumptions for ANOVA but the additional assumptions shown in Box 5.7 must also be met.

Box 5.7 Additional assumptions for ANCOVA

The following assumptions for ANCOVA must be met in addition to the assumptions shown in Box 5.1 for ANOVA:
- the measurement of the covariate is reliable
- if there is more than one covariate, there is low collinearity between covariates
- the association between the covariate and the outcome is linear
- there is homogeneity of the regression, that is the slopes across the data in each cell are the same as the slope in the total sample
- there is no interaction between the covariate and the factors
- there are no multivariate outliers

In building the ANCOVA model, the choice of covariates must be made carefully and should be limited to covariates that can be measured reliably.

Few covariates are measured without any error but unreliable covariates lead to a loss of statistical power. Covariates such as age and height can be measured reliably but other covariates such as reported hours of sleep or time spent exercising may be subject to significant reporting bias.

It is also important to limit the number of covariates to variables that are not significantly related to one another. As in all multivariate models, collinearity, that is a significant association or correlation between explanatory variables, can result in an unstable model and unreliable estimates of effect, which can be difficult to interpret. Ideally, the correlation (r) between covariates should be low.

Research question

Weight is related to the length of a baby and therefore it makes sense to use ANCOVA to test whether the significant differences in weight between gender and parity groups are maintained after adjusting for length. In testing this, length is added into the model as a covariate. The SPSS commands for running an ANCOVA model are shown in Box 5.8. Maternal education has been omitted from this model because the previous three-way ANOVA showed that this variable does not have a significant relationship with babies' weights.

Box 5.8 SPSS commands for obtaining an ANCOVA model

SPSS commands
weights – SPSS Data Editor
        Analyze → General Linear Model → Univariate
Univariate
        Click on Reset
        Highlight Weight and click into Dependent Variable
        Highlight Gender and Parity recoded (3 levels) and click into Fixed Factors
        Highlight Length, click into Covariate(s)
        Click on Model
Univariate: Model
        Click on Custom
        Under Build Term(s) pull down menu and click on Main effects
        Highlight gender, parity1 and length and click over into Model
        Sum of squares: Type III on pull down menu (default)
        Tick Include intercept in model (default), click Continue
Univariate
        Click on Contrasts
Univariate Contrasts
        Factors: Highlight parity1
        Change Contrast: pull down menu, highlight Polynomial, click Change,
        click Continue
Univariate
        Click on Options
Univariate: Options

> *Highlight gender and Parity1, click into 'Display Means for'*
> Tick 'Compare main effects'
> *Confidence interval adjustment: using LSD (none)(default)*
> *Click Continue*
> *Univariate*
> *Click OK*

Tests of Between-Subject Effects
Dependent Variable: Weight (Kg)

Source	Type III sum of squares	df	Mean square	F	Sig.
Corrected model	111.164[a]	4	27.791	172.747	0.000
Intercept	20.805	1	20.805	129.322	0.000
GENDER	8.378	1	8.378	52.074	0.000
PARITY1	1.929	2	0.965	5.996	0.003
LENGTH	79.155	1	79.155	492.024	0.000
Error	87.678	545	0.161		
Total	10684.926	550			
Corrected total	198.842	549			

[a] R squared = 0.559 (adjusted R squared = 0.556).

Custom Hypothesis Tests

Contrast Results (K matrix)

Parity re-coded (three levels) Polynomial contrast[a]		Dependent variable Weight (kg)
Linear	Contrast estimate	0.098
	Hypothesised value	0
	Difference (estimate − hypothesised)	0.098
	Std. error	0.030
	Sig.	0.001
	95% confidence interval Lower bound	0.039
	for difference Upper bound	0.157
Quadratic	Contrast estimate	−0.035
	Hypothesised value	0
	Difference (estimate − hypothesised)	−0.035
	Std. error	0.029
	Sig.	0.238
	95% confidence interval Lower bound	−0.092
	For difference Upper bound	0.023

[a] Metric = 1.000, 2.000, 3.000.

The Tests of Between-Subject Effects table shows that by adding a strong covariate, the explained variation has increased from 16.4% to 55.9% as indicated by the R square value. All three factors in the model are statistically significant but parity is now less significant at $P = 0.003$ compared to $P = 0.001$ in the former three-way ANOVA model. These P values, which are adjusted for the covariate, are more accurate than the P values from the previous one-way and three-way ANOVA models. The Contrast Results table shows that the linear trend for weight to increase with increasing parity remains significant, but slightly less so at $P = 0.001$.

Estimated Marginal Means

Estimates
Dependent Variable: Weight (kg)

Gender	Mean	Std. error	95% confidence interval	
			Lower bound	Upper bound
Male	4.494[a]	0.025	4.445	4.542
Femal	4.238[a]	0.025	4.190	4.287

[a] Covariates appearing in the model are evaluated at the following values: length (cm) = 54.841.

Pairwise Comparisons
Dependent Variable: Weight (kg)

(I) gender	(J) gender	Mean difference (I − J)	Std. error	Sig.[a]	95% confidence interval for difference[a]	
					Lower bound	Upper bound
Male	Female	0.255*	0.035	0.000	0.186	0.325
Female	Male	−0.255*	0.035	0.000	−0.325	−0.186

Based on estimated marginal means.
*The mean difference is significant at the 0.05 level.
[a] Adjustment for multiple comparisons: least significant difference (equivalent to no adjustments).

Univariate Tests
Dependent Variable: Weight (kg)

	Sum of squares	df	Mean square	F	Sig.
Contrast	8.378	1	8.378	52.074	0.000
Error	87.678	545	0.161		

*The F tests the effect of gender. This test is based on the linearly independent pairwise comparisons among the estimated marginal means.

When there is a significant covariate in the model, the marginal means are calculated with the covariate held at its mean value. Thus, the marginal means are predicted means and not observed means. In this model, the marginal means are calculated at the mean value of the covariate length, that is 54.841 as shown in the footnote of the Estimates table. In this situation, the marginal means need to be treated with caution because they may not correspond with any situation in real life where the covariate is held at its mean value and is balanced between groups. In observational studies, the marginal means from such analyses often have no interpretation apart from group comparisons.

Testing the model assumptions

It is important to conduct tests to check that the assumptions of any ANOVA model have been met. By re-running the model with different options, statistics can be obtained to test that the residuals are normally distributed, that there are no influential multivariate outliers, that the variance is homogeneous and that there are no interactions between the covariate and the factors. Here, the assumptions are being tested only when final model is obtained but in practice the assumptions would be tested at each stage in the model building process. The SPSS commands shown in Box 5.9 can be used to test the model assumptions.

Box 5.9 SPSS commands for testing the model assumptions

SPSS Commands
weights – SPSS Data Editor
  Analyze → General Linear Model → Univariate
Univariate
  Click on Reset
  Highlight Weight and click into Dependent Variable
  Highlight Gender and Parity recoded (3 levels) and click into Fixed Factors
  Highlight Length, click into Covariate(s)
  Click on Model
Univariate: Model
  Click on Custom
  Under Build Term(s) pull down menu and click on Main effects
  Highlight gender, parity1 and length and click over into Model
  Pull down menu, click on All 2-way
  Highlight gender, parity1 and length, click over into Model
  Sum of squares: type III on pull down menu (default)
  Tick Include intercept in model (default), click Continue
Univariate
  Click on Save
Univariate: Save
  Under Predicted Values tick Unstandardized
  Under Residuals tick Standardized

> *Under Diagnostics tick Cook's distances and Leverage values*
> > *Click Continue*
> *Univariate*
> > *Click on Options*
> *Univariate Options*
> > *Tick on Estimates of effect size, Homogeneity tests, Spread vs level plot*
> > *Residual plot, and Lack of fit, click Continue*
> *Univariate*
> > *Click OK*

Univariate analysis of variance

Levene's Test of Equality of Error Variances[a]
Dependent Variable: Weight (kg)

F	df1	df2	Sig.
1.947	5	544	0.085

Tests the null hypothesis that the error variance
of the dependent variable is equal across groups.
[a] Design.
Intercept+GENDER+PARITY1+LENGTH+GENDER *
PARITY1+GENDER * LENGTH+PARITY1 * LENGTH

In Levene's Test of Equality of Error Variances table, Levene's test indicates that the differences in variances are not significantly different with a P value of 0.085. If the P value had been significant at < 0.05, regression would be the preferred method of analysis. Other options would be to halve the critical P values for any between-group differences say to $P = 0.025$ instead of $P = 0.05$. This is an arbitrary decision but would reduce the type I error rate. A less rigorous option would be to select a post-hoc test that adjusts for unequal variances.

Tests of Between-Subject Effects
Dependent Variable: Weight (kg)

Source	Type III sum of squares	df	Mean square	F	Sig.	Partial eta squared
Corrected model	114.742[a]	9	12.749	81.862	0.000	0.577
Intercept	18.697	1	18.697	120.056	0.000	0.182
GENDER	2.062	1	2.062	13.237	0.000	0.024
PARITY1	0.898	2	0.449	2.884	0.057	0.011
LENGTH	73.731	1	73.731	473.425	0.000	0.467
GENDER * PARITY1	0.230	2	0.115	0.739	0.478	0.003

Continued

Source	Type III sum of squares	df	Mean square	F	Sig.	Partial eta squared
GENDER * LENGTH	2.434	1	2.434	15.631	0.000	0.028
PARITY1 * LENGTH	0.793	2	0.397	2.547	0.079	0.009
Error	84.099	540	0.156			
Total	10684.926	550				
Corrected total	198.842	549				

[a] R squared = 0.577 (adjusted R squared = 0.570).

The Sig. column in the Tests of Between-Subject Effects table shows that gender and length are significant predictors of weight with $P < 0.0001$ and that parity is a marginal predictor with $P = 0.057$. However, there is a significant interaction between gender and length at $P < 0.0001$ although there are no significant interactions between gender and parity ($P = 0.478$) or parity and length ($P = 0.079$).

When interactions are present in any multivariate model, the main effects of the variables involved in the interaction are no longer of interest because it is the interaction that describes the relationship between the variables and the outcome. However, the main effects must always be included in the model even though they are no longer of interest. The interaction between gender and length violates the ANCOVA model assumption that there is no interaction between the covariate and the factors. In this case, regression would be the preferred analysis. Alternatively, the ANCOVA could be conducted for males and females separately although this will reduce the precision around the estimates of effect simply because the sample size in each model is halved.

In the Tests of Between-Subject Effects table, an estimate of partial eta squared is reported for each effect. This statistic gives an estimate of the proportion of the variance that can be attributed to each factor. In ANCOVA, this statistic is calculated as the sum of squares for the effect divided by the sum of squares for the effect plus the sum of squares for the error. These partial eta squared values for each factor can be directly compared but cannot be added together to indicate how much of the variance of the outcome variable is accounted for by the explanatory variables.

Lack of Fit Tests
Dependent Variable: Weight (kg)

Source	Sum of squares	df	Mean square	F	Sig.	Partial eta squared
Lack of fit	20.907	114	0.183	1.236	0.070	0.249
Pure error	63.192	426	0.148			

The lack of fit test divides the total variance into the variance due to the interaction terms not included in the model (lack of fit) and the variance in the model (pure error). An F value that is not significant as in this table at $P = 0.070$ indicates that the model cannot be improved by adding further interaction terms, which in this case would have been the three-way interaction term between gender, parity and length. However, any significant interaction that includes the covariate would violate the assumption of the model.

It is important to examine the variance across the model using a spread-vs-level plot because the cell sizes in the model are unequal. The spread-vs-level plot shows one point for each cell. If the variance is not related to the cell means then unequal variances will not be a problem. However, if there is a relation such as the variance increasing with the mean of the cell, then unequal variances will bias the F value.

The Spread-vs-Level plot shown in Figure 5.7 indicates that the standard deviation on the y-axis increases with the mean weight of each gender and parity cell as shown on the x-axis. However, the range in standard deviations is relatively small, that is from approximately 0.45 to 0.65. This ratio of less than 1:2 for standard deviation, or 1:4 for variance, will not violate the ANOVA assumptions.

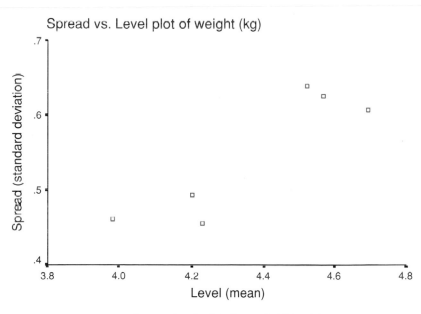

Groups: Gender * Parity recoded (3 levels)

Figure 5.7 Spread (standard deviation) by level (mean) plot of weight for each gender and parity group.

If the variances are widely unequal, it is sometimes possible to reduce the differences by transforming the measurement. If there is a linear relation between the variance and the means of the cells and all the data values are positive, taking the square root or logarithm of the measurements may be helpful.

Transforming variables into units that are not easy to communicate are last resort methods to avoid violating the assumptions of ANOVA or ANCOVA. In practice, the use of a different statistical test such as multiple regression analysis may be preferable because the assumptions are not as restrictive.

Testing residuals: unbiased and normality

One assumption of ANOVA and ANCOVA is that the residuals are unbiased. This means that the differences between the observed and predicted values for each participant are not systematically different from one another. If the plot of the observed against predicted values, as shown in the centre of the top row, were funnel shaped or deviated markedly from the line of identity, which is a diagonal line across the plot, this assumption would be violated.

Using the commands in Box 5.9 the matrix plot shown in Figure 5.8 can be obtained. This plot shows that the observed and predicted values have a linear relationship with no systematic differences across the range. In addition, the negative and positive residuals balance one another with a random scatter around a horizontal centre line.

Dependent variable: Weight (kg)

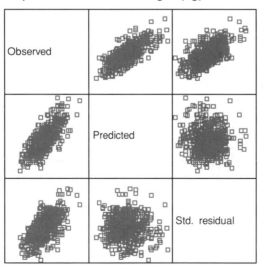

Model: Intercept + GENDER + PARITY1 + LENGTH + GENDER*PARITY1 + G

LENGTH + PARITY1*LENGTH

Figure 5.8 Matrix plot of observed and predicted values by standardised residuals for weight.

The assumption that the residuals, that is the within-group differences, have a normal distribution can be tested when running the ANOVA model. It is important that this assumption is met especially if the sample size is relatively small because the effect of non-normally distributed residuals or of multivariate outliers is to bias the P values.

When residuals are requested in *Save* as shown in Box 5.9, the residual for each case is created as a new variable at the end of the spreadsheet. Thus, the distribution of the residuals can be explored in more detail using standard tests of normality in *Analyze → Descriptive Statistics → Explore* as shown in Box 2.2 in Chapter 2, with the new variable Standardised Residual for weight as the dependent variable.

Descriptives

			Statistic	Std. error
Standardised residual for WEIGHT	Mean		0.0000	0.04229
	95% confidence interval for mean	Lower bound	−0.0831	
		Upper bound	0.0831	
	5% trimmed mean		0.0014	
	Median		−0.0295	
	Variance		0.984	
	Std. deviation		0.99177	
	Minimum		−2.69	
	Maximum		3.16	
	Range		5.85	
	Inter-quartile range		1.3246	
	Skewness		0.069	0.104
	Kurtosis		0.178	0.208

Extreme Values

			Case number	Value
Standardised residual for WEIGHT	Highest	1	256	3.16
		2	101	3.08
		3	404	3.03
		4	32	2.80
		5	447	2.73
	Lowest	1	252	−2.69
		2	437	−2.48
		3	311	−2.37
		4	35	−2.37
		5	546	−2.34

Tests of Normality

	Kolmogorov–Smirnov[a]			Shapiro-Wilk		
	Statistic	*df*	Sig.	Statistic	*df*	Sig.
Standardised residual for WEIGHT	0.020	550	0.200*	0.995	550	0.069

*This is a lower bound of the true significance.
[a] Lilliefors significance correction.

The descriptive statistics and the tests of normality show that the standardised residuals are normally distributed with a mean residual of zero and a standard deviation very close to unity at 0.992, as expected. The histogram and normal Q–Q plot shown in Figure 5.9 indicate only small deviations from normality in the tails of the distribution.

For an approximately normal distribution, 99% of standardised residuals will by definition fall within three standard deviations of the mean. Therefore, 1% of the sample is expected to be outside this range. In this sample size of 550 children, it would be expected that 1% of the sample, that is five children, would have a standardised residual outside the area that lies between −3 and +3 standard deviations from the mean. The Extreme Values table shows that residual scores for three children are more than 3 standard deviations from the mean and the largest standardised residual is 3.16. The number of outliers is less than would be expected by chance. In addition, all three outliers have values that are just outside the cut-off range and therefore are not of concern.

Identifying multivariate outliers: Leverage and discrepancy

To identify multivariate outliers, statistics such as leverage and discrepancy for each data point can be calculated. Leverage measures how far or remote a data point is from the remaining data but does not indicate whether the remote data point is on the same line as other cases or far away from the line. Thus, leverage does not provide information about the direction of the distance from the other data points[7]. Discrepancy indicates whether the remote data point is in line with other data points. Figure 5.10 shows how remote points or outliers can have a high leverage and/or a high discrepancy.

Cook's distances are a measure of influence, that is a product of leverage and discrepancy. Influence measures the change in regression coefficients (Chapter 6) if the data point is removed[6]. A recommended cut-off for detecting influential cases is a Cook's distance greater than $4/(n - k - 1)$, where n is the sample size and k is the number of explanatory variables in the model. In this example, any distance that is greater than $4/(550 - 3 - 1)$, or 0.007, should be investigated. Obviously the larger the sample size the smaller the cook's

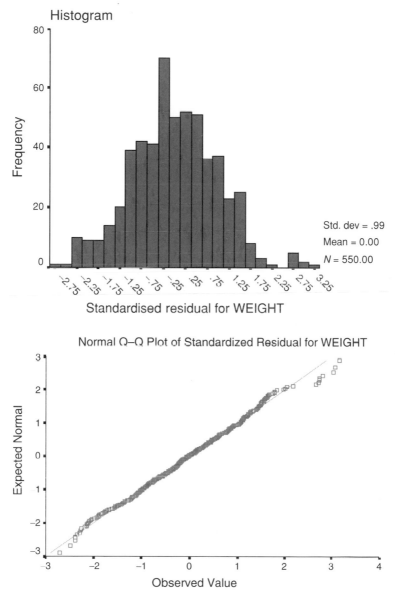

Figure 5.9 Plots of standardised residuals by weight.

distance becomes. Therefore in practice, Cook's distances above 1 should be investigated because these cases are regarded as influential cases or outliers.

A leverage value that is greater than $2(k+1)/n$, where k is the number of explanatory variables in the model and n is the sample size, is of concern. In the working example, this value would be $2 \times (3+1)/550$, or 0.015. As with Cook's distance, this leverage calculation is also influenced by sample size

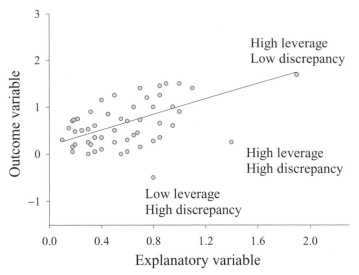

Figure 5.10 Distribution of data points and outliers.

and the number of explanatory variables in the model. In practice, leverage values less than 0.2 are acceptable and leverage values greater than 0.5 need to be investigated. Leverage is also related to Mahalanobis distance, which is another technique to identify multivariate outliers when regression is used[6] (Chapter 6).

Cook's distances can be plotted in a histogram using the SPSS commands shown Box 5.10. These commands can be repeated for leverage values.

Box 5.10 SPSS commands to examine potential multivariate outliers

SPSS Commands
weights – SPSS Data Editor
        Graphs → Histogram
Histogram
        Highlight Cook's distance for weight, click into Variable
        Click OK

The plots shown in Figure 5.11 indicate that there are no multivariate outliers because there are no Cook's distances greater than 1 or leverage points greater than 0.2.

Deciding whether points are problematic will always be context specific and several factors need to be taken into account including sample size and diagnostic indicators. If problematic points are detected, it is reasonable to remove them, re-run the model and decide on an action depending on their influence on the results. Possible solutions are to re-code values to remove

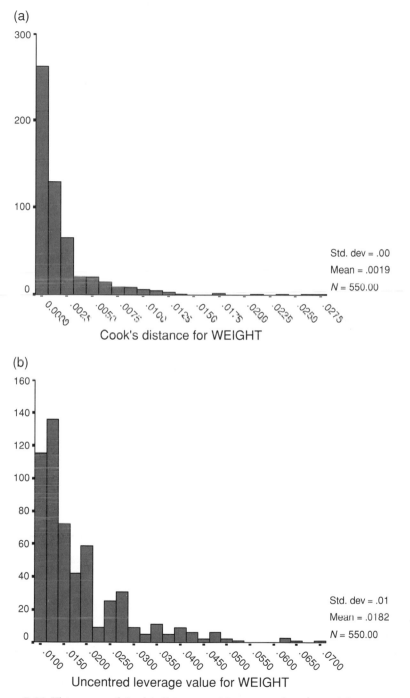

Figure 5.11 Histograms of Cook's distance and leverage values for weight.

their undue influence, to recruit a study sample with a larger sample size if the sample being tested is small or to limit the generalisability of the model.

Reporting the results

If the model assumptions had all been met, the results of the final ANCOVA model could be reported in a similar way to reporting the three-way ANOVA. The statistics reported should include information to assure readers that all ANCOVA assumptions had been met and should include values of partial eta squared to convey the relative contribution of each factor to the model. Other statistics to report are the total amount of variation explained and the significance of each factor in the model.

In the present ANCOVA model, because there was a significant interaction between factors, it is better to analyse the data using regression as described in Chapter 6.

Notes for critical appraisal

There are many assumptions for ANOVA and ANCOVA and it is important that all assumptions are tested and met to avoid inaccurate P values. Some of the most important questions to ask when critically appraising a journal article in which ANOVA or ANCOVA is used to analyse the data are shown in Box 5.11.

Box 5.11 Questions for critical appraisal

The following questions should be asked when appraising published results from analyses in which ANOVA or ANCOVA has been used:
- Have any repeated measures been treated as independent observations?
- Is the outcome variable normally distributed?
- Does each cell have an adequate number of participants?
- Are the variances between cells fairly similar?
- Are the residuals normally distributed?
- Are there any outliers that would tend to inflate or reduce differences between groups or that would distort the model and the standard errors, and therefore the P values?
- Does the model include any unreliable covariates or covariates that do not have a linear relationship with the outcome?
- If there is an increase in means across the range of a factor, has a trend test been used?
- Have tests of homogeneity and collinearity been included?
- Would regression have been a more appropriate statistical test to use?
- Do the P values reflect the differences between cell means and the group sizes?

References

1. Stevens, J. Applied multivariate statistics for the social sciences (3rd edition). Mahwah, NJ: Lawrence Erlbaum Associates, 1996; pp 6–9.
2. Altman DG, Bland JM. Comparing several groups using analysis of variance. BMJ 1996; 312: 1472–1473.
3. Norman GR, Streiner DL. One-way ANOVA. In: Biostatistics. The bare essentials. Missouri, USA: Mosby, 1994; pp 64–72.
4. Bland JM, Alman DG. Multiple significance tests: the Bonferroni method. BMJ 1995; 310: 170.
5. Perneger TV. What's wrong with Bonferroni adjustments. BMJ 1998; 316: 1236–1238.
6. Norman GR, Streiner DL. Biostatistics. The bare essentials. Missouri, USA: Mosby Year Book Inc, 1994: p. 168.
7. Tabachnick BG, Fidell LS. Using multivariate statistics (4th edition). Boston, USA: Allyn and Bacon, 2001; pp 68–70.

CHAPTER 6
Continuous data analyses: correlation and regression

Angling may be said to be so like mathematics that it can never be fully learnt.
IZAAK WALTON (1593–1683)

Objectives

The objectives of this chapter are to explain how to:
- explore a linear relation between two continuous variables
- interpret parametric and non-parametric correlation coefficients
- build a regression model that conforms to satisfies assumptions of regression assumptions
- use a regression model as a predictive equation
- include binary and dummy group variables in a multivariate model
- plot regression equations that include binary group variables
- include more than one continuous variable in a multivariate model
- test for collinearity and interactions
- identify and deal with outliers and remote points
- explore non-linear fits for regression models
- critically appraise the literature when regression models are reported

---

Correlation coefficients

A correlation coefficient describes how closely two variables are related, that is the amount of variability in one measurement that is explained by another measurement. The range of a correlation coefficient is from -1 to $+1$, where $+1$ and -1 indicate that one variable has a perfect linear association with the other variable and that both variables are measuring the same entity without error. In practice, this rarely occurs because even if two instruments are intended to measure the same entity both usually have some degree of measurement error.

A correlation coefficient of zero indicates a random relationship and the absence of a linear association. A positive coefficient value indicates that both variables increase in value together and a negative coefficient value indicates that one variable decreases in value as the other variable increases. It is important to note that a significant association between two variables does not imply that they have a causal relationship. Also, a correlation coefficient that is not significant does not imply that there is no relationship between the variables because there may be a non-linear relationship such as a curvilinear or cyclical relationship.

Correlation coefficients are rarely used as important statistics in their own right. An inherent limitation is that correlation coefficients reduce complex relationships to a single number that does not adequately explain the relationship between the two variables. Another inherent problem is that the statistical significance of the test is often over-interpreted. The P value is an estimate of whether the correlation coefficient is significantly different from zero so that a small correlation of no clinical importance can become statistically significant, especially when the sample size is large. In addition, the range of the data as well as the relationship between the two variables influences the correlation coefficient.

There are three types of bivariate correlations and the type of correlation that is used to examine a linear relation is determined by the nature of the variables.

Pearson's correlation coefficient (r) is a parametric correlation coefficient that is used to measure the association between two continuous variables that are both normally distributed. The correlation coefficient (r) can be squared to give the coefficient of determination (r^2), which is an estimate of the per cent of variation in one variable that is explained by the other variable.

The assumptions for using Pearson's correlation coefficient are shown in Box 6.1.

Box 6.1 Assumptions for using Pearson's correlation coefficient

The assumptions that must be satisfied to use Pearson's correlation coefficient are:
- both variables must be normally distributed
- the sample must have been selected randomly from the general population
- the observations are independent of one another
- the relation between the two variables is linear
- the variance is constant over the length of the data

If the assumption of random selection is not met, the correlation coefficient does not describe the true association between two variables that would be found in the general population. In this case, it would not be valid to generalise the association to other populations or to compare the r value with results from other studies.

Spearman's ρ (rho) is a rank correlation coefficient that is used for two ordinal variables or when one variable has a continuous normal distribution and the other variable is categorical or non-normally distributed. When this statistic is computed, the categorical or non-normally distributed variable is ranked, that is sorted into ascending order and numbered sequentially, and then a correlation of the ranks with the continuous variable that is equivalent to Pearson's r is calculated.

Kendall's τ (tau) is used for correlations between two categorical or non-normally distributed variables. In this test, Kendall's τ is calculated as the number of concordant pairs minus the number of disconcordant pairs divided by the total number of pairs. Kendall's tau-b is adjusted for the number of pairs that are tied.

Research question

The spreadsheet **weights.sav**, which was used in Chapter 5, contains the data from a population sample of 550 term babies who had their weight recorded at 1 month of age.

Question:	Is there an association between the weight, length and head circumference of 1 month old babies?
Null hypothesis:	That there is no association between weight, length and head circumference of babies at 1 month of age.
Variables:	Weight, length and head circumference (continuous)

All three variables of weight, length and head circumference are continuous variables that have a normal distribution and therefore their relationships to one another can be examined using Pearson's correlation coefficients. Before computing any correlation coefficient, it is important to obtain scatter plots to obtain an understanding of the nature of the relationships between the variables. Box 6.2 shows the SPSS commands to obtain the scatter plots.

Box 6.2 SPSS commands to obtain scatter plots between variables

SPSS Commands
weights – SPSS Data Editor
   Graphs → Scatter
Scatterplot
   Click on Matrix and click on Define
Scatterplot Matrix
   Highlight Weight, Length, Head circumference, click over into Matrix
    Variables
   Click OK

The matrix in Figure 6.1 shows each of the variables plotted against one another. The number of rows and columns is equal to the number of variables selected. Each variable is shown once on the x-axis and once on the y-axis to give six plots, three of which are mirror images of the other three. In Figure 6.1, the scatter plot between weight and length is shown in the middle box on the top row, the scatter plot between weight and head circumference is in the right hand box on the top row, and the scatter plot between length and head

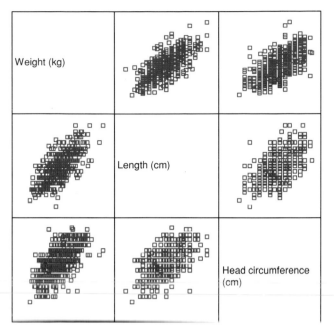

Figure 6.1 Scatter plot of weight by length by head circumference.

circumference is in the third column of the middle row. All scatter plots in Figure 6.1 slope upwards to the right indicating a positive association between the two variables. If an association was negative, the scatter plot would slope downwards to the right.

The plots shown in Figure 6.1 indicate that there is a reasonable, positive linear association for all bivariate combinations of the three variables. It is clear that weight has a closer relationship with length than with head circumference in that the scatter around the plot is narrower. Box 6.3 shows the SPSS commands to obtain the correlation coefficients between the three variables. Normally only one type of coefficient would be requested but to illustrate the difference between coefficients, all three are requested in this example.

Box 6.3 SPSS commands to obtain correlation coefficients

SPSS Commands
weights – SPSS Data Editor
    Analyze → Correlate → Bivariate
Bivariate Correlations
    Highlight Weight, Length, Head circumference, click over into Variables
    Under Correlation Coefficients, tick Pearson (default), Kendall's tau-b and
        Spearman
    Under Test of Significance, tick Two-Tailed (default)
    Click OK

Correlations

Correlations

		Weight (kg)	Length (cm)	Head circumference (cm)
Weight (kg)	Pearson correlation	1	0.713**	0.622**
	Sig. (two-tailed)	.	0.000	0.000
	N	550	550	550
Length (cm)	Pearson correlation	0.713**	1	0.598**
	Sig. (two-tailed)	0.000	.	0.000
	N	550	550	550
Head circumference (cm)	Pearson correlation	0.622**	0.598**	1
	Sig. (two-tailed)	0.000	0.000	.
	N	550	550	550

** Correlation is significant at the 0.01 level (two-tailed).

A comparison of the Pearson correlations (r values) in the Correlations table shows that the best predictor of weight is length with an r value of 0.713 compared to a weaker, but moderate association between weight and head circumference with an r value of 0.622. Head circumference is related to length with a slightly lower r value of 0.598. Despite their differences in magnitude, the correlation coefficients are all highly significant at the $P < 0.0001$ level emphasising the insensitive nature of the P values for selecting the most important predictors of weight.

Non-parametric Correlations

Correlations

			Weight (kg)	Length (cm)	Head circumference (cm)
Kendall's tau_b	Weight (kg)	Correlation coefficient	1.000	0.540**	0.468**
		Sig. (two-tailed)	.	0.000	0.000
		N	550	550	550
	Length (cm)	Correlation coefficient	0.540**	1.000	0.454**
		Sig. (two-tailed)	0.000	.	0.000
		N	550	550	550
	Head circumference (cm)	Correlation coefficient	0.468**	0.454**	1.000
		Sig. (two-tailed)	0.000	0.000	.
		N	550	550	550

Continued

			Weight (kg)	Length (cm)	Head circumference (cm)
Spearman's rho	Weight (kg)	Correlation coefficient	1.000	0.711**	0.626**
		Sig. (two-tailed)	.	0.000	0.000
		N	550	550	550
	Length (cm)	Correlation coefficient	0.711**	1.000	0.596**
		Sig. (two-tailed)	0.000	.	0.000
		N	550	550	550
	Head circumference (cm)	Correlation coefficient	0.626**	0.596**	1.000
		Sig. (two-tailed)	0.000	0.000	.
		N	550	550	550

**Correlation is significant at the 0.01 level (two-tailed).

In the Non-parametric Correlations table, Kendall's tau-b coefficients are all lower than the Pearson's coefficients in the previous table but Spearman's coefficients are similar in magnitude to Pearson's coefficients.

The influence on *r* values when using a selected sample rather than a random sample can be demonstrated by repeating the analysis using only part of the data set. Using *Analyze → Descriptive Statistics → Descriptives* shows that length ranges from a minimum value of 48.0 cm to a maximum value of 62.0 cm. To examine the correlation in a selected sample, the data set can be restricted to babies less than 55.0 cm in length using the commands shown in Box 6.4.

Box 6.4 SPSS commands to calculate a correlation coefficient for a subset of the data

SPSS Commands
weights – SPSS Data Editor
        Data → Select Cases
Select Cases
        Tick 'If condition is satisfied' → Click on 'If' box
Select Cases: If
        Highlight Length and click over into white box
        Type in '<55' following length
        Click Continue
Select Cases
        Click OK

When *Select Cases* is used, the line numbers of cases that are unselected appear in Data View with a diagonal line through them indicating that they will be excluded from any analysis. In addition, a filter variable to indicate the status of each case in the analysis is generated at the end of the spreadsheet and the text *Filter On* is shown in the bottom right hand side of the Data View screen.

To examine the relationship between the variables for only babies less than 55.0 cm in length, Pearson's correlation coefficients can be obtained using the commands shown in Box 6.2.

Correlations

Correlations

		Weight (kg)	Length (cm)	Head circumference (cm)
Weight (kg)	Pearson correlation	1	0.494**	0.504**
	Sig. (two-tailed)	.	0.000	0.000
	N	272	272	272
Length (cm)	Pearson correlation	0.494**	1	0.390**
	Sig. (two-tailed)	0.000	.	0.000
	N	272	272	272
Head circumference (cm)	Pearson correlation	0.504**	0.390**	1
	Sig. (two-tailed)	0.000	0.000	.
	N	272	272	272

** Correlation is significant at the 0.01 level (two-tailed).

When compared with Pearson's r values from the full data set, the correlation coefficient between weight and length is substantially reduced from 0.713 to 0.494 when the upper limit of length is reduced from 62 cm to 55 cm. However, the top centre plot in Figure 6.1 shows that the relationship between weight and length in the lower half of the data is similar to the total sample. In general, r values are higher when the range of the explanatory variable is wider even though the relationship between the variables is the same. For this reason, only the coefficients from random population samples have an unbiased value and can be compared with one another.

Once the correlation coefficients are obtained, the full data set can be reselected using the command sequence *Data* → *Select Cases* → *All cases*.

Regression models

Regression models are used to measure the extent to which one or more explanatory variables predict an outcome variable. In this, a regression model is used to fit a straight line through the data, where the regression line is the best predictor of the outcome variable using one or more explanatory variables.

There are two principal purposes for building a regression model. The most common purpose is to build a predictive model, for example in situations in which age and gender are used to predict normal values in lung size or body mass index (BMI). Normal values are the range of values that occur naturally in the general population. In developing a model to predict normal values, the emphasis is on building an accurate predictive model.

The second purpose of using a regression model is to examine the effect of an explanatory variable on an outcome variable after adjusting for other important explanatory factors. These types of models are used for hypothesis testing. For example, a regression model could be built using age and gender to predict BMI and could then be used to test the hypothesis that groups with different exercise regimes have different BMI values.

The mathematics of regression are identical to the mathematics of analysis of covariance (ANCOVA). However, regression provides more information than ANCOVA in that a linear equation is generated that explains the relationship between the explanatory variables and the outcome. By using regression, more information about the relationships between variables and the between-group differences is obtained. Regression can also be a more flexible approach because some of the assumptions such as those relating to cell and variance ratios are not as restrictive as the assumptions for ANCOVA. However, in common with ANCOVA, it is important to remember that regression gives a measure of association at one point in time only, that is, at the time the measurements were collected, and a significant association does not infer causality.

Although the mathematics of regression are similar to ANOVA in that the explained and unexplained variations are compared, some terms are labelled differently. In regression, the distance between an observed value and the overall mean is partitioned into two components – the variation about the regression, which is also called the residual variation, and the variation due to the regression[1]. Figure 6.2 shows how the variation for one data point, shown as a circle, is calculated.

The variation about the regression is the explained variation and the variation due to the regression is the unexplained variation. As in ANOVA, these distances are squared and summed and the mean square is calculated. The F value, which is calculated as the regression mean square divided by the residual mean square, ranges from 1 to a large number. If the two sources of variance are similar, there is no association between the variables and the F value is close to 1. If the variation due to the regression is large compared to the variation about the regression, then the F value will be large indicating a strong association between the outcome and explanatory variables.

When there is only one explanatory variable, the equation of the best fit for the regression line is as follows:

$$y = a + bx$$

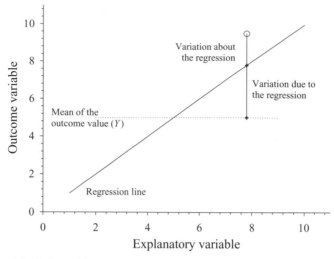

Figure 6.2 Calculation of the variation in regression.

where 'y' is the value of the outcome variable, 'x' is the value of the explanatory variable, 'a' is the intercept of the regression line and 'b' is the slope of the regression line. When there is only one explanatory variable, this is called a simple linear regression.

In practice, the slope of the line, as estimated by 'b', represents the unit change in the outcome variable 'y' with each unit change in the explanatory variable 'x'. If the slope is positive, 'y' increases as 'x' increases and if the slope is negative, 'y' decreases as 'x' increases. The intercept is the point at which the regression line intersects with the y-axis when the value of 'x' is zero. This value is part of the regression equation but does not usually have any clinical meaning. The fitted regression line passes through the mean values of both the explanatory variable 'x' and the outcome variable 'y'.

When using regression, the research question must be framed so that the explanatory and outcome variables are classified correctly. An important concept is that regression predicts the mean y value given the observed x value and the error around the explanatory variable is not taken into account. Therefore, measurements that can be taken accurately, such as age and height, make good explanatory variables. Measurements that are difficult to measure accurately or are subject to bias, such as birth weight recalled by parents when the baby has reached school age, should be avoided as explanatory variables.

Assumptions for regression

To avoid bias in a regression model or a lack of precision around the estimates, the assumptions for using regression that are shown in Box 6.5 must be tested and met. In regression, mean values are not compared as in ANOVA so that any bias between groups as a result of non-normal distributions is not as problematic. Regression models are robust to moderate degrees of non-normality provided that the sample size is large and that there are few multivariate outliers in the final model. In general, the residuals but not the outcome variable has to be normally distributed. Also, the sample does not have to be selected randomly because the regression equation describes the relation between the variables and is not influenced by the spread of the data. However, it is important that the final prediction equation is only applied to populations with the same characteristics as the study sample.

Box 6.5 Assumptions for using regression

The assumptions that must be met when using regression are as follows:

Study design
- the sample is representative of the population to which inference will be made
- the sample size is sufficient to support the model
- the data have been collected in a period when the relationship between the outcome and the explanatory variable/s remains constant
- all important explanatory variables (covariates) are included

Independence
- all observations are independent of one another
- there is low collinearity between explanatory variables

Model building
- the relation between the explanatory variable/s and the outcome variable is approximately linear
- the explanatory variables correlate with the outcome variable
- the residuals are normally distributed
- the variance is homoscedastic, that is constant over the length of the model
- there are no multivariate outliers that bias the regression estimates

---

Under the study design assumptions shown in Box 6.5, the assumption that the data are collected in a period when the relationship remains constant is important. For example, in building a model to predict normal values for blood pressure the data must be collected when the participants have been resting rather than exercising and participants taking anti-hypertensive medications should be excluded. It is also important that all known covariates are included in the model before testing the effects of new variables added to the model.

The two assumptions of independence between observations and explanatory variables are important. When explanatory variables are significantly related to each other, a decision needs to be made about which variable to include and which variable to exclude.

The remaining assumptions about the nature of the data can be tested when building the model. In this chapter, the assumptions are tested after obtaining a parsimonious model but in practice the assumptions should be tested at each step in the model building process.

Research question

Using the spreadsheet **weights.sav,** regression analysis can be used to answer the following research question:

Question:	Can body length be used to predict weight at 1 month of age?
Null hypothesis:	That there is no relation between length and weight at 1 month.
Variables:	Outcome variable = weight (continuous)
	Explanatory variable = length (continuous)

The SPSS commands to obtain a regression equation for the relation between length and weight are shown in Box 6.6.

Box 6.6 SPSS commands to obtain regression estimates

SPSS Commands
weights – SPSS Data Editor
          Analyze → Regression → Linear
Linear Regression
          Highlight Weight, click into Dependent box
          Highlight Length, click into Independent(s) box
          Method = Enter (default)
          Click OK

Regression

Model Summary

Model	R	R square	Adjusted R square	Std. error of the estimate
1	0.713[a]	0.509	0.508	0.42229

[a] Predictors: (constant), length (cm).

ANOVA[b]

Model		Sum of squares	df	Mean square	F	Sig.
1	Regression	101.119	1	101.119	567.043	0.000[a]
	Residual	97.723	548	0.178		
	Total	198.842	549			

[a] Predictors: (constant), length (cm).
[b] Dependent variable: weight (kg).

In linear regression, the R value in the Model Summary table is the multiple correlation coefficient and is the correlation between the observed and predicted values of the outcome variable. The value of R will range between 0 and 1. R can be interpreted in a similar way to Pearson's correlation coefficient. In simple linear regression, R is the absolute value of Pearson's correlation coefficient between the outcome and explanatory variable.

The R square value is the square of the R value, that is 0.713×0.713, and is often called the coefficient of determination. R square has a valuable interpretation in that it indicates the per cent of the variance in the outcome variable that can be explained or accounted for by the explanatory variables. The R square value of 0.509 indicates a modest relationship in that 50.9% of the variation in weight is explained by length. The adjusted R square value is the R value adjusted for the number of explanatory variables included in the model and can therefore be compared between models that include different numbers of explanatory variables. The standard error of the estimate of 0.42229 is the standard error around the outcome variable weight at the mean value of the explanatory variable length and as such gives an indication of the precision of the model.

In the ANOVA table, the F value is calculated as the unexplained variation due to the regression divided by the explained variation about the regression, or the residual variation. Thus, F is the regression mean square of 101.119 divided by the residual mean square of 0.178, or 568.08. The resulting F value of 567.043 in the table is slightly different as a result of rounding errors and is highly significant at $P < 0.0001$ indicating that there is a significant linear relation between length and weight.

Coefficients[a]

Model		Unstandardised coefficients		Standardised coefficients		
		B	Std. error	Beta	t	Sig.
1	(Constant)	−5.412	0.411		−13.167	0.000
	Length (cm)	0.178	0.007	0.713	23.813	0.000

[a] Dependent variable: weight (kg).

The Coefficients table shows the unstandardised coefficients that are used to formulate the regression equation in the form of $y = a + bx$ as follows:

Weight $= -5.412 + (0.178 \times$ Length$)$

Because length is the only explanatory variable in the model, the standardised coefficient, which indicates the relative contribution of a variable to the model, is the same as the R value shown in the first table. The t values, which are calculated by dividing the beta values (unstandardised coefficient B) by their standard errors, are a test of whether each regression coefficient is significantly different from zero. In this example, both the constant (intercept) and slope of the regression line are significantly different from zero at $P < 0.0001$ which is shown in the column labelled 'sig'. For length, the square of the t value is equal to the F value in the ANOVA table, that is the square of 23.813 is equal to 567.043.

Regression equations can only be generalised to samples with the same characteristics as the study sample. Thus, this regression model only describes the relation between weight and length in 1 month old babies who were term births because premature birth was an exclusion criterion for study entry. The model could not be used to predict normal population values because they are not from a random population sample, which would include premature births. However, the model could be used to predict normal values for term babies.

Plotting the regression

The commands shown in Box 6.7 can be used to obtain a scatter plot, plot the observed values of weight against length and to draw the regression line with prediction intervals.

Box 6.7 SPSS commands to obtain a scatter plot

SPSS Commands
weights – SPSS Data Editor
         Graphs → Interactive → Scatterplot
Create Scatterplot
         Highlight Length, hold left hand mouse button and drag into x-axis box
         Highlight Weight, hold left hand mouse button and drag into y-axis box
         Click on Fit
         Pull down menu under Method and highlight Regression
         Prediction Lines: tick Mean and Individual
         Click OK

In Figure 6.3, the 95% mean prediction interval around the regression line is a 95% confidence interval, that is the area in which there is 95% certainty that

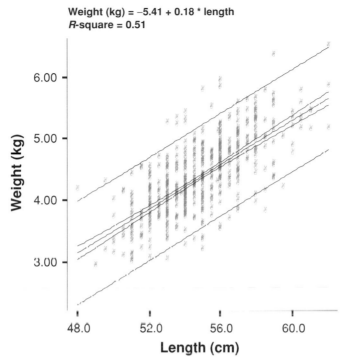

Figure 6.3 Scatter plot of weight on length with regression line and 95% confidence interval.

the true regression line lies. This interval band is slightly curved because the errors in estimating the intercept and the slope are included in addition to the error in predicting the outcome variable[2]. The error in estimating the slope increases as the difference between the predicted value and the actual value of the explanatory variable increases, resulting in a curved 95% confidence band around the sample regression line. In Figure 6.3, the 95% confidence interval is narrow as a result of the large sample size.

The 95% individual prediction interval is the larger band around the regression line in Figure 6.3. This interval in which 95% of the data points lie is the distance between the 2.5 and 97.5 percentiles. This interval is used to predict normal values. Clearly, any definition of normality is specific to the context but normal values should only be based on large sample sizes, preferably of at least 200 participants[3].

Multiple linear regression

A regression model in which the outcome variable is predicted from two or more explanatory variables is called a multiple linear regression. Explanatory variables may be continuous or categorical. For example, it is common to use height and age, both of which are continuous variables, to predict lung size or to use age and gender, a continuous and a categorical variable, to predict BMI. For multiple regression, the equation that explains the line of best fit, i.e. the regression line, is

$$y = a + b_1x_1 + b_2x_2 + b_3x_3 + \cdots$$

where 'a' is the intercept and 'b_i' is slope for each explanatory variable. In effect, b_1, b_2, b_3, etc. are the weights assigned to each of the explanatory variables in the model. In multiple regression models, the coefficient for a variable can be interpreted as the unit change in the outcome variable with each unit change in the explanatory variable when all of the other explanatory variables are held constant.

Multiple regression is used when there are several explanatory variables that predict an outcome or when the effect of a factor that can be manipulated is being tested. For example, height, age and gender could be used to predict lung function and then the effects of other potential explanatory variables such as current respiratory symptoms or smoking history could be tested. In multiple regression models, all explanatory variables that have an important association with the outcome should be included.

Multiple linear regression models should be built up gradually through a series of univariate bivariate, and multivariate methods. In multiple regression, each explanatory variable should ideally have a significant correlation with the outcome variable but the explanatory variables should not be significantly correlated with one another, that is collinear. Models should not be over-fitted with a large number of variables that increase the R square by small amounts. In over-fitted models, the R square may decrease when the model is applied to other data.

Decisions about which variables to remove or include in a model should be based on expert knowledge and biological plausibility in addition to statistical considerations. These decisions often need to take cost, measurement error and theoretical constructs into account in addition to the strength of association indicated by R values, P values and standardised coefficients. The ideal model should be parsimonious, that is comprising of the smallest number of variables that predict the largest amount of variation.

Once a decision has been made about which explanatory variables to test in a model, the distribution of both the outcome and the continuous explanatory variables should be examined using methods outlined in Chapter 2, largely to identify any univariate outliers. Also, the order in which the explanatory variables are entered into the model is important because this can make a difference to the amount of variance that is explained by each explanatory variable, especially when explanatory variables are significantly related to each other[4].

There are three different methods of entering the explanatory variables that is standard, stepwise or sequential[5]. In standard multiple regression, called the enter method in SPSS, all variables are entered into the model together and the unique contribution of each variable to the outcome variable is calculated. However, an explanatory variable that is correlated with the outcome variable may not be a significant predictor when the other explanatory variables have accounted for a large proportion of the variance so that the remaining variance is small[5].

In stepwise multiple regression, the order of the explanatory variables is determined by the strength of their correlation with the outcome variable or by predetermined statistical criteria. The stepwise procedure can be forward selection, backward deletion or stepwise, all of which are available options in SPSS. In forward selection, variables are added one at a time until the addition of another variable accounts only for a small amount of variance. In backward selection, all variables are entered and then are deleted one at a time if they do not contribute significantly to the prediction of the outcome. Forward selection and backward deletion may not result in the same regression equation[2]. Stepwise is a combination of both forward selection and backward deletion in which variables are added one at a time and retained if they satisfy set statistical criteria but are deleted if they no longer contribute significantly to the model[3].

In sequential multiple regression, which is also called hierarchical regression, the order of entering the explanatory variables is determined by the researcher using logical or theoretical factors, or by the strength of the correlation with the outcome variable. When each new variable is entered, the variance contributed by the variable, possible collinearity with other variables and the influence of the variable on the model are assessed. Variables can be entered one at a time or together in blocks and the significance of each variable, or each variable in the block, is assessed at each step. This method delivers a stable and reliable model and provides invaluable information about the inter-relationships between the explanatory variables.

Sample size considerations

For multiple regression, it is important to have an adequate sample size. A simple rule that has been suggested for predictive equations is that the minimum number of cases should be at least 100 or, for stepwise regression, that the number of cases should be at least $40 \times m$, where m is the number of variables in the model[5]. More precise methods for calculating sample size and power are available[6]. To avoid underestimating the sample size for regression, sample size calculations should be based on the regression model itself and not on correlation coefficients.

It is important not to include too many explanatory variables in the model relative to the number of cases because this can inflate the R^2 value. When the sample size is very small, the R^2 value will be artificially inflated, the adjusted R^2 value will be reduced and the imprecise regression estimates may have no sensible interpretation. If the sample size is too small to support the number of explanatory variables being tested, the variables can be tested one at a time and only the most significant included in the final model. Alternatively, a new explanatory variable can be created that is a composite of the original variables, for example BMI could be included instead of weight and height.

A larger sample size increases the precision around the estimates by reducing standard errors and often increases the generalisability of the results. The sample size needs to be increased if a small effect size is anticipated or if there is substantial measurement error in any variable, which tends to reduce statistical power to demonstrate significant associations between variables.

It is important to achieve a balance in the regression model with the number of explanatory variables and sample size, because even a small R value will become statistically significant when the sample size is very large. Thus, when the sample size is large it is prudent to be cautious about type I errors. When the final model is obtained, the clinical importance of estimates of effect size should be used to interpret the coefficients for each variable rather than reliance on P values.

Collinearity

Collinearity is a term that is used when two or more of the explanatory variables are significantly related to one another. The issue of collinearity is only important for the relationships between explanatory variables and naturally does not need to be considered in relationships between the explanatory variables and the outcome.

Regression is more robust to some degrees of collinearity than ANOVA but the smaller the sample size and the larger the number of variables in the model, the more problematic collinearity becomes. Important degrees of collinearity need to be reconciled because they can distort the regression coefficients and lead to a loss of precision, that is inflated standard errors of the beta coefficients, and thus to an unstable and unreliable model. In extreme cases of collinearity, the direction of effect, that is the sign, of a regression coefficient may change.

Correlations between explanatory variables cause logical as well as statistical problems. If one variable accounts for most of the variation in another explanatory variable, the logic of including both explanatory variables in the model needs to be considered since they are approximate measures of the same entity. The correlation (r) between explanatory variables in a regression model should not be greater than 0.70.[7] For this reason, the decision of which variables to include should be based on theoretical constructs rather than statistical considerations based on regression estimates. Variables that can be measured with reliability and with minimum measurement error are preferred whereas measurements that are costly, invasive, unreliable or removed from the main causal pathway are less useful in predictive models.

The amount of collinearity in a model is estimated by the variance inflation factor (VIF), which is calculated as $1/(1 - R^2)$ where R^2 is the squared multiple correlation coefficient. In essence, VIF measures how much the variance of the regression coefficient has been inflated due to collinearity with other explanatory variables[8]. In regression models, P values rely on an estimate of variance around the regression coefficients, which is proportional to the VIF and thus if the VIF is inflated, the P value may be unreliable. A VIF that is large, say greater than or equal to 4, is a sign of collinearity and the regression coefficients, their variances and their P values are likely to be unreliable.

In SPSS, collinearity is estimated by tolerance, that is $1 - R^2$. Tolerance has an inverse relationship to VIF in that VIF $= 1/$tolerance. Tolerance values close to zero indicate collinearity[8]. In regression, tolerance values less than 0.2 are usually considered to indicate collinearity. The relation between R, tolerance and VIF is shown in Table 6.1. A tolerance value below 0.5, which corresponds with an R value above 0.7 is of concern.

Table 6.1 Relation between R, tolerance and variance inflation factor (VIF)

R	Tolerance	VIF
0.25	0.94	1.07
0.50	0.75	1.33
0.70	0.51	1.96
0.90	0.19	5.26
0.95	0.10	10.26

Collinearity can be estimated from examining the standard errors and from tolerance values as described in the examples below, or collinearity statistics can be obtained in the *Statistics* options under the *Analyze → Regression→ Linear* commands.

Multiple linear regression: testing for group differences

Regression can be used to test whether the relation between the outcome and explanatory variables is the same across categorical groups, say males and females. Rather than split the data set and analyse the data from males and females separately, it is often more useful to incorporate gender as a binary explanatory variable in the regression model. This process maintains statistical power by maintaining sample size and has the advantage of providing an estimate of the size of the difference between the gender groups.

The spreadsheet **weights.sav** used previously in this chapter will be used to answer the following research questions.

Research question

Question: Is the prediction equation of weight using length different for males and females or for babies with siblings?

Variables: Outcome variable = weight (continuous)
Explanatory variables = length (continuous), gender (category, two levels) and parity (category, two levels)

In this model, length is included because it is an important predictor of weight. In effect, the regression model is used to adjust weight for differences in length between babies and then to test the null hypothesis that there is no difference in weight between groups defined by gender and parity.

It is simple to include a categorical variable in a regression model when the variable is binary, that is, has two levels only. Binary regression coefficients have a straight forward interpretation if the variable is coded 0 for the comparison group, for example a factor that is absent or reply of no, and 1 for the group of interest, for example a factor that is present or a reply that is coded yes.

The *Transform → Recode* commands shown in Box 1.10 in Chapter 1 can be used to re-code gender into a new variable labelled gender2 with values 0 and 1, making an arbitrary decision to code male gender as the comparison group.

Similarly, parity can be re-coded into a new variable, parity2 with the value 0 for singletons unchanged and with values of 1 or greater re-coded to 1 using the *Range* option from *1 through 3*. Once re-coded, values and labels for both variables need to be added in the Variable View screen and the numbers in each group verified as correct using the frequency commands shown in Box 1.7 in Chapter 1. It is important to always have systems in place to check for possible re-coding errors and to document re-coded group numbers in any new variables.

In this chapter, regression equations are built using the sequential method. To add variables to the regression model in blocks, the commands shown in Box 6.8 can be used with the enter method and block option. Prior bivariate analysis using *t*-tests for gender and one-way ANOVA for parity (not shown) indicated that the association between gender and weight is stronger than the association between parity and weight. Therefore, gender is added in the model before parity. Using the sequential method, the statistics of the two models are easily compared, collinearity between variables can be identified and reasons for any inflation in standard errors and loss of precision become clear.

Box 6.8 SPSS commands to generate a regression model with a binary explanatory variable

SPSS Commands
weights – SPSS Data Editor
       Analyze → Regression → Linear
Linear Regression
       Highlight Weight, click into Dependent box
       Highlight Length, click into Independent(s) box
       Under Block 1 of 1, click Next
       Highlight Gender recoded, click into Independent(s) box in Block 2 of 2
       Method = Enter (default)
       Click OK

Regression

Model Summary

Model	R	R square	Adjusted R square	Std. error of the estimate
1	0.713[a]	0.509	0.508	0.42229
2	0.741[b]	0.549	0.548	0.40474

[a] Predictors: (constant), length (cm).
[b] Predictors: (constant), length (cm), gender re-coded.

ANOVA[c]

Model		Sum of squares	df	Mean square	F	Sig.
1	Regression	101.119	1	101.119	567.043	0.000[a]
	Residual	97.723	548	0.178		
	Total	198.842	549			
2	Regression	109.235	2	54.617	333.407	0.000[b]
	Residual	89.607	547	0.164		
	Total	198.842	549			

[a] Predictors: (constant), length (cm).
[b] Predictors: (constant), length (cm), gender re-coded.
[c] Dependent variable: weight (kg).

Coefficients[a]

Model		Unstandardised coefficients B	Std. error	Standardised coefficients Beta	t	Sig.
1	(Constant)	−5.412	.0411		−13.167	0.000
	Length (cm)	0.178	0.007	0.713	23.813	0.000
2	(Constant)	−4.563	0.412		−11.074	0.000
	Length (cm)	0.165	0.007	0.660	22.259	0.000
	Gender re-coded	−0.251	0.036	−0.209	−7.039	0.000

[a] Dependent variable: weight (kg).

Excluded Variables[b]

Model		Beta In	t	Sig.	Partial correlation	Collinearity statistics Tolerance
1	Gender re-coded	−0.209[a]	−7.039	0.000	−0.288	0.936

[a] Predictors in the model: (constant), length (cm).
[b] Dependent variable: weight (kg).

The Model Summary table indicates the strength of the predictive or explanatory variables in the regression model. The first model contains length and the second model contains length and gender. Because there are a different number of variables in the two models, the adjusted R square value is used when making direct comparisons between the models. The adjusted R square value can be used to assess whether the fit of the model improves with inclusion of the additional variable, that is whether the amount of explained variation increases. By comparing the adjusted R square of Model 1 generated in Block 1 with the adjusted R square of Model 2 generated in Block 2, it is clear that adding gender improves the model fit because the adjusted R square increases from 0.508 to 0.548. This indicates that 54.8% of the variation is now explained. If it is important to know whether the R square increases by a significant amount, a P value for the change can be obtained by using the following commands *Regression* → *Linear* → *Statistics* → *R squared change*.

In the ANOVA table, the regression mean square decreases from 101.119 in Model 1 to 54.617 in Model 2 when gender is added because more of the unexplained variation is now explained. With high F values, both models are clearly significant as expected.

In the Coefficients table, the standard error around the beta coefficient for length (B) remains at 0.007 in both models indicating that the model is stable. An increase of more than 10% in a standard error indicates collinearity between the variables in the model and the variable being added.

With two explanatory variables in the model, the regression line will be of the form of $y = a + b_1x_1 + b_2x_2$, where x_1 is length and x_2 is gender. Substituting the variables and the unstandardised coefficients from the Coefficients table, the equation for model is as follows:

Weight $= -4.563 + (0.165 \times \text{Length}) - (0.251 \times \text{Gender})$

Because males are coded zero, the final term in the equation is removed for males. The term for gender indicates that, after adjusting for length, females are 0.251 kg lighter than males. In effect this means that the y intercept is –4.563 for males and –4.814 (i.e. –4.563 – 0.251) for females. Thus the lines for males and females are parallel but females have a lower y-axis intercept.

The unstandardised coefficients cannot be directly compared to assess their relative importance because they are in the original units of the measurements. However, the standardised coefficients indicate the relative importance of each variable in comparable standardised units (z scores). The Coefficients table shows that length with a standardised coefficient of 0.660 is a more significant predictor of weight than gender with a standardised coefficient of –0.209. As with an R value, the negative sign is an indication of the direction of effect only. The standardised coefficients give useful additional information because they show that although both predictors have the same P values, they are not of equal importance in predicting weight.

The Excluded Variables table shows the model with gender omitted. The beta In is the standardised coefficient that would result if gender is included in the model and is identical to the standardised coefficient in the Coefficients table above. The partial correlation is the unique contribution of gender to predicting weight after the effect of length is removed and is an estimate of the relative importance of this predictive variable in isolation from length. The collinearity statistic tolerance is close to 1 indicating that the predictor variables are not closely related to one another and that the regression assumption of independence between predictive variables is not violated.

Plotting a regression line with categorical explanatory variables

To plot a regression equation, it is important to ascertain the range of the explanatory variable values because the line should never extend outside the absolute range of the data. To obtain the minimum and maximum values of length for males and females the commands *Analyze* → *Compare Means* → *Means* can be used with length as the dependent variable and gender2 as the independent variable, and *Options* clicked to request minimum and maximum values. This provides the information that the length of male babies ranges from 50 to 62 cm and that the length of female babies ranges from 48 to 60.5 cm.

Table 6.2 shows how an Excel spreadsheet can be used to compute the coordinates for the beginning and end of the regression line for each gender. The regression coefficients from the equation are entered in the first three columns, and the minimum and maximum values for length and indicators of gender are entered in the next two columns. Weight is then calculated using the equation of the regression line and the calculation function in Excel.

Table 6.2 Excel spreadsheet to calculate regression line coordinates

Column 1 a	Column 2 b1	Column 3 b2	Column 4 length	Column 5 gender2	Column 6 predicted weight
−4.563	0.165	−0.251	50	0	3.687
−4.563	0.165	−0.251	62	0	5.667
−4.563	0.165	−0.251	48	1	3.106
−4.563	0.165	−0.251	60.5	1	5.169

The line coordinates from columns 4 and 6 can be copied and pasted into SigmaPlot to draw the graph using the commands shown in Box 6.9. The SigmaPlot spreadsheet should have the lower and upper coordinates for males in columns 1 and 2 and the lower and upper coordinates for females in columns 3 and 4 as follows:

Column 1	Column 2	Column 3	Column 4
50.0	3.69	48.0	3.11
62.0	5.67	60.5	5.17

Box 6.9 SigmaPlot commands to plot regression lines

SigmaPlot Commands
SigmaPlot – [Data 1*]
       Graph → Create Graph
Create Graph – Type
       Highlight 'Line Plot', click Next
Create Graph – Style
       Highlight 'Simple Straight Line', click Next
Create Graph – Data Format
       Data format = Highlight 'XY Pair', click Next
Create Graph – Select Data
       Highlight Column 1, click into Data for X
       Highlight Column 2, click into Data for Y
       Click Finish

The second line for females can be added using *Graph → Add Plot* and using the same command sequence shown in Box 6.9, except that the *Data for X* is column 3 and the *Data for Y* is column 4. The resulting graph can then be customised using the many options in *Graph → Graph Properties*. The completed graph, as shown in Figure 6.4, is a useful tool for presenting summary results

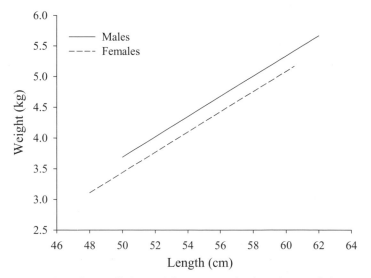

Figure 6.4 Equations for predicting weight at 1 month of age in term babies.

in a way that shows the relationship between weight and length and the size of the difference between the genders.

Regression models with two explanatory categorical variables

Having established the relation between weight, length and gender, the re-coded binary variable parity2 can be added to the model. Using the commands shown in Box 6.8, length and gender re-coded can be added as independent variables into Block 1 of 1 and parity re-coded (binary) as an independent variable into Block 2 of 2 to obtain the following output.

Regression

Model Summary

Model	R	R square	Adjusted R square	Std. error of the estimate
1	0.741[a]	0.549	0.548	0.40474
2	0.747[b]	0.559	0.556	0.40088

[a] Predictors: (constant), gender re-coded, length (cm).
[b] Predictors: (constant), gender re-coded, length (cm), parity re-coded.

Coefficients[a]

Model		Unstandardised coefficients		Standardised coefficients		
		B	Std. error	Beta	t	Sig.
1	(Constant)	−4.563	0.412		−11.074	0.000
	Length (cm)	0.165	0.007	0.660	22.259	0.000
	Gender re-coded	−0.251	0.036	−0.209	−7.039	0.000
2	(Constant)	−4.572	0.408		−11.203	0.000
	Length (cm)	0.164	0.007	0.655	22.262	0.000
	Gender re-coded	−0.255	0.035	−0.212	7.200	0.000
	Parity re-coded (binary)	0.124	0.036	0.097	3.405	0.001

[a] Dependent variable: weight (kg).

Excluded Variables[b]

Model		Beta In	t	Sig.	Partial correlation	Collinearity statistics Tolerance
1	Parity re-coded (binary)	0.097[a]	3.405	0.001	0.144	0.997

[a] Predictors in the model: (constant), gender re-coded, length (cm).
[b] Dependent variable: weight (kg).

The Model Summary table shows that adding parity to the model improves the adjusted R square value only slightly from 0.548 in Model 1 to 0.556 in Model 2, that is 55.6% of the variation is now explained.

In the ANOVA table, the mean square decreases from 54.617 in Model 1 to 37.033 in Model 2 because more of the unexplained variation is now explained.

In the Coefficients table, the standard error for length remains at 0.007 in both models and the standard error for gender reduces slightly from 0.036 in Model 1 to 0.035 in Model 2 indicating that the model is stable. The unstandardised coefficients indicate that the equation for the regression model is now as follows:

$$\text{Weight} = -4.572 + (0.164 \times \text{Length}) - (0.255 \times \text{Gender}) + (0.124 \times \text{Parity})$$

When parity status is singleton, i.e. parity equals zero, the final term of the regression equation will return a zero value and will therefore be removed for singleton babies. Therefore, the model indicates that, after adjusting for length and gender, babies who have siblings are on average 0.124 kg heavier than singleton babies.

The standardised coefficients in the Coefficients table show that length and gender are more significant predictors than parity in that their standardised coefficients are larger. These coefficients give a useful estimate of the size of effect of each variable when, as in this case, the P values are similar.

The Excluded Variables table shows that tolerance remains high at 0.997 indicating that there is no collinearity between variables.

Plotting regression lines with two explanatory categorical variables

Figure 6.4 shows regression lines plotted for a single binary explanatory variable. To include the second binary explanatory variable of sibling status in the graph, two line coordinates are computed for each of the four groups, that is males with no siblings; males with one or more siblings; females with no siblings and females with one or more siblings. To obtain the minimum and maximum values for each of these groups, the data can be split by gender using the *Split File* command shown in Box 4.8 in Chapter 4 and then the commands *Analyze→Compare Means→Means* can be used with length as the dependent variable and parity2 as the independent variable and *Options* clicked to request minimum and maximum values.

Again, Excel can be used to calculate the regression coordinates using the regression equation and with an indicator for parity included in an additional column. The Excel spreadsheet from Table 6.3 and the commands from Box 6.9 can be used to plot the figure in SigmaPlot with additional lines included under *Graph→Add Plot*.

Table 6.3 Excel spreadsheet for calculating coordinates for regression lines with two binary explanatory variables

Column 1 a	Column 2 b1	Column 3 b2	Column 4 b3	Column 5 length	Column 6 gender2	Column 7 parity2	Column 8 predicted weight
−4.572	0.164	−0.255	0.124	50	0	0	3.63
−4.572	0.164	−0.255	0.124	62	0	0	5.60
−4.572	0.164	−0.255	0.124	49	1	0	3.21
−4.572	0.164	−0.255	0.124	58.5	1	0	4.77
−4.572	0.164	−0.255	0.124	50	0	1	3.75
−4.572	0.164	−0.255	0.124	62	0	1	5.72
−4.572	0.164	0.255	0.124	48	1	1	3.17
−4.572	0.164	−0.255	0.124	60.5	1	1	5.22

The coordinates from columns 5 and 8 can be copied and pasted into SigmaPlot and then split and rearranged to form the following spreadsheet of line coordinates.

Line 1 – X	Line 1 – Y	Line 2 – X	Line 2 – Y	Line 3 – X	Line 3 – Y	Line 4 – X	Line 4 – Y
50.0	3.63	49.0	3.21	50.0	3.75	48.0	3.17
62.0	5.60	58.5	4.77	62.0	5.72	60.5	5.22

The SigmaPlot commands shown in Box 6.9 but with 'multiple straight lines' selected under Graph Styles can be used to draw the four regression lines as shown in Figure 6.5. Plotting the lines is a useful method to indicate the size of the differences in weight between the four groups.

Including multi-level categorical variables

The previous model includes categorical variables with only two levels, that is binary explanatory variables. A categorical explanatory variable with three or more levels can also be included in a regression model but first needs to be transformed into a series of binary variables. Simply adding a variable with three or more levels would produce a regression coefficient that indicates the effect for each level of the variable. If the effects for each level are unequal, the regression assumption that there is an equal (linear) effect across each level of the variable will be violated. Thus, multi-level categorical variables can only be used when there is a linearity of effect over the categories. This assumption of linearity is not required for ANOVA.

When there are different effects across three or more levels of a variable, the problem of non-linearity can be resolved by creating dummy variables, which are also called indicator variables. It is not possible to include a dummy variable for each level of the variable because the dummy variables would

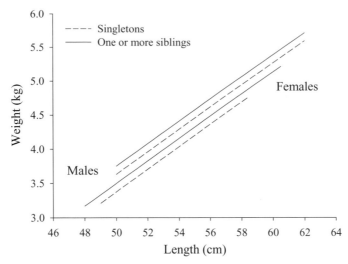

Figure 6.5 Regression lines by gender and parity status for predicting weight at 1 month of age in term babies.

lack independence and create collinearity. Therefore for k levels of a variable, there will be $k - 1$ dummy variables, for example for a variable with three levels two dummy variables will be created. It is helpful in interpreting the results if each dummy variable has a binary coding of 0 or 1.

The variable parity1 with three levels from Chapter 5, that is parity coded as babies with 0, 1 or 2 or more siblings, can be re-coded into dummy variables using *Transform → Recode → Into Different Variables.*

parityd1:   Old Value = 1 → New Value = copy old value (1 sibling);
*   Old Value: All other values → New Value = 0*
parityd2:   Old Value = 2 → New Value = 1 (2 or more siblings)
*   Old Value: All other values → New Value = 0*

Clearly a dummy variable for singletons is not required because if the values of parityd1 and parityd2 are both coded 0, the case is singleton. Dummy variables are invaluable for testing the effects of ordered groups that are likely to be different, for example lung function in groups of non-smokers, ex-smokers and current smokers. It is essential that dummy variables are used when groups are non-ordered, for example when marital status is categorised as single, married or divorced.

Using the SPSS commands shown in Box 6.8, length and gender2 can be added into the model as independent variables into Block 1 of 1 and the dummy variables parityd1 and parityd2 added in Block 2 of 2. Related dummy variables must always be included in a model together because they cannot be treated independently. If one dummy variable is significant in the model and a related dummy variable is not, they must both be left in the model together.

Regression

Model Summary

Model	R	R square	Adjusted R square	Std. error of the estimate
1	0.741[a]	0.549	0.548	0.40474
2	0.748[b]	0.559	0.556	0.40109

[a] Predictors: (constant), gender recoded, length (cm).
[b] Predictors: (constant), gender recoded, length (cm) dummy variable – parity = 1, dummy variable – parity >=2.

Coefficients[a]

Model		Unstandardised coefficients		Standardised coefficients		
		B	Std. error	Beta	t	Sig.
1	(Constant)	−4.563	0.412		−11.074	0.000
	Length (cm)	0.165	0.007	0.660	22.259	0.000
	Gender recoded	−0.251	0.036	−0.209	−7.039	0.000
2	(Constant)	−4.557	0.409		−11.144	0.000
	Length (cm)	0.164	0.007	0.654	22.182	0.000
	Gender recoded	−0.255	0.035	−0.212	−7.216	0.000
	Dummy variable – parity = 1	0.111	0.042	0.088	2.678	0.008
	Dummy variable – parity >= 2	0.138	0.043	0.108	3.249	0.001

[a] Dependent variable: weight (kg).

Excluded Variables[b]

Model		Beta In	t	Sig.	Partial correlation	Collinearity statistics Tolerance
1	Dummy variable – parity = 1	0.034[a]	1.188	0.236	0.051	0.999
	Dummy variable – parity >= 2	0.063[a]	2.183	0.029	0.093	0.994

[a] Predictors in the model: (constant), gender re-coded, length (cm).
[b] Dependent variable: weight (kg).

In the Model Summary table, the adjusted R square value shows that the addition of the dummy variables for parity improves the fit of the model only slightly from 0.548 to 0.556, that is by 0.8%. In the Coefficients table, the P values for the unstandardised coefficients show that both dummy variables are significant predictors of weight with P values of 0.008 and 0.001 respectively. However, the low standardised coefficients and the small partial correlations in the Excluded Variables table show that the dummy variables contribute little to the model compared to length and gender.

The regression equation shown in the Coefficients table is now as follows:

$$\text{Weight} = -4.557 + (0.164 \times \text{Length}) - (0.255 \times \text{Gender})$$
$$+(0.111 \times \text{Parityd1}) + (0.138 \times \text{Parityd2})$$

Because of the binary coding used, the final two terms in the model are rendered zero for singletons because both dummy variables are coded zero. The coefficients for the final two terms indicate that after adjusting for length and gender, babies with one sibling are on average 0.111 kg heavier than singletons, and babies with two or more siblings are on average 0.138 kg heavier than singletons.

Multiple linear regression with two continuous variables and two categorical variables

Any combination of continuous and categorical explanatory variables can be included in a multiple linear regression model. The previous regression model with one continuous and two categorical variables, that is length, gender and parity, can be further extended with the addition of second continuous explanatory variable, that is head circumference.

Research question

Using the file **weights.sav**, the research question can be extended to examine whether head circumference contributes to the prediction of weight in 1 month old babies after adjusting for length, gender and parity. The final predictive equation could be used to generate normal values for term babies, to calculate z scores for babies' weights, or to calculate per cent predicted weights.

The regression model obtained previously can be built on to test the influence of the variable, head circumference. The model in which parity2 was included as a binary variable is used because including parity with three levels coded as dummy variables did not substantially improve the fit of the model. Using the SPSS commands shown in Box 6.8, length, gender2 and parity2 can be added in Block 1 of 1and head circumference in Block 2 of 2 to generate the following output.

Regression

Model Summary

Model	R	R square	Adjusted R square	Std. error of the estimate
1	0.747[a]	0.559	0.556	0.40088
2	0.772[b]	0.596	0.593	0.38406

[a] Predictors: (constant), parity re-coded, gender re-coded, length (cm).
[b] Predictors: (constant), parity re-coded, gender re-coded, length (cm), head circumference (cm).

Coefficients[a]

Model		Unstandardised coefficients		Standardised coefficients		
		B	Std. error	Beta	t	Sig.
1	(Constant)	−4.572	0.408		−11.203	0.000
	Length (cm)	0.164	0.007	0.655	22.262	0.000
	Gender re-coded	−0.255	0.035	−0.212	−7.200	0.000
	Parity re-coded (binary)	0.124	0.036	0.097	3.405	0.001
2	(Constant)	−6.890	0.511		−13.496	0.000
	Length (cm)	0.130	0.009	0.520	15.243	0.000
	Gender re-coded	−0.196	0.035	−0.163	−5.624	0.000
	Parity re-coded (binary)	0.093	0.035	0.073	2.638	0.009
	Head circumference (cm)	0.110	0.016	0.249	7.061	0.000

[a] Dependent variable: weight (kg).

Excluded Variables[b]

Model		Beta In	t	Sig.	Partial correlation	Collinearity statistics Tolerance
1	Head circumference (cm)	0.249[a]	7.061	0.000	0.290	0.598

[a] Predictors in the model: (constant), parity re-coded (binary), gender re-coded, length (cm).
[b] Dependent variable: weight (kg).

The Model Summary table shows that the adjusted R square increases slightly from 55.6% to 59.3% with the addition of head circumference. In the Coefficients table, all predictors are significant and the standardised co-efficients show that length contributes to the model to a greater degree than head circumference, but that head circumference makes a larger contribution than gender or parity. However, the tolerance statistic in the Excluded Variables has fallen to 0.598 indicating some collinearity in the model. This is expected because the initial Pearson's correlations showed a significant association between length and head circumference with an r value of 0.598. As a result of the collinearity, the standard error for length has inflated from 0.007 in Model 1 to 0.009 in Model 2, a 29% increase. The benefit of explaining an extra 3.7% of the variation in length has to be balanced with this loss of precision.

Deciding which variables to include in a model can be difficult. Head circumference is expected to vary with length as a result of common factors that influence body size and growth. In this situation, head circumference should be classified as an alternative outcome rather than an independent explanatory variable because it is on the same developmental pathway as length.

Each model building situation will be different but it is important that the relationships between the variables and the purpose of building the model are always carefully considered.

Interactions

An interaction occurs when there is a multiplicative rather than additive relationship between two variables. An additive effect of a binary variable was shown in Figure 6.4 where the lines for each gender had the same slopes so that they were parallel. If an interactive effect is present, the two lines would have different slopes and would cross over or intersect at some point[9].

Again, coding of binary variables as 0 and 1 is helpful for interpreting interactions. In the following equation, which shows an interaction between length and gender, the third and fourth terms in the model will be zero when gender is coded 0. When gender is coded as 1, the third term will add a fixed amount to the prediction of the outcome variable and the fourth interactive term will add an amount that increases as length increases thereby causing the regression lines for each gender to increasingly diverge.

$$\text{Weight} = a + (b_1 \times \text{Length}) + (b_2 \times \text{Gender}) + (b_3 \times \text{Length} \times \text{Gender})$$

It is preferable to explore evidence that an interaction is present rather than testing for all possible interactions in the model. Testing for all interactions will almost certainly throw up some spurious but significant P values[10]. Interactions naturally introduce collinearity into the model because the interaction term correlates with both of its derivatives. This will result in an unstable model, especially when the sample size is small.

Interactions between variables can be identified by plotting the dependent variable against the explanatory variable for each group within a factor. The regression plots can then be inspected to assess whether there is a different linear relationship across the groups. To obtain the plots shown in Figure 6.6, the SPSS commands shown in Box 6.7 can be used with gender2 highlighted and dragged into the *Panel Variables* box and accepted for conversion to a categorical variable. Prediction lines are not requested.

The regression equations shown in Figure 6.6 indicate that the y intercept is different for males and females as expected from the former regression equations. When they values of the data points are a long way from zero, as in these plots, the intercept has no meaningful interpretation although they can indicate that the slopes are different. However, the slope of the line through the points is similar at 0.19 for males and 0.13 for females. This similarity of slopes suggests that there is no important interaction between length and gender in predicting weight. The graphs can be repeated to investigate a possible interaction between head circumference and gender.

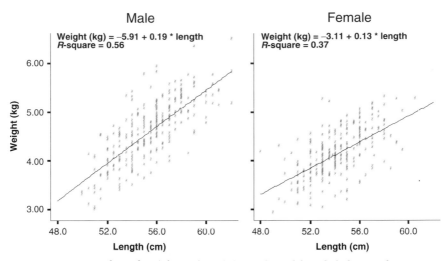

Figure 6.6 Scatter plots of weight on length for male and female babies with regression line.

The plots in Figure 6.7 show that the intercept is different between the genders at −6.75 for males and −3.22 for females. Moreover, the slope of 0.30 for males is 50% higher than the slope of 0.20 for females as shown by the different slopes of the regression lines through the plots. If plotted on the same figure, the two regression lines would intersect at some point indicating an interaction between head circumference and gender. The interaction term can be computed for inclusion in the model as shown in Box 6.10.

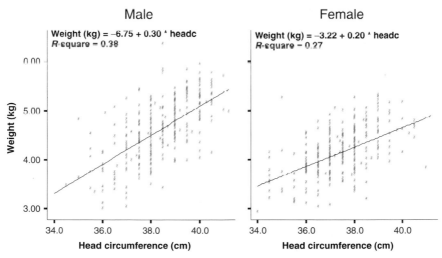

Figure 6.7 Scatter plots of weight on head circumference for male and female babies with regression line.

> **Box 6.10** SPSS command to compute an interaction term
>
> *SPSS Commands*
> *weights – SPSS Data Editor*
> *   Transform → Compute*
> *Compute Variable*
> *   Target Variable = headxgen*
> *   Numeric Expression = Head circumference * Gender recoded*
> *   Click OK*

In practice, head circumference would be omitted from the model because of its collinearity with length but it is included in this model solely for demonstrating the effect of an interaction term. The model is obtained using the commands shown in Box 6.8 and by adding length, gender2, parity2 and head circumference into Block 1 of 1 and the interaction term headxgen into Block 2 of 2.

Regression

Model Summary

Model	R	R square	Adjusted R square	Std. error of the estimate
1	0.772[a]	0.596	0.593	0.38406
2	0.775[b]	0.601	0.597	0.38211

[a] Predictors: (constant), head circumference (cm), parity re-coded (binary), gender re-coded, length (cm).
[b] Predictors: (constant), head circumference (cm), parity re-coded (binary), gender re-coded, length (cm), head by gender interaction.

Coefficients[a]

Model		Unstandardised coefficients		Standardised coefficients		
		B	Std. error	Beta	t	Sig.
1	(Constant)	−6.890	0.511		−13.496	0.000
	Length (cm)	0.130	0.009	0.520	15.243	0.000
	Gender re-coded	−0.196	0.035	−0.163	−5.624	0.000
	Parity re-coded (binary)	0.093	0.035	0.073	2.638	0.009
	Head circumference (cm)	0.110	0.016	0.249	7.061	0.000
2	(Constant)	−8.086	0.689		−11.731	0.000
	Length (cm)	0.128	0.009	0.512	15.034	0.000
	Gender re-coded	2.282	0.966	1.898	2.362	0.019
	Parity re-coded (binary)	0.093	0.035	0.073	2.651	0.008
	Head circumference (cm)	0.144	0.020	0.326	7.063	0.000
	Head by gender interaction	−0.065	0.025	−2.040	−2.567	0.011

[a] Dependent variable: weight (kg).

Excluded Variables[b]

Model		Beta In	t	Sig.	Partial correlation	Collinearity statistics Tolerance
1	Head by gender interaction	−2.040[a]	−2.567	0.011	−0.109	0.001

[a] Predictors in the model: (constant), head circumference (cm), parity re-coded (binary), gender re-coded, length (cm).
[b] Dependent variable: weight (kg).

The Model Summary table shows that the interaction term only slightly improves the fit of the model by increasing the adjusted R square from 0.593 to 0.597. In the Coefficients table, the interaction term in Model 2 is significant with a P value of 0.011 and therefore must be included because it helps to describe the true relationship between weight, head circumference and gender. If an interaction term is included then both derivative variables, that is head circumference and gender, must be retained in the model regardless of their statistical significance. Once an interaction is present, the coefficients for the derivative variables have no interpretation except that they form an integral part of the mathematical equation.

The Coefficients table shows that inclusion of the interaction term inflates the standard error for head circumference from 0.016 in Model 1 to 0.02 in Model 2 and significantly inflates the standard error for gender from 0.035 to 0.966. These standard errors have inflated as a result of the collinearity with the interaction term and, as a result, the tolerance value in the Excluded Variables table is very low and unacceptable at 0.001, also a sign of collinearity. This example highlights the trade off between building a stable predictive model and deriving an equation that describes an interaction between variables. Collinearity caused by interactions can be removed by a technique called centreing[7], which is described later in this chapter but is rarely used in the literature.

Model of best fit

The final model with all variables and the interaction term included could be considered to be over-fitted. By including variables that explain little additional variation and by including the interaction term, the model not only becomes complex but the precision around the estimates is sacrificed and the regression assumptions of independence are violated. Head circumference should be omitted because of its relation with length and because it explains only a small additional amount of variation in weight. Thus the interaction term is also omitted. The final model with only length, gender and parity is parsimonious. Once the final model is reached, the remaining regression assumptions should be confirmed.

Residuals

The residuals are the distances between each data point and the value predicted by the regression equation, that is the variation about the regression line shown in Figure 6.2. The residual distances are converted to standardised residuals that are in units of standard deviations from the regression. Standardised residuals are assumed to be normal or approximately normally distributed with a mean of zero and a standard deviation of 1.

Given the characteristics of a normal distribution, it is expected that 5% of standardised residuals will be outside the area that lies between −1.96 and +1.96 standard deviations from the mean (see Figure 2.2). In addition, 1% of standardised residuals are expected to be outside the area that lies between −3 and +3 standard deviations from the mean.

As the sample size increases, there will be an increasing number of potential outliers. In this sample size of 550 babies, it is expected that 5 children will have a standardised residual that will be outside the area that lies between −3 and +3 standard deviations from the mean.

An assumption of regression is that the residuals are normally distributed. The residual for each case can be saved to a data column using the *Save* option and the plots of the residuals can be obtained while running the model as shown in Box 6.11. The normality of the residuals can then be inspected using *Analyze → Descriptive Statistics → Explore* as discussed in Chapter 2.

Box 6.11 SPSS commands to test the regression assumptions

SPSS Commands
weights – SPSS Data Editor
    Analyze → Regression → Linear
Linear Regression
    Highlight Weight, click into the Dependent box
    Highlight Length, Gender recoded, Parity recoded (binary), click into
      the Independent(s) box
    Click on Statistics
Linear Regression: Statistics
    Under Regression Coefficients, tick Estimates (default)
    Tick Model fit (default) and Collinearity diagnostics
    Under Residuals, tick Casewise diagnostics – Outliers outside 3 standard
      deviations (default), click Continue
Linear Regression
    Click Plots
Linear Regression: Plots
    Under Scatter 1 of 1, highlight *ZPRED and click into X; highlight
      *ZRESID and click into Y
    Under Standardized Residual Plots, tick Histogram and Normal
      probability plot
    Click Continue

Linear Regression
        Click on Save
Linear Regression: Save
        Under Predicted Values, tick Standardized
        Under Residuals, tick Standardized
        Under Distances, tick Mahalanobis, Cook's and Leverage values
        Click Continue
Linear Regression
        Click OK

Regression

Coefficients[a]

Model		B	Std. error	Beta	t	Sig.	Tolerance	VIF
		Unstandardised coefficients		Standardised coefficients			Collinearity statistics	
1	(Constant)	−4.572	0.408		−11.203	0.000		
	Length (cm)	0.164	0.007	0.655	22.262	0.000	0.933	1.071
	Gender re-coded	−0.255	0.035	−0.212	−7.200	0.000	0.935	1.069
	Parity re-coded	0.124	0.036	0.097	3.405	0.001	0.997	1.003

[a] Dependent variable: weight (kg).

Casewise diagnostics[a]

Case number	Std. residual	Weight (kg)	Predicted value	Residual
243	3.122	5.23	3.9783	1.2517

[a] Dependent variable: weight (kg).

Residual Statistics[a]

	Minimum	Maximum	Mean	Std. deviation	N
Predicted value	3.1594	5.7069	4.3664	0.44985	550
Std. predicted value	−2.683	2.980	0.000	1.000	550
Standard error of predicted value	0.02687	0.06017	0.03365	0.00604	550
Adjusted predicted value	3.1413	5.7047	4.3665	0.44988	550
Residual	−1.0791	1.2517	0.0000	0.39978	550
Std. residual	−2.692	3.122	0.000	0.997	550
Stud. residual	−2.706	3.130	0.000	1.001	550
Deleted residual	−1.0904	1.2581	−0.0001	0.40276	550
Stud. deleted residual	−2.722	3.156	0.000	1.003	550
Mahal. distance	1.469	11.372	2.995	1.529	550
Cook's distance	0.000	0.028	0.002	0.003	550
Centred leverage value	0.003	0.021	0.005	0.003	550

[a] Dependent variable: weight (kg).

The Coefficients table shows the variables in the model and the high tolerance values confirm their lack of collinearity. The Casewise Diagnostics table
shows the cases that are more than three standard deviations from the regression line. There is only one case that has a standardised residual that is more
than three standard deviations from the regression, that is case number 243
which is a baby with a weight of 5.23 kg compared with a predicted value of
3.9783 kg and with a standardised residual of 3.122.

The Residuals Statistics table shows the minimum and maximum predicted
values. The predicted values range from 3.159 to 5.707 kg and the unstandardised residuals range from 1.079 kg below the regression line to 1.252 kg
above the regression line. This is the minimum and maximum distances of
babies from the equation, which is the variation about the regression.

The standardised predicted values and standardised residuals shown in the
Residuals Statistics table are expressed in units of their standard deviation and
have a mean of zero and a standard deviation of approximately or equal to 1,
as expected when they are normally distributed.

The histogram and normal P–P plot shown in Figure 6.8 indicate that the
distribution of the residuals deviates only slightly from a classically bell shaped
distribution.

The variance around the residuals can also be used to test whether the model
violates the assumption of homoscedasticity, that is equal variance over the
length of the regression model. Residual plots are a good method for examining
the spread of variance. The scatter plot in Figure 6.8 shows that there is an
equal spread of residuals across the predicted values indicating that the model
is homoscedastic.

Outliers and remote points

Outliers are data points that are more than three standard deviations from
the regression line. Outliers in regression are identified in a similar manner
to outliers in ANOVA. Univariate outliers should be identified before fitting
a model but multivariate outliers, if present, are identified once the model
of best fit is obtained. Outliers that cause a poor fit degrade the predictive
value of the regression model; however, this has to be balanced with loss of
generalisability if the points are omitted.

Multivariate outliers are data values that have an extreme value on a combination of explanatory variables and exert too much leverage and/or discrepancy (see Figure 5.10 in Chapter 5). Data points with high leverage and low
discrepancy have no effect on the regression line but tend to increase the R
square value and reduce the standard errors. On the other hand, data points
with low leverage and high discrepancy tend to influence the intercept but
not the slope of the regression or the R square value and tend to inflate the
standard errors. Data points with both a high leverage and a high discrepancy
influence the slope, the intercept and the R square value. Thus, a model that

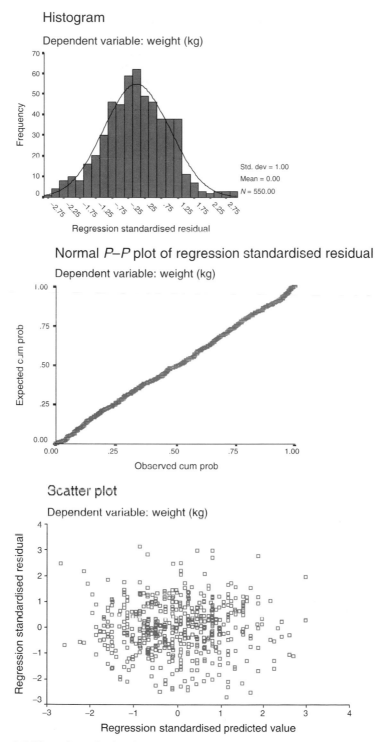

Figure 6.8 Plots of standardised residuals for regression on weight.

contains problematic data points with high leverage and/or high discrepancy values may not generalise well to the population.

Multivariate outliers can be identified using Cook's distances and leverage values as discussed in Chapter 5. The Residuals Statistics table shows that the largest Cook's distance is 0.028, which is below the critical value of 1, and the largest leverage value is 0.021, which is below the critical value of 0.05 indicating that there are no influential outliers in this model. In regression, Mahalanobis distances can also be inspected. Mahalanobis distances are evaluated using critical values of chi-square with degrees of freedom equal to the number of explanatory variables in the model. To adjust for the number of variables being tested, Mahalanobis distances are usually considered unacceptable at the $P < 0.001$ level, although the influence of any values with $P < 0.05$ should be examined.

To plot the Mahalanobis distances, which have been saved to a column at the end of the data sheet, the commands Graphs → Histogram can be used to obtain Figure 6.9. Any Mahalanobis distance that is greater than 16.266, that is a chi-square value for $P < 0.001$ with three degrees of freedom (because there are three explanatory variables in the model), would be problematic. The graph shows that no Mahalanobis distances are larger than this. This is confirmed in the Residual Statistics table, which shows that the maximum Mahalanobis distance is 11.372.

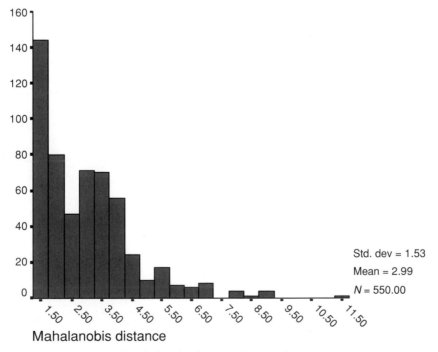

Figure 6.9 Histogram of Mahalanobis distances for weight.

If multivariate outliers are detected they can be deleted but it is not reasonable to remove troublesome data points simply to improve the fit of the model. In addition, when one extreme data point is removed another may take its place so it is important to recheck the data after deletion to ensure that there are no further multivariate outliers. Alternatively, the data can be transformed to reduce the influence of the multivariate outlier or the extreme data point can be re-coded to a less extreme value. However, a multivariate outlier depends on a combination of explanatory variables and therefore the scores would have to be adjusted for each variable. Any technique that is used to deal with multivariate outliers should be recorded in the study handbook and described in any publications.

Validating the model

If the sample size is large enough, the model can be built using one-half of the data and then validated with the other half. If this is the purpose, the sample should be split randomly. Other selections of 60% to 80% for building the model and 40% to 20% for validation can be used. A model built using one part of the data and validated using the other part of the data provides good evidence of stability and reliability. However, both models must have an adequate sample size and must conform to the assumptions for regression to minimise collinearity and maximise precision and stability.

Non-linear regression

If scatter plots suggest that there is a curved relationship between the explanatory and outcome variables, then a linear model may not be the best fit. Other non-linear models that may be more appropriate for describing the relationship can be examined using the SPSS commands shown in Box 6.12. Logarithmic, quadratic and exponential fits are the most common transformations

---

Box 6.12 SPSS commands for examining the equation that best fits the data

SPSS Commands
weights – SPSS Data Editor
    Analyze → Regression → Curve Estimation
Curve Estimation
    Highlight Weight, click into Dependent(s) box
    Highlight Length, click into Independent Variable box
    Under Models, tick Linear (default), Logarithmic, Quadratic
        and Exponential
    Click OK

used in medical research when data are skewed or when a relationship is not linear.

Curve fit

```
Independent:    LENGTH

  Dependent  Mth   Rsq   d.f.        F  Sigf        b0       b1      b2

    WEIGHT   LIN  .509    548   567.04  .000   -5.4121    .1783
    WEIGHT   LOG  .508    548   566.40  .000  -34.875   9.8019
    WEIGHT   QUA  .509    547   283.03  .000   -6.6256    .2224  -.0004
    WEIGHT   EXP  .503    548   555.23  .000     .4578    .0409
```

In the Curve Fit table, b0 is the intercept which is the coefficient labelled 'a' in previous models. The equations of the models are as follows:

$$\text{Linear:} \quad \text{Weight} = b_0 + (b_1 \times \text{Length})$$
$$\text{Logarithmic:} \quad \text{Weight} = b_0 + (b_1 \times \log_e \text{Length})$$
$$\text{Quadratic:} \quad \text{Weight} = b_0 + (b_1 \times \text{Length}) + (b_2 \times \text{Length}^2)$$
$$\text{Exponential:} \quad \text{Weight} = b_0 + (b_1 \times e^{\text{length}})$$

The R square values, denoted as Rsq in the Curve Fit table, show that the linear and the quadratic models have the best fit with R square values of 0.509 closely followed by the logarithmic model with an R square of 0.508. The plots in Figure 6.10 show that the curves for the four models only deviate at the extremities of the data points, which are the regions in which prediction

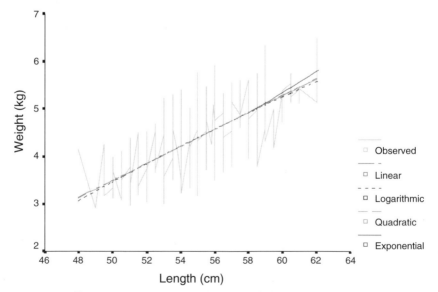

Figure 6.10 Different curve estimates of weight on length.

is less certain. Because the linear model is easier to communicate, in practice it would be the preferable model to use.

If it was important to use the quadratic model, say to compare with other quadratic models in the literature, then the square of length can be computed as lensq in the menu *Transform → Compute* using the formula lensq = length × length. The quadratic equation can be obtained using the commands shown in Box 6.8, with length added as independent variable into Block 1 of 1 and the square of length (lensq) into Block 2 of 2.

Model Summary

Model	R	R square	Adjusted R square	Std. error of the estimate
1	0.713[a]	0.509	0.508	0.42229
2	0.713[b]	0.509	0.507	0.42266

[a] Predictors: (constant), length (cm).
[b] Predictors: (constant), length (cm), length squared.

Coefficients[a]

Model		Unstandardised coefficients		Standardised coefficients		
		B	Std. error	Beta	t	Sig.
1	(Constant)	−5.412	0.411		−13.167	0.000
	Length (cm)	0.178	0.007	0.713	23.813	0.000
2	(Constant)	−6.626	7.053		−0.939	0.348
	Length (cm)	0.222	0.256	0.890	0.868	0.386
	Length squared	0.000	0.002	−0.177	−0.172	0.863

[b] Dependent variable: weight (kg).

Excluded Variables[b]

Model		Beta In	t	Sig.	Partial correlation	Collinearity statistics Tolerance
1	Length squared	−0.177[a]	−0.172	0.863	−0.007	0.001

[a] Predictors in the model: (constant), length (cm).
[b] Dependent variable: weight (kg).

The Model Summary and Coefficients tables show that the R square and the regression coefficients are as indicated in the curve fit procedure. However, the standard error for length has increased from 0.007 in Model 1 to 0.256 in Model 2. In addition, length is no longer significant in Model 2 and the Excluded Variables table shows that tolerance is very low at 0.001 indicating that the explanatory variables are highly related to one other.

Collinearity can occur naturally when a quadratic term is included in a regression equation because the variable and its square are related. A scatter plot using the SPSS commands *Graphs → Scatter → Simple* to plot length squared against length demonstrates the direct relationship between the two variables as shown in Figure 6.11.

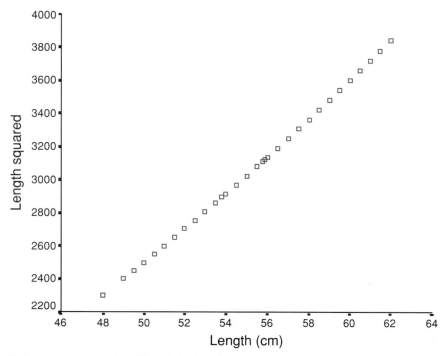

Figure 6.11 Scatter plot of length by length squared.

Centreing

To avoid collinearity in quadratic equations, a simple mathematical trick of centreing, that is subtracting a constant from the data values, can be applied[11]. The constant that minimises collinearity most effectively is the mean value of the variable. Using *Descriptive Statistics → Descriptives* in SPSS indicates that the mean of length is 54.841 cm. Using the commands *Transform → Compute* the mean value is used to compute a new variable for length centred (lencent) as length – 54.841 and then to compute another new variable which is the square of lencent (lencntsq).

A scatter plot of length centred and its square in Figure 6.12 shows that the relationship is no longer linear simply because subtracting the mean value gives half of the values a negative value but then squaring all values returns a positive value again. The relation is thus U-shaped and no longer linear.

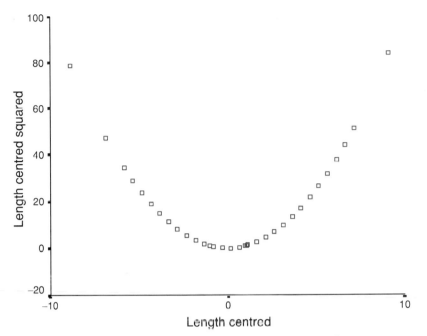

Figure 6.12 Scatter plot of length squared by length centred squared.

The regression can now be re-run using the commands shown in Box 6.8 but with length centred in Block 1 of 1 and its square in Block 2 of 2.

Model Summary

Model	R	R square	Adjusted R square	Std. error of the estimate
1	0.713[a]	0.509	0.508	0.42229
2	0.713[b]	0.509	0.507	0.42266

[a] Predictors: (constant), length centred.
[b] Predictors: (constant), length centred, length centred squared.

Coefficients[a]

Model		Unstandardised coefficients		Standardised coefficients	t	Sig.
		B	Std. error	Beta		
1	(Constant)	4.366	0.018		242.494	0.000
	Length centred	0.178	0.007	0.713	23.813	0.000
2	(Constant)	4.369	0.022		194.357	0.000
	Length centred	0.179	0.008	0.714	23.499	0.000
	Length centred squared	0.000	0.002	−0.005	0.172	0.863

[a] Dependent variable: weight (kg).

Excluded Variables[b]

Model		Beta In	t	Sig.	Partial correlation	Collinearity statistics Tolerance
1	Length centred squared	−0.005[a]	−0.172	0.863	−0.007	0.973

[a] Predictors in the model: (constant), length centred.
[b] Dependent variable: weight (kg).

The Model Summary table shows that when length is centred, the R square value remains unchanged and the Coefficients table shows the standard error for length is similar at 0.007 in Model 1 and 0.008 in Model 2. In addition, the unstandardised coefficients are now significant and the tolerance value is high at 0.973. The unstandardised coefficient for the square term is close to zero with a non-significant P value indicating its negligible contribution to the model. The equation for this regression model is as follows:

$$\text{Weight} = 4.369 + (0.179 \times (\text{Length} - 54.841)) + (0.0001 \times (\text{Length} - 54.841)^2)$$

This centred model is a more stable quadratic model than the model given by the curve fit option and is therefore more reliable for predicting weight or for testing the effects of other factors on weight.

The technique of centreing can also be used to remove collinearity caused by interactions which are naturally related to their derivatives[7].

Notes for critical appraisal

Box 6.13 shows the questions that should be asked when critically appraising a paper that reports linear or multiple regression analyses.

Box 6.13 Questions to ask when critically appraising a regression analysis

The following questions should be asked when appraising published results from analyses in which regression has been used:
- Was the sample size large enough to justify using the model?
- Are the axes the correct way around with the outcome on the y-axis and the explanatory variable on the x-axis?
- Were any repeated measures from the same participants treated as independent observations?
- Were all of the explanatory variables measured independently from the outcome variable?
- Have the explanatory variables been measured reliably?

- Is there any collinearity between the explanatory variables that could reduce the precision of the model?
- Are there any multivariate outliers that could influence the regression estimates?
- Is evidence presented that the residuals are normally distributed?
- Are there sufficient data at the extremities of the regression or should the prediction range be shortened?

References

1. Simpson J, Berry G. Simple regression and correlation. In: Handbook of public health methods, Kerr C, Taylor R, Heard G (editors). Roseville, Australia: McGraw-Hill Companies Inc, 1998: pp 288–295.
2. Kachigan, SK. Multivariate statistical analysis (2nd edition). New York: Radius Press, 1991; pp 172–174.
3. Altman DG. Reference intervals. In: Practical statistics for medical research, London, pp 419–423.
4. Stevens J. Applied multivariate statistics for the social sciences (3rd edition). Boston, USA: Lawrence Erlbaum Associates 1996; pp 101–103.
5. Tabachnick BG, Fidell LS. Using multivariate statistics (4th edition). Boston, MA: Allyn and Bacon, 2001; pp 131–138.
6. Dupont WD, Plummer WD. Power and sample size calculations for studies involving linear regression. Control Clin Trials 1998; 19:589–601.
7. Tabachnick BG, Fidell LS. Testing hypotheses in multiple regression. In: Using multivariate statistics. Boston, USA: Allyn and Bacon, 2001; pp 136–159.
8. Van Steen K, Curran D, Kramer J, Molenberghs G, Van Vreckem A, Bottomley A, Sylvester R. Multicollinearity in prognostic factor analyses using the EORTC QLQ-C30: identification and impact on model selection. Stat Med 2002; 21:3865–3884.
9. Peat JK, Mellis CM, Williams K, Xuan W. Confounders and effect modifiers. In: Health science research. A handbook of quantitative methods. Crows Nest: Allen and Unwin, 2001; pp 90–104.
10. Altman DG, Matthews JNS. Interaction 1: heterogeneity of effects. BMJ 1996; 313:486.
11. Kleinbaum DG, Kupper LL, Muller KE, Nizam A. Applied regression analysis and other multivariable methods. Pacific Grove, California: Duxbury Press, 1998; pp 237–245.

CHAPTER 7

Categorical variables: rates and proportions

When the methods of statistical inference were being developed in the first half of the twentieth century, calculations were done using pencil, paper, tables, slide rules and with luck a very expensive adding machine[1].

MARTIN BLAND STATISTICIAN

Objectives

The objectives of this chapter are to explain how to:
- use the correct summary statistics for rates and proportions
- present categorical baseline characteristics correctly
- crosstabulate categorical variables and obtain meaningful percentages
- choose the correct chi-square value
- plot percentages and interpret 95% confidence intervals
- manage cells with small numbers
- use trend tests for ordered exposure variables
- convert continuous variables with a non-normal distribution into categorical variables
- calculate the number needed to treat
- calculate significance and estimate effect size for paired categorical data
- critically appraise the literature in which rates and proportions are reported

---

Categorical variables are summarised using statistics called rates and proportions. A rate is a number used to express the frequency of a characteristic of interest in the population, such as 1 case per 10 000. In some cases, the rate is applied to a time period such as per annum. Frequencies can also be described using summary statistics such as a percentage e.g. 20% or a proportion e.g. 0.2. Rates, percentages and proportions are frequently used for summarising information that is collected with tick box options on questionnaires.

Obtaining information about the distribution of the categorical variables in a study provides a good working knowledge of the characteristics of the sample. The spreadsheet **surgery.sav** contains data from a sample of 141 consecutive babies who were admitted to hospital to undergo surgery. The SPSS commands shown in Box 7.1 can be used to obtain frequencies and histograms for the categorical variables prematurity (1 = Premature; 2 = Term) and gender2 (1 = Male and 2 = Female). The frequencies for place of birth were obtained in Chapter 1.

> **Box 7.1** SPSS commands to obtain frequencies and histograms
>
> **SPSS Commands**
> *surgery – SPSS Data Editor*
> *Analyze → Descriptive Statistics → Frequencies*
> *Frequencies*
> *Highlight Prematurity and Gender recoded, click into Variable(s) box*
> *Click on Charts*
> *Frequencies: Charts*
> *Chart Type: Tick Bar charts, Click Continue*
> *Frequencies*
> *Click Ok*

Frequency Table

Prematurity

		Frequency	Per cent	Valid per cent	Cumulative per cent
Valid	Premature	45	31.9	31.9	31.9
	Term	96	68.1	68.1	100.0
	Total	141	100.0	100.0	

Gender Recoded

		Frequency	Per cent	Valid per cent	Cumulative per cent
Valid	Male	82	58.2	58.2	58.2
	Female	59	41.8	41.8	100.0
	Total	141	100.0	100.0	

The valid per cent column in the first Frequency table indicates that 31.9% of babies in the sample were born prematurely and that 68.1% of babies in the sample were term births. The per cent and valid per cent columns are identical because all children in the sample have information of their birth status, that is there are no missing data. In journal articles and scientific reports when the sample size is greater than 100, percentages such as these are reported with one decimal place only. When the sample size is less than 100, no decimal places are used. If the sample size was less than 20 participants, percentages would not be reported (Chapter 1) although SPSS includes them on the output.

The valid per cent column in the second Frequency table indicates that there are more males than females in the sample (58.2% vs 41.8%).

The bar charts shown in Figure 7.1 are helpful for comparing the frequencies visually and are often useful for a poster or a talk. However, charts are not suitable for presenting sample characteristics in journal articles or other

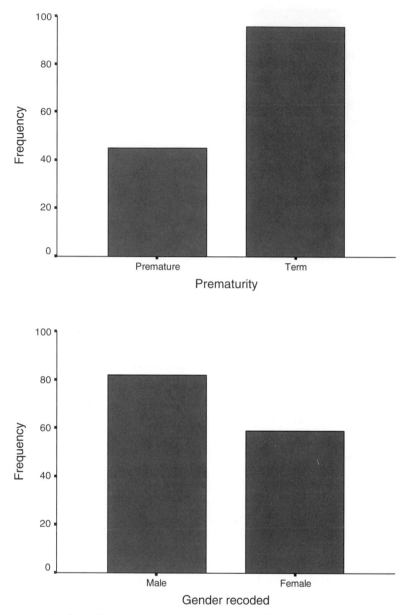

Figure 7.1 Number of babies by prematurity status and by gender.

publications because accurate frequency information cannot be read from them and they are 'space hungry' for the relatively small amount of information provided.

Baseline characteristics

The baseline characteristics of the sample could be described as shown in Table 7.1 or Table 7.2. If the percentage of male children is included, it is not necessary to report the percentage of female children because this is the complement that can be easily calculated. Similarly, it is not necessary to include percentages of both term and premature birth since one can be calculated from the other. In most cases, observed numbers are not included in addition to percentages because the numbers can be calculated from the percentages and the total number of the sample. However, some journals request that the number of cases and the sample size, e.g. 82/141, are reported in addition to percentages.

Table 7.1 Baseline characteristics

Characteristic	Per cent
Total number	*141*
Male	58.2%
Place of birth	
Local	63.8%
Regional	23.4%
Overseas	6.4%
No information	6.4%
Premature birth	31.9%

Although confidence intervals around percentage figures can be computed, these statistics are more appropriate for comparing rates in two or more different groups, as discussed later in this chapter, and not for describing the sample characteristics.

Table 7.2 Baseline characteristics

Characteristic	Sample size (N)	Per cent
Male	141	58.2%
Place of birth	132	
Local		68.2%
Regional		25.0%
Overseas		6.8%
Premature birth	141	31.9%

Describing categorical data

When describing frequencies, it is important to use the correct term. A common mistake is to describe prevalence as incidence, or vice versa, although these terms have different meanings and cannot be used interchangeably.

Incidence is a term used to describe the number of new cases with a condition divided by the population at risk. Prevalence is a term used to describe the total number of cases with a condition divided by the population at risk. The population at risk is the number of people during the specified time period who were susceptible to the condition. The prevalence of an illness in a specified period is the number of incident cases in that period plus the previous prevalent cases and minus any deaths or remissions.

Both incidence and prevalence are usually calculated for a defined time period, for example for a 1 or 5 year period. When the number of cases of a condition is measured at a specified point in time, the term point prevalence is used. The terms incidence and prevalence should only be used when the sample is selected randomly. When the sample has not been selected randomly from the population, the terms percentage, proportion, or frequency are more appropriate.

Chi-square tests

A chi-square test is used to assess whether the frequency of a condition is significantly different between two or more groups, for example groups who received different treatments or who have different exposures. Thus, chi-square tests would be used to assess whether there is a significant between-group difference in the frequency of participants with a certain condition. For example, chi-square could be used to test whether the absence or presence of an illness is independent of whether a child was or was not immunised.

The data for chi-square tests are summarised using crosstabulations as shown in Table 7.3. These tables are sometimes called frequency or contingency tables. Table 7.3 is called a 2×2 table because each variable has two levels, but tables can have larger dimensions when either the exposure or the disease has more than two levels.

Table 7.3 Crosstabulation for estimating chi-square

	Disease absent	Disease present	Total
Exposure absent	d	c	$c + d$
Exposure present	b	a	$a + b$
Total	$b + d$	$a + c$	Total

In a contingency table, one variable (usually the exposure) forms the rows and the other variable (usually the disease) forms the columns. In the above example, the exposure immunisation (no, yes) would form the rows and the illness (present, absent) would form the columns. The four internal cells of the table show the counts for each of the disease/exposure groups, for example cell '*a*' shows the number who satisfy exposure present (immunised) and disease present (illness positive).

The assumptions for using a chi-square test are shown in Box 7.2.

Box 7.2 Assumptions for using chi-square tests

The assumptions that must be met when using a chi-square test are that:
- each observation must be independent
- each participant is represented in the table once only
- 80% of the expected cell frequencies should exceed 5 and all expected cell frequencies should exceed 1

A major assumption of chi-square tests is independence, that is each participant must be represented in the analysis once only. Thus, if repeat data have been collected, for example if data have been collected from hospital inpatients and some patients have been re-admitted, a decision must be made about which data, for example, from the first admission or the last admission, are used in the analyses.

The expected frequency in each cell, which is discussed later in this chapter, is an important concept in determining *P* values and deciding the validity of a chi-square test. For each cell, a certain number of participants would be expected given the frequencies of each of the characteristics in the sample.

When a chi-square test is requested, most statistics programs provide a number of chi-square values on the output. The chi-square statistic that is conventionally used depends on both the sample size and the expected cell counts as shown in Table 7.4. However, these guidelines are quite conservative and if the result from a Fisher's exact test is available, it could be used in

Table 7.4 Type and application of chi-square tests

Statistic	Application
Pearsons' chi-square	Used when the sample size is very large, say over 1000
Continuity correction	Applied to 2 × 2 tables only and is an approximation to Pearson's for a smaller sample size, say less than 1000
Fisher's exact test	Must always be used when one or more cells in a 2 × 2 table have a small expected number of cases
Linear-by-linear	Used to test for a trend in the frequency of the outcome across an ordered exposure variable

all situations because it is a gold standard test, whereas Pearson's chi-square and the continuity correction tests are approximations. Fisher's exact test is generally printed for 2×2 tables and, depending on the program used, may also be produced for crosstabulations larger than 2×2. The linear-by-linear test is most appropriate in situations in which an ordered exposure variable has three or more categories and the outcome variable is binary.

As in all analyses, it is important to identify which variable is the outcome variable and which variable is the explanatory variable. This is important for setting up the crosstabulation table to display the percentages that are appropriate for answering the research question. This can be achieved by either:

- entering the explanatory variable in the rows, the outcome in the columns and using row percentages, or
- entering the explanatory variable in the columns, the outcome in the rows and using column percentages

A table set up in either of these ways will display the per cent of participants with the outcome of interest in each of the explanatory variable groups. In most study designs, the outcome is a disease and the explanatory variable is an exposure or an experimental group. However, in case–control studies in which cases are selected on the basis of their disease status, the disease may be treated as the explanatory variable and the exposure as the outcome variable.

Research question

The data set **surgery.sav** contains data from babies who were admitted to hospital for surgery. This sample was not selected randomly and therefore only percentages will apply and the terms incidence and prevalence cannot be used. However, chi-square tests are valid to assess whether there are any between-group differences in the proportion of babies with certain characteristics.

Question:	Are males who are admitted for surgery more likely than females to have been born prematurely?
Null hypothesis:	That the proportion of males in the premature group is equal to the proportion of females in the premature group.
Variables:	Outcome variable = prematurity (categorical, two levels)
	Explanatory variable = gender (categorical, two levels)

The command sequence to obtain a crosstabulation and chi-square test is shown in Box 7.3.

Box 7.3 SPSS commands to obtain a chi-square test

SPSS Commands
surgery – SPSS Data Editor
   Analyze → Descriptive Statistics → Crosstabs

> *Crosstabs*
> > *Highlight Gender recoded and click into Row(s)*
> > *Highlight Prematurity and click into Column(s)*
> > *Click Statistics*
> *Crosstabs: Statistics*
> > *Tick Chi-square, click Continue*
> *Crosstabs*
> > *Click Cells*
> *Crosstabs: Cell Display*
> > *Counts: tick Observed (default),*
> > *Percentages: tick Row*
> > *Click Continue*
> *Crosstabs*
> > *Click OK*

Crosstabs

Gender Re-coded * Prematurity Crosstabulation

			Prematurity		
			Premature	Term	Total
Gender re-coded	Male	Count	33	49	82
		% within gender re-coded	40.2%	59.8%	100.0%
	Female	Count	12	47	59
		% within gender re-coded	20.3%	79.7%	100.0%
Total		Count	45	96	141
		% within gender re-coded	31.9%	68.1%	100.0%

Chi-Square Tests

	Value	df	Asymp. sig. (two-sided)	Exact sig. (two-sided)	Exact sig. (one-sided)
Pearson chi-square	6.256[b]	1	0.012		
Continuity correction[a]	5.374	1	0.020		
Likelihood ratio	6.464	1	0.011		
Fisher's exact test				0.017	0.009
Linear-by-linear association	6.212	1	0.013		
N of valid cases	141				

[a] Computed only for a 2 × 2 table.
[b] 0 cell (0.0%) has expected count less than 5. The minimum expected count is 18.83.

The first Crosstabulation table shows that the two variables each have two levels to create a 2 × 2 table with four cells. The table shows that 40.2% of males in the sample were premature compared with 20.3% of females, that is the rate of prematurity in the males is almost twice that in the females.

Chi-square values are calculated from the number of observed and expected frequencies in each cell of the crosstabulation. The observed numbers are the numbers shown in each cell of the crosstabulation. The expected number for each cell is calculated as

Row total × Column total/Grand total

For cell a in Table 7.3, the expected number is $((a + b) \times (a + c))$/Total

The above formula is an estimate of how many cases would be expected in any one cell given the frequencies of the outcome and the exposure in the sample. The Pearson chi-square value is then calculated by the following summation from all cells:

$$\text{Chi-square value} = \frac{\Sigma(\text{Observed count} - \text{Expected count})^2}{\text{Expected count}}$$

The continuity corrected chi-square is calculated in a similar way but with a correction made for a smaller sample size. Obviously, if the observed and expected values are similar, then the chi-square value will be close to zero and therefore will not be significant. The more different the observed and expected values are from one another, the larger the chi-square value becomes and the more likely the P value will be significant.

In the Crosstabulation, the smallest cell has an observed count of 12. The expected number for this cell is $59 \times 45/141$, or 18.83 as shown in the footnote of the Chi-Square Tests table.

In the Chi-Square Tests table, the continuity correction chi-square of 5.374 is conventionally used because the sample size is only 141 children. This value indicates that the difference in rates of prematurity between the genders is statistically significant at $P = 0.02$. This result would be reported as 'there was a significant difference in prematurity between males and females (40.2% vs 20.3%, $P = 0.02$)'.

Confidence intervals

When between-group differences are compared, the summary percentages are best shown with 95% confidence intervals. As discussed in Chapter 3, it is useful to include the 95% confidence intervals when results are shown as figures because the degree of overlap between them provides an approximate significance of the differences between groups.

Many statistics programs do not provide confidence intervals around frequency statistics. However, 95% confidence intervals can be easily computed using an Excel spreadsheet. The standard error around a proportion is calculated as $\sqrt{[p(1 - p)/n]}$ where p is the proportion expressed as a decimal number and n is the number of cases in the group from which the proportion is calculated. The standard error around a proportion is rarely reported but is commonly converted into a 95% confidence interval which is $p \pm (SE \times 1.96)$.

An Excel spreadsheet in which the percentage is entered as its decimal equivalent in the first column and the number in the group is entered in the second column can be used to calculate confidence intervals as shown in Table 7.5.

Table 7.5 Excel spreadsheet to compute 95% confidence intervals around proportions

	Proportion	N	SE	Width	CI lower	CI upper
Male	0.402	82	0.054	0.106	0.296	0.508
Female	0.203	59	0.052	0.103	0.100	0.306

The formula for the standard error (SE) is entered into the formula bar of Excel as sqrt $(p \times (1 - p)/n)$ and the formula for the width of the confidence interval is entered as $1.96 \times SE$. This width, which is the dimension of the 95% confidence interval that is entered into SigmaPlot to draw bar charts with error bars, can then be both subtracted and added to the proportion to calculate the 95% confidence interval values shown in the last two columns of Table 7.5.

The calculations are undertaken in proportions (decimal numbers) but are easily converted back to percentages by moving the decimal point two places to the right. Using the converted values, the result could be reported as 'the percentage of male babies born prematurely was 40.2% (95% CI 29.6 to 50.8%). This was significantly higher than the percentage of female babies born prematurely which was 20.3% (95% CI 10.0 to 30.6%) ($P = 0.02$)'. The P value of 0.02 for this comparison is derived from the Chi-Square Tests table.

Creating a figure using SigmaPlot

The summary statistics from Table 7.5 can be entered into SigmaPlot by first using the commands $File \rightarrow New$ and then entering the percentages in column 1 and the width of the confidence interval, also converted to a percentage in column 2.

Column 1	Column 2
40.2	10.6
20.3	10.3

The SigmaPlot commands for plotting these summary statistics as a figure are shown in Box 7.4.

Box 7.4 SigmaPlot commands to draw simple histograms

SigmaPlot Commands
Sigmaplot – [Data 1]
        Graph → Create Graph
Create Graph - Type
        Highlight Horizontal Bar Chart, click Next
Create Graph - Style
        Highlight Simple Error Bars, click Next
Create Graph – Error Bars
        Symbol Values = Worksheet Columns (default), click Next
Create Graph – Data Format
        Highlight Single X, click Next
Create Graph – Select Data
        Data for Bar = use drop box and select Column 1
        Data for Error = use drop box and select Column 2
        Click Finish

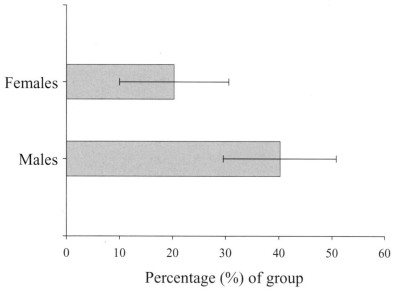

Figure 7.2 Per cent of male and female babies born prematurely.

The graph can then be customised using the options under *Graph → Properties* to produce Figure 7.2. The lack of overlap between the confidence intervals is an approximate indication of a statistically significant difference between the two groups.

2 × 3 chi-square tables

In addition to the common application of analysing 2 × 2 tables, chi-square tests can also be used for larger 2 × 3 tables in which one variable has two levels and the other variable has three levels.

Research question

Question: Are the babies born in regional centres (away from the hospital or overseas) more likely to be premature than babies born in local areas?

Null hypothesis: That the proportion of premature babies in the group born locally is not different to the proportion of premature babies in the groups born regionally or overseas.

Variables: Place of birth (categorical, three levels and) prematurity (categorical, two levels)

In this research question, there is no clear outcome or explanatory variable because both variables in the analysis are characteristics of the babies. This type of question is asked when it is important to know about the inter-relationships between variables in the data set. If prematurity has an important association with place of birth, this may need to be taken into account in multivariate analyses.

The SPSS commands shown in Box 7.3 can be used with place of birth recoded entered into the rows, prematurity entered into the columns and row percentages requested.

Crosstabs

Place of birth (re-coded) * Prematurity Crosstabulation

			Prematurity		Total
			Premature	Term	
Place of birth (re-coded)	Local	Count	29	61	90
		% within place of birth (re-coded)	32.2%	67.8%	100.0%
	Regional	Count	6	27	33
		% within place of birth (re-coded)	18.2%	81.8%	100.0%
	Overseas	Count	5	4	9
		% within place of birth (re-coded)	55.6%	44.4%	100.0%
Total		Count	40	92	132
		% within place of birth (re-coded)	30.3%	69.7%	100.0%

Chi-Square Tests

	Value	df	Asymp. sig. (two-sided)
Pearson chi-square	5.170[a]	2	0.075
Likelihood ratio	5.146	2	0.076
Linear-by-linear association	0.028	1	0.866
N of valid cases	132		

[a] 1 cell (16.7%) has expected count less than 5. The minimum expected count is 2.73.

The row percentages in the Crosstabulation table show that there is a difference in the frequency of prematurity between babies born at different locations. The per cent of babies who are premature is 32.2% from local centres, 18.2% from regional centres and 55.6% from overseas centres. This difference in percentages fails to reach significance with a Pearson's chi-square value of 5.170 and a P value of 0.075. For tables such as this that are larger than 2×2, an exact chi-square test that is used when an expected count is low has to be requested and is not a default option (see next section).

In the crosstabulation, the absolute difference in per cent of premature babies between regional and overseas centres is quite large at $55.6\% - 18.2\%$, or 37.4%. The finding of a non-significant P value in the presence of this large between-group difference could be considered a type II error as a consequence of the small sample size. In this case, the sample size is too small to demonstrate statistical significance when a large difference of 37.4% exists. If the sample size had been larger, then the P value for the same between-group difference would be significant. Conversely, the difference between the groups may have been due to chance and a larger sample size might show a smaller between-group difference.

A major problem with this analysis is the small numbers in some of the cells. There are only nine babies in the overseas group. The row percentages illustrate the problem that arises when some cells have small numbers. The five premature babies born overseas are 55.6% of their group because each baby is $1/9^{th}$ or 11.1% of the group. When a group size is small, adding or losing a single case from a cell results in a large change in frequency statistics. Because of these small group sizes, the footnote in the Chi-Square Tests table indicates that one cell in the table has an expected count less than five.

Using the formula shown previously, the expected number of premature babies referred from overseas is $9 \times 40/132$ or 2.73. This minimum expected cell count is printed in the footnote below the Chi-Square Tests table. If a table has less than five expected observations in more than 20% of cells, the assumptions for the chi-square test are not met. The warning message suggests that the P value of 0.075 is unreliable and probably an overestimate of significance.

Cells with small numbers

Small cells cannot be avoided at times, for example when a disease is rare. However, cells and groups with small numbers are a problem in all types of analyses because their summary statistics are often unstable and difficult to interpret. When calculating a chi-square statistic, most packages will give a warning message when the number of expected cases in a cell is low.

Chi-square tests may be valid when the number of observed counts in a cell is zero as long as the expected number is greater than 5 in 80% of the cells and greater than 1 in all cells. If expected numbers are less than this, then an exact chi-square based on alternative assumptions can be used. An exact chi-square can be obtained for the 3×2 table above by clicking on the *Exact* button in the bottom left hand corner of the *Crosstabs* dialogue box. The following table is obtained when the Monte Carlo method of computing the exact chi-square is requested. The Monte Carlo P value is based on a random sample of a probability distribution rather than a chi-square distribution which is an approximation. When the Monte-Carlo option is selected, the P value will vary each time the test is run on the same data set because it is based on a random sample of probabilities.

The Chi-Square Tests table shows that the asymptotic significance value of $P = 0.075$ is identical to the exact significance value obtained previously i.e. $P = 0.075$. The two-sided test should be used because the direction of effect could have been either way, that is the proportion of premature babies could have been higher or lower in any of the groups.

An alternative to using exact methods is to merge the group with small cells with another group but only if the theory is valid. Alternatively, the group can be omitted from the analyses although this will reduce the generalisability of the results. It is usually sensible to combine groups when there are less than 10 cases in a cell. The number of viable cells for statistical analysis usually depends on sample size. As a rule of thumb, the maximum number of cells that can be tested using chi-square is the sample size divided by 10. Thus, a sample size of 160 could theoretically support 16 cells such as an 8×2 table, a 5×3 table or a 4×4 table. However, this relies on an even distribution of cases over the cells, which rarely occurs. In practice, the maximum number of cells is usually the sample size divided by 20. In this data set this would be 141/20 or approximately seven cells which would support a 2×2 or 2×3 table. These tables would be viable as long as no cell size is particularly small.

The pathway for analysing categorical variables when some cells have small numbers is shown in Figure 7.3.

Chi-Square Tests

	Value	df	Asymp. sig. (two-sided)	Monte Carlo sig. (two-sided)				Monte Carlo sig. (one-sided)		
				Sig.	95% confidence interval			Sig.	95% confidence interval	
					Lower bound	Upper bound			Lower bound	Upper bound
Pearson chi-square	5.170[a]	2	0.075	0.075[b]	0.070	0.081				
Likelihood ratio	5.146	2	0.076	0.100[b]	0.094	0.106				
Fisher's exact test	5.072			0.075[b]	0.070	0.081				
Linear-by-linear association	0.028[c]	1	0.866	0.879[b]	0.872	0.885		0.481[b]	0.472	0.491
N of valid cases	132									

[a] One cell (16.7%) has expected count less than 5. The minimum expected count is 2.73.
[b] Based on 10 000 sampled tables with starting seed 624387341.
[c] The standardized statistic is −0.168.

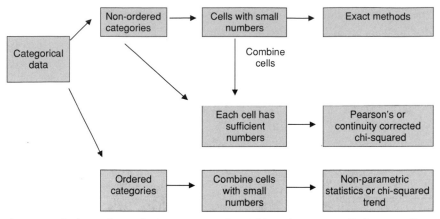

Figure 7.3 Pathway for analysing categorical variables when some cells have small numbers.

Re-coding to avoid small cell numbers

Groups can easily be combined to increase cell size if the re-coding is intuitive. However, if two or more unrelated groups need to be combined, they could be described with a generic label such as 'other' if neither group is more closely related to one of the other groups in the analysis. In the data set **surgery.sav**, it makes sense to combine the regional group with the overseas group because both are distinct from the local group. The SPSS commands to transform a variable into a new variable were shown in Box 1.10 in Chapter 1 and can be used to transform place2 with three levels into a binary variable called place3 (local, regional/overseas). To ensure that all output is self-documented, it is important to label each new variable in Variable View after re-coding and to verify the frequencies of place3 using the commands shown in Box 1.9.

Frequencies

Place of Birth (Binary)

		Frequency	Per cent	Valid per cent	Cumulative per cent
Valid	Local	90	63.8	68.2	68.2
	Regional or overseas	42	29.8	31.8	100.0
	Total	132	93.6	100.0	
Missing	System	9	6.4		
Total		141	100.0		

Having combined the small overseas group of nine children with the regional group of 33 children, the new combined group has 42 children. The crosstabulation to answer the research question can then be repeated using the command sequence shown in Box 7.3 to compute a 2 × 2 table with the binary place of birth variable entered into the rows.

Crosstabs

Place of Birth (Binary) * Prematurity Crosstabulation

			Prematurity		
			Premature	Term	Total
Place of birth (binary)	Local	Count	29	61	90
		% within place of birth (binary)	32.2%	67.8%	100.0%
	Regional or overseas	Count	11	31	42
		% within place of birth (binary)	26.2%	73.8%	100.0%
Total		Count	40	92	132
		% within place of birth (binary)	30.3%	69.7%	100.0%

Chi-Square Tests

	Value	df	Asymp. sig. (two-sided)	Exact sig. (two-sided)	Exact sig. (one-sided)
Pearson chi-square	0.493[b]	1	0.482		
Continuity correction[a]	0.249	1	0.618		
Likelihood ratio	0.501	1	0.479		
Fisher's exact test				0.546	0.312
Linear-by-linear association	0.490	1	0.484		
N of valid cases	132				

[a] Computed only for a 2 × 2 table.
[b] 0 cell (0.0%) has expected count less than 5. The minimum expected count is 12.73.

   The Crosstabulation shows that 32.2% of babies in the sample from local areas were premature compared to 26.2% of babies from regional centres or overseas. The Chi-Square Tests table shows the continuity corrected P value of 0.618 which is not significant. This value, which is very different from the P value of 0.075 for the 3 × 2 table, is more robust because all cells have adequate sizes. With the small cells combined with larger cells, the footnote shows that no cell has an expected count less than five and thus the assumptions for chi-square are met.
   Using the Excel spreadsheet created previously in Table 7.5, the percentages can be added as proportions and the confidence intervals calculated as shown in Table 7.6.

Table 7.6 Excel spreadsheet to compute confidence intervals around proportions

	Proportion	N	SE	Width	CI lower	CI upper
Local	0.322	90	0.049	0.097	0.225	0.419
Regional or overseas	0.262	42	0.068	0.133	0.129	0.395

Presenting the results: crosstabulated information

When presenting crosstabulated information of the effects of explanatory factors for a report, journal article or presentation, it is appropriate to use tables with the outcome variable presented in the columns and the risk factors or explanatory variables presented in the rows as shown in Table 7.7.

The chi-square analyses show that the number of males and females referred for surgery is significantly different but that the per cent of premature babies from regional or overseas areas is not significantly different from the per cent of premature babies in the group born locally. The results of these analyses could be presented as shown in Table 7.7.

Table 7.7 Factors associated with prematurity in 141 children attending hospital for surgery

Risk factor	Per cent premature and 95% CI	P value
Male	40.2% (95% CI 29.6, 50.8)	0.02
Female	20.3% (95% CI 10.0, 30.6)	
Born in local area	32.2% (95% CI 22.5, 41.9)	0.62
Born in regional area or overseas	26.2% (95% CI 12.9, 39.5)	

The overlap of the 95% confidence intervals in this table is consistent with the P values and shows that there is only a minor overlap of 95% confidence intervals between genders but a large overlap of 95% confidence intervals between regions.

Differences in proportions

When comparing proportions between two groups, it can be useful to express the size of the absolute difference in proportions between the groups. A 95% confidence interval around this difference is invaluable in interpreting the significance of the difference because if the interval does not cross the line of no difference (zero value) then the difference between groups is statistically significant.

The Excel spreadsheet shown in Table 7.8 can be used to calculate the differences in proportions, the standard error around the differences and the width of the confidence intervals. The difference in proportions is calculated

Table 7.8 Excel spreadsheet to compute confidence intervals around a difference in proportions

	p1	n1	p2	n2	1–p1	1–p2	Difference	SE	Width	CI lower	CI upper
Gender	0.402	82	0.203	59	0.598	0.797	0.199	0.075	0.148	0.051	0.347
Place	0.322	90	0.262	42	0.678	0.738	0.06	0.084	0.164	−0.104	0.224

as $p_1 - p_2$ and the standard error of the difference as $\sqrt{((p_1 \times (1 - p_1)/n_1) + (p_2 \times (1 - p_2)/n_2))}$, where p_1 is the proportion and n_1 is the number of cases in one group and p_2 is the proportion and n_2 is the number of cases in the other group. The width of the confidence interval is calculated as before as SE × 1.96.

Presenting the results: differences in percentages

The results from the above analyses can be presented as shown in Table 7.9 as an alternative to the presentation shown in Table 7.7. In Table 7.7, the precision in both groups could be compared but Table 7.9 shows the absolute difference between the groups. This type of presentation is useful for example when comparing percentages between two groups that were studied in different time periods and the outcome of interest is the change over time.

Table 7.9 Risk factor for prematurity in 141 children attending for surgery

Risk factor	Per cent premature	Difference and 95% confidence interval	P value
Male	40.2%	19.9% (95% CI 5.1, 34.7)	0.02
Female	20.3%		
Born locally	32.2%	6.0% (95% CI −10.4, 22.4)	0.62
Born regionally/overseas	26.2%		

The 95% confidence interval for the difference between genders does not contain the zero value of no difference as expected because the *P* value is significant. On the other hand, the confidence interval for the difference between places of birth contains the zero value indicating there is little difference between groups and that the *P* value is not significant.

When using larger crosstabulations, such as 2 × 3 tables, it can be difficult to interpret the *P* value without further sub-analyses, as shown when answering the following research question.

Research question

Question: Are babies who are born prematurely more likely to require different types of surgical procedures than term babies?

Null hypothesis: That the proportion of babies who require each type of surgical procedure in the group born prematurely is the same as in the group of term babies.

Variables: Outcome variable = procedure performed (categorical, three levels)

Explanatory variable = prematurity (categorical, two levels)

In situations such as this where the table is 3×2 because the outcome has three levels, both the row and column cell percentages can be used to provide useful summary statistics for between-group comparisons. The commands shown in Box 7.3 can be used with prematurity as the explanatory variable entered in the rows and procedure performed as the outcome variable in the columns. In addition, the column percentages can be obtained by ticking the column option in *Cells*.

Crosstabs

Prematurity * Procedure Performed Crosstabulation

			Procedure performed			
			Abdominal	Cardiac	Other	Total
Prematurity	Premature	Count	9	23	13	45
		% within prematurity	20.0%	51.1%	28.9%	100.0%
		% within procedure performed	17.0%	41.1%	40.6%	31.9%
	Term	Count	44	33	19	96
		% within prematurity	45.8%	34.4%	19.8%	100.0%
		% within procedure performed	83.0%	58.9%	59.4%	68.1%
Total		Count	53	56	32	141
		% within prematurity	37.6%	39.7%	22.7%	100.0%
		% within procedure performed	100.0%	100.0%	100.0%	100.0%

Chi-Square Tests

	Value	df	Asymp. sig. (two-sided)
Pearson chi-square	8.718[a]	2	0.013
Likelihood ratio	9.237	2	0.010
Linear-by-linear association	6.392	1	0.011
N of valid cases	141		

[a] 0 cell (0.0%) has expected count less than 5. The minimum expected count is 10.21.

The row percentages in the Crosstabulation show that fewer of the premature babies required abdominal procedures than the term babies (20.0% vs 45.8%) and that more of the premature babies had cardiac procedures than the term babies (51.1% vs 34.4%). In addition, more of the premature babies than the term babies had other procedures (28.9% vs 19.8%). The significance of these differences from the Chi-Square Tests table is $P = 0.013$. However, this P value does not indicate the specific between-group comparisons that are significantly different from one another. In practice, the P value indicates that there is a significant difference in percentages within the table but does indicate which groups are significantly different from one another. In this situation where there is no ordered explanatory variable, the linear by linear association has no interpretation.

The column percentages shown in the Crosstabulation table can be used to interpret the 2 × 2 comparisons. These percentages show that rates of surgery types in premature babies are abdominal vs cardiac surgery 17.0% vs 41.1%, abdominal vs other surgery 17.0% vs 40.6% and cardiac vs other surgery 41.1% vs 40.6%. To obtain P values for these comparisons, the *Data* → *Select Cases* → *If condition is satisfied* option can be used to select two groups at a time and compute three separate 2 × 2 tables. For the three comparisons above, this provides P values of 0.011, 0.031 and 1.0 respectively. Thus, the original P value from the 2 × 3 table was significant because the rate of prematurity was significantly lower in the abdominal surgery group compared to both the cardiac and other surgery groups. However, there was no significant difference between the cardiac vs other surgery group. This process of making multiple comparisons increases the chance of a type I error, that is finding a significant difference when one does not exist. A preferable method is to compute confidence intervals as shown in the Excel spreadsheet in Table 7.5 and then examine the degree of overlap. The computed intervals are shown in Table 7.10.

Table 7.10 Excel spreadsheet to compute confidence intervals around proportions

	Proportion	N	SE	Width	CI lower	CI upper
Abdominal-premature	0.17	53	0.052	0.101	0.069	0.271
Cardiac-premature	0.411	56	0.066	0.129	0.282	0.540
Other-premature	0.406	32	0.087	0.170	0.236	0.576
Abdominal-term	0.83	53	0.052	0.101	0.729	0.931
Cardiac-term	0.589	56	0.066	0.129	0.460	0.718
Other-term	0.594	32	0.087	0.170	0.424	0.764

The rates and their confidence intervals can then be plotted using SigmaPlot as shown in Box 7.5. The data sheet has the proportions and confidence interval widths converted into percentages for the premature babies in columns 1 and 2 and for the term babies in columns 3 and 4 as follows.

Column 1	Column 2	Column 3	Column 4
17.0	10.1	83.0	10.1
41.1	12.9	58.9	12.9
40.6	17.0	59.4	17.0

Box 7.5 SigmaPlot commands for plotting multiple bars

SigmaPlot Commands
SigmaPlot – [Data 1]*
        Graph → Create Graph
Create Graph - Type
        Highlight Horizontal Bar Chart, click Next
Create Graph - Style
        Highlight Grouped Error Bars, click Next
Create Graph – Error Bars
        Symbol Values – Worksheet Columns (default), click Next
Create Graph – Data Format
        Highlight Many X, click Next
Create Graph – Select Data
        Data for Set 1 = used drop box and select Column 1
        Data for Error 1 = used drop box and select Column 2
        Data for Set 2 = used drop box and select Column 3
        Data for Error 2 = used drop box and select Column 4
        Click Finish

Figure 7.4 shows clearly that the 95% confidence intervals of the bars for the per cent of the abdominal surgery group who are term or premature babies do not overlap either of the other groups and therefore the percentages are significantly different as described by the *P* values. The sample percentages of term and premature babies in the cardiac surgery and other procedure groups are almost identical as described by the *P* value of 1.0.

Larger chi-square tables

In addition to 2 × 2 and 2 × 3 tables, chi-square tests can also be used to analyse tables of larger dimensions as shown in the following research question. However, the same assumptions apply and the sample size should be sufficient to support the table without creating small cells with few expected counts.

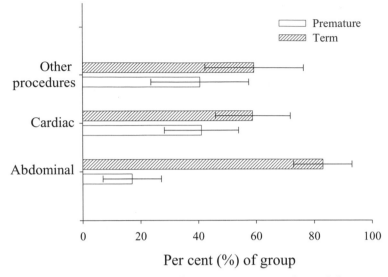

Figure 7.4 Percentage of surgical procedures in premature and term babies.

Research question

Question: Do babies who have a cardiac procedure stay in hospital
                longer than babies who have other procedures?
Null hypothesis: That length of stay is not different between children who
                undergo different procedures
Variables: Outcome variable = length of stay (categorised into
                quintiles)
                Explanatory variable = procedure performed
                (categorical, three levels)

In the data set, length of stay is a right skewed continuous variable. As an alternative to using rank-based non-parametric tests, it is often useful to divide non-normally distributed variables such as this into categories. Box 7.6 shows the SPSS commands that can be used to divide length of stay into quintiles, that is five groups with approximately equal cell sizes.

Box 7.6 SPSS commands to categorise variables

SPSS Commands
surgery – SPSS Data Editor
         Transform → Categorize Variables
Categorize Variables
         Highlight Length of stay and click into 'Create Categories for' box
         Enter the number 5 into the 'Number of categories' box
         Click OK

Once this new variable is obtained, it should be labelled in the Variable View window, for example this variable has been labelled 'Length of stay quintiles'. The SPSS commands to obtain information about the sample size of each quintile and the range of values in each quintile band are shown in Box 7.7.

Box 7.7 SPSS commands to obtain statistics for each quintile

SPSS Commands
surgery – SPSS Data Editor
    Data → Split file
Split File
    Click option 'Organize output by groups'
    Highlight Length of stay quintiles and click into 'Groups based on'
    Click OK
surgery – SPSS Data Editor
    Analyze→ Descriptive Statistics →Descriptives
Descriptives
    Highlight Length of stay and click into Variable(s) box
    Click OK

Descriptives

Length of stay quintiles = 1

Descriptive Statistics[a]

	N	Minimum	Maximum	Mean	Std. deviation
Length of stay	25	0	18	13.52	4.556
Valid N (listwise)	25				

[a] Length of stay quintiles = 1.

Length of stay quintiles = 2

Descriptive Statistics[a]

	N	Minimum	Maximum	Mean	Std. deviation
Length of stay	29	19	22	20.86	1.060
Valid N (listwise)	29				

[a] Length of stay quintiles = 2.

Length of stay quintiles = 3

Descriptive Statistics[a]

	N	Minimum	Maximum	Mean	Std. deviation
Length of stay	26	23	30	26.96	2.720
Valid N (listwise)	26				

[a] Length of stay quintiles = 3.

Length of stay quintiles = 4

Descriptive Statistics[a]

	N	Minimum	Maximum	Mean	Std. deviation
Length of stay	26	31	44	39.31	3.813
Valid N (listwise)	26				

[a] Length of stay quintiles = 4.

Length of stay quintiles = 5

Descriptive Statistics[a]

	N	Minimum	Maximum	Mean	Std. deviation
Length of stay	26	45	244	90.65	52.092
Valid N (listwise)	26				

[a] Length of stay quintiles = 5.

The output shows the number of cases, the mean, and the minimum and maximum days of each quintile. This information is important for labelling the quintile groups in Variable View so that the output is self-documented. The information of quintile ranges is also important for describing the quintile values when reporting the results. The number of cases in some quintiles are unequal because there are some ties in the data.

The SPSS commands for obtaining crosstabulations shown in Box 7.3 can now be used to answer the research question. Before running the crosstabulation, the *Data → Split File* command needs to be reversed using the option *Analyze all cases, do not create groups* in *Split File*. In the crosstabulation, the procedure performed is entered into the rows as explanatory variable and length of stay quintiles are entered in the columns as the outcome variable. The row percentages are selected in *Cells*.

It is very difficult to interpret large tables such as this 3×5 table. The crosstabulation has 15 cells, each with fewer than 20 observed cases. Although some cells have only two or three cases, the Chi-Square Tests footnote shows that no cells have an expected number less than 5, so that the analysis and the P value are valid. Although the P value is significant at $P = 0.004$, no clear trends are apparent in the table. If the cardiac and abdominal patients are compared, the abdominal group has fewer babies in the lowest quintile and the cardiac group has slightly fewer babies in the highest quintile. In the group of babies who had other procedures, most babies are either in the lowest or in the highest quintiles of length of stay. Thus, the P value is difficult to interpret without any further sub-group analyses and the interpretation of the statistical significance of the results is difficult to communicate. Again, in a table such as this with a non-ordered explanatory variable, the linear-by-linear statistic has no interpretation and should not be used. A solution to removing small cells would be to divide length of stay into two groups only, perhaps above and below the median value or above and below a clinically

Procedure Performed * Length of Stay Quintiles Crosstabulation

| | | | Length of stay quintiles | | | | | |
			0–18 days	19–22 days	23–30 days	31–44 days	45–244 days	Total
Procedure performed	Abdominal	Count	2	11	15	11	9	48
		% within procedure performed	4.2%	22.9%	31.3%	22.9%	18.8%	100.0%
	Cardiac	Count	15	13	7	12	6	53
		% within procedure performed	28.3%	24.5%	13.2%	22.6%	11.3%	100.0%
	Other	Count	8	5	4	3	11	31
		% within procedure performed	25.8%	16.1%	12.9%	9.7%	35.5%	100.0%
Total		Count	25	29	26	26	26	132
		% within procedure performed	18.9%	22.0%	19.7%	19.7%	19.7%	100.0%

Chi-Square Tests

	Value	df	Asymp. sig. (two-sided)
Pearson chi-square	22.425[a]	8	0.004
Likelihood ratio	24.341	8	0.002
Linear-by-linear association	0.676	1	0.411
N of valid cases	132		

[a] 0 cells (0.0%) has expected count less than 5. The minimum expected count is 5.87.

important threshold, and to examine the per cent of babies in each procedure group who have long or short stays.

Chi-square trend test for ordered variables

Chi-square trend tests, which in SPSS are called linear-by-linear associations, work well when the exposure variable can be categorised into ordered groups, such as quintiles for length of stay, and the outcome variable is binary. The linear-by-linear statistic then indicates whether there is a trend for the outcome to increase or decrease as the exposure increases.

Research question

Question: Is there a trend for babies who stay longer in hospital to have a higher infection rate?
Null hypothesis: That infection rates do not change with length of stay
Variables: Outcome variable = infection (categorical, two levels)
                     Explanatory/exposure variable = length of stay
                     (categorised into quintiles, ordered)

In this research question, it makes sense to test whether there is a trend for the per cent of babies with infection to increase significantly with an increase in length of stay. The SPSS commands shown in Box 7.3 can be used with length of stay quintiles in the rows, infection in the columns and the row percentages requested.

Crosstabs

Length of Stay Quintiles * Infection Crosstabulation

			Infection		
			No	Yes	Total
Length of stay quintiles	0–18 days	Count	19	6	25
		% within length of stay quintiles	76.0%	24.0%	100.0%
	19–22 days	Count	21	8	29
		% within length of stay quintiles	72.4%	27.6%	100.0%
					Continued

| | | Infection | | Total |
		No	Yes	
23–30 days	Count	17	9	26
	% within length of stay quintiles	65.4%	34.6%	100.0%
31–44 days	Count	12	14	26
	% within length of stay quintiles	46.2%	53.8%	100.0%
45–244 days	Count	11	15	26
	% within length of stay quintiles	42.3%	57.7%	100.0%
Total	Count	80	52	132
	% within length of stay quintiles	60.6%	39.4%	100.0%

Chi-Square Tests

	Value	df	Asymp. sig. (two-sided)
Pearson chi-square	10.344[a]	4	0.035
Likelihood ratio	10.433	4	0.034
Linear-by-linear association	9.551	1	0.002
N of valid cases	132		

[a] 0 cell (0.0%) has expected count less than 5. The minimum expected count is 9.85.

The Crosstabulation table shows that the per cent of children with infection increases with length of stay quintile, from 24.0% in the lowest length of stay quintile group to 57.7% in the highest quintile group. The Pearson chi-square indicates that there is a significant difference in percentages between some groups in the table with $P = 0.035$. From this, it can be inferred that the lowest rate of infection in the bottom quintile is significantly different from the highest rate in the top quintile but not that any other rates are significantly different from one other. More usefully, the linear-by-linear association indicates that there is a significant trend for infection to increase with length of stay at $P = 0.002$.

Presenting the results

When presenting the effects of an ordered exposure variable on several outcomes in a scientific table, the exposure groups are best shown in the columns and the outcomes in the rows. This is the reverse presentation to Table 7.9. Using this layout the per cent of babies in each exposure group can be compared across a line of the table. The data from the Crosstabulation above can be presented as shown in Table 7.11. If other outcomes associated with length of stay were also investigated, further rows could be added to the table.

Table 7.11 Rates of infection by length of stay

	Length of stay in quintiles						
	1	2	3	4	5		*P* value
Range (days)	0–18	19–22	23–30	31–44	45–244	*P* value	for trend
Number in group	25	29	26	26	26		
Percentage with infection	24.0%	27.6%	34.6%	53.8%	57.7%	0.035	0.002

To obtain a graphical indication of the magnitude of the trend across the data, a clustered bar chart can be requested using the SPSS commands shown in Box 7.8. If the number of cases in each group is unequal, as in this data set, then percentages rather than numbers must be selected in the *Bars Represent* option so that the height of each bar is standardised for the different numbers in each group and can be directly compared.

Box 7.8 SPSS commands to obtain a clustered bar chart

SPSS Commands
surgery – SPSS Data Editor
      Graphs → Bar
Bar Charts
      Click Clustered, click Define
Define Clustered Bar: Summaries for Groups of Cases
      Bars Represent: Tick % of cases box
      Highlight Infection and click into Category Axis
      Highlight Length of stay quintiles and click into Define Clusters by
      Click Options
Options
      Omit default check for Display groups defined by missing variables
          Click Continue
Define Clustered Bar: Summaries for Groups of Cases
      Click OK

In Figure 7.5, the group of bars on the left hand side of the graph shows the decrease in the per cent of babies who did not have infection across length of stay quintiles. The group of bars on the right hand side shows the complement of the data, that is the increase across quintiles of the per cent of babies who did have infection. A way of presenting the data to answer the research question would be to draw a bar chart of the per cent of children with infection only as shown on the right hand side of Figure 7.5. This chart can be drawn in SigmaPlot using the commands shown in Box 7.4 with a vertical bar chart rather than a horizontal bar chart selected. Using the SigmaPlot commands *Statistics → Linear Regression → All data in plot* will provide a plot that is more useful for presenting the results in that a trend line across exposures is shown as in Figure 7.6.

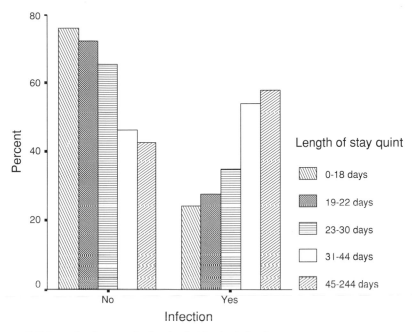

Figure 7.5 Length of stay quintiles for babies by infection status.

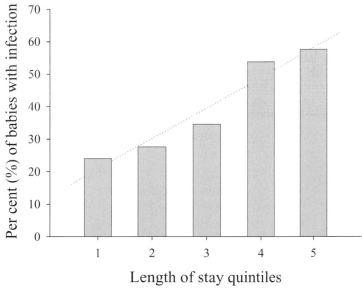

Figure 7.6 Rate of infection across length of stay quintiles.

Number needed to treat

In interpreting the results from clinical trials, clinicians are often interested in how many patients need to be administered a treatment to prevent one adverse event. This statistic, which is called number needed to treat (NNT), can be calculated from clinical studies in which the effectiveness of an intervention is compared in two groups, for example a standard treatment group and a new treatment group. For 2×2 crosstabulations, a chi-square test is used to indicate significance between the groups or a difference in proportions is used to indicate whether the new treatment group has a significantly lower rate of adverse events than the standard treatment group. However, in clinical situations, these statistics, which describe the general differences between two groups, may not be the major results of interest. In a clinical setting, the statistic NNT provides a number that can be directly applied to individual patients and may therefore be more informative.

To calculate NNT, two categorical variables each with two levels are required in order to compute a 2×2 crosstabulation. One variable must indicate the presence or absence of the adverse event, for example, an outcome such as death or disability, and the other variable must indicate group status (exposure), for example whether patients are in the intervention or control group.

The file **therapy.sav** contains data for 200 patients, half of whom were randomised to receive standard therapy and half of whom were randomised to receive a new therapy. The two outcomes that have been collected are the presence or absence of stroke and the presence or absence of disability. Each outcome variable is a binary yes/no response. Using the commands shown in Box 7.3, the following 2×2 tables for each outcome can be obtained. To calculate NNT, the outcome is entered as the rows, the treatment group is entered in the columns and column percentages are requested.

Crosstabs

Stroke * Treatment Group Crosstabulation

			Treatment group		Total
			New therapy	Standard treatment	
Stroke	No complications	Count	85	79	164
		% within treatment group	85.0%	79.0%	82.0%
	Stroke	Count	15	21	36
		% within treatment group	15.0%	21.0%	18.0%
Total		Count	100	100	200
		% within treatment group	100.0%	100.0%	100.0%

Chi-Square Tests

	Value	df	Asymp. sig. (two-sided)	Exact sig. (two-sided)	Exact sig. (one-sided)
Pearson chi-square	1.220[b]	1	0.269		
Continuity correction[a]	0.847	1	0.357		
Likelihood ratio	1.224	1	0.269		
Fishers exact test				0.358	0.179
Linear-by-linear association	1.213	1	0.271		
N of valid cases	200				

[a] Computed only for a 2 × 2 table.
[b] 0 cell (0.0%) has expected count less than 5. The minimum expected count is 18.00.

The first Crosstabulation shows that the rate of stroke is 15% in the new treatment group compared to 21.0% in the standard treatment group. The Chi-Square Tests table shows the continuity corrected chi square value with $P = 0.357$ which indicates that this difference in rates is not statistically significant. However, statistical significance, which depends largely on sample size, may not be of primary interest in a clinical setting.

From the table, NNT is calculated from the absolute risk reduction (ARR), which is simply the difference in the per cent of patients with the outcome of interest between the groups. From the Crosstabulation for stroke:

$$ARR = 21.0\% - 15.0\% = 6.0\%$$

ARR is then converted to a proportion, which in decimal format is 0.06, and the reciprocal is taken to obtain NNT:

$$NNT = 1/ARR = 1/0.06 = 16.67$$

Obviously, NNT is always rounded to the nearest whole number. This indicates that 17 people will need to receive the new treatment to prevent one extra person from having a stroke.

Crosstabs

Disability * Treatment Group Crosstabulation

			Treatment group		
			New therapy	Standard treatment	Total
Disability	No disability	Count	82	68	150
		% within treatment group	82.0%	68.0%	75.0%
	Disability	Count	18	32	50
		% within treatment group	18.0%	32.0%	25.0%
Total		Count	100	100	200
		% within treatment group	100.0%	100.0%	100.0%

Chi-Square Tests

	Value	df	Asymp. sig. (two-sided)	Exact sig. (two-sided)	Exact sig. (one-sided)
Pearson chi-square	5.227[b]	1	0.022		
Continuity correction[a]	4.507	1	0.034		
Likelihood ratio	5.281	1	0.022		
Fishers exact test				0.033	0.017
Linear-by-linear association	5.201	1	0.023		
N of valid cases	200				

[a] Computed only for a 2 × 2 table.
[b] 0 cell (0.0%) has expected count less than 5. The minimum expected count is 25.00.

The second Crosstabulation shows that the rate of disability is 18% in the new treatment group compared to 32.0% in the standard treatment group. The continuity corrected chi-square value with $P = 0.034$ shows that this new treatment achieves a significant reduction in rate of disability. The calculation of NNT is as follows:

ARR $= 32.0\% - 18.0\% = 14.0\%$

NNT $= 1/ARR = 1/0.14 = 7.14$

This indicates that seven people will need to receive the new treatment to prevent one extra person having a major disability. The larger the difference between groups as shown by a larger ARR, the fewer the number of patients who need to receive the treatment to prevent occurrence of one additional adverse event. Methods for calculating confidence intervals for NNT, which must be a positive number, are reported in the literature[2].

If nothing goes wrong, is everything OK?

Occasionally in clinical trials there may be no events in one group. If the *Crosstabs* procedure is repeated again, with the variable indicating survival entered as the outcome in the rows, the following table is produced.

Crosstabs

Death * Treatment Group Crosstabulation

			Treatment group New therapy	Treatment group Standard treatment	Total
Death	Survived	Count	100	92	192
		% within treatment group	100.0%	92.0%	96.0%
	Died	Count	0	8	8
		% within treatment group	0.0%	8.0%	4.0%
Total		Count	100	100	200
		% within treatment group	100.0%	100.0%	100.0%

Chi-Square Tests

	Value	df	Asymp. sig. (two-sided)	Exact sig. (two-sided)	Exact sig. (one-sided)
Pearson chi-square	8.333[b]	1	0.004		
Continuity correction[a]	6.380	1	0.012		
Likelihood ratio	11.424	1	0.001		
Fishers exact test				0.007	0.003
Linear-by-linear association	8.292	1	0.004		
N of valid cases	200				

[a] Computed only for a 2 × 2 table.
[b] 2 cells (50.0%) have expected count less than 5. The minimum expected count is 4.00.

When no adverse events occur in a group, as for deaths in the new treatment group this does not mean that no deaths will ever occur in patients who receive the new treatment. One way to estimate the proportion of patients in this group who might die is to calculate the upper end of the confidence interval around the zero percentage. To compute a confidence interval around a percentage that is less than 1% requires exact methods based on a binomial distribution. However, a rough estimate of the upper 95% confidence interval around a zero percentage is 3/n where n is the number of participants in the group. From the Crosstabulation, the upper 95% confidence interval around no deaths in the new therapy group would then be 3/100, or 3%. This is an approximate calculation only and may yield a conservative estimate. For more accurate estimates, Web programs are available (see Useful Web sites).

Paired categorical variables

Paired categorical measurements taken from the same participants on two occasions or matched categorical data collected in matched case – control studies must be analysed using tests for repeated data.

The measurements collected in these types of study designs are not independent and therefore chi-square tests cannot be used because the assumptions would be violated. In this situation, McNemar's test is used to assess whether there is a significant change in proportions over time for paired data or whether there is a significant difference in proportions between matched cases and controls. In this type of analysis, the outcome of interest is the within-person changes or the within-pair differences and there are no explanatory variables.

Research question

The file **health-camp.sav** contains the data from 86 children who attended a camp to learn how to self manage their illness. The children were asked whether they knew how to manage their illness appropriately and whether they knew when to use their rescue medication appropriately at both the start and completion of the camp.

Question: Did attendance at the camp increase the number of
                     children who knew how to manage their illness
                     appropriately?
Null hypothesis: That there was no change in children's knowledge of
                     illness management between the beginning and
                     completion of the health camp.
Variables: Appropriate knowledge (categorical, binary) at the
                     beginning and completion of the camp.

In this research question the explanatory variable is time which is built
into the analysis method and knowledge at both Time 1 and Time 2 are the
outcome variables.

The assumptions for using paired categorical tests are shown in Box 7.9.

Box 7.9 Assumptions for a paired McNemar's test

For a paired McNemar's test the following assumptions must be met:
• the outcome variable has a categorical scale
• each participant is represented in the table once only
• the difference between the paired proportions is the outcome of interest

---

The relation between the measurements is summarised using a paired 2×2
contingency table and McNemar's test can be obtained using the commands
shown in Box 7.10.

Box 7.10 SPSS commands to obtain McNemar's test

SPSS Commands
health-camp – SPSS Data Editor
        Analyze → Descriptive Statistics → Crosstabs
Crosstabs
        Highlight Knowledge-Time1 and click into Row(s)
        Highlight Knowledge-Time2 and click into Column(s)
        Click on Statistics
Crosstabs: Statistics
        Tick McNemar, click Continue
Crosstabs
        Click on Cells
Crosstabs: Cell Display
        Tick Observed under Counts (default), tick Total under Percentages
        Click Continue
Crosstabs
        Click OK

Crosstabs

Knowledge–Time1 * Knowledge–Time2 Crosstabulation

			Knowledge–Time2		
			No	Yes	Total
Knowledge–Time1	No	Count	27	29	56
		% of total	31.4%	33.7%	65.1%
	Yes	Count	6	24	30
		% of total	7.0%	27.9%	34.9%
Total		Count	33	53	86
		% of total	38.4%	61.6%	100.0%

Chi-Square Tests

	Value	Exact sig. (two-sided)
McNemar test		0.000[a]
N of valid cases	86	

[a] Binomial distribution used.

In the Crosstabulation, the total column and total row cells indicate that 34.9% of children had appropriate knowledge at the beginning of the camp (Yes at Time 1) and 61.6% at the end of the camp (Yes at Time 2). More importantly, the internal cells of the table show that 31.4% of children did not have appropriate knowledge on both occasions and 27.9% did have appropriate knowledge on both occasions. The percentages also show that 33.7% of children improved their knowledge (i.e. went from No at Time 1 to Yes at Time 2) and only 7.0% of children reduced their knowledge (i.e. went from Yes at Time 1 to No at Time 2). The Chi-Square Tests table shows a McNemar P value of <0.0001 indicating a significant increase in the proportion of children who improved their illness management knowledge.

When reporting paired information, summary statistics that reflect how many children improved their knowledge compared to how many children reduced their knowledge are used. This difference in proportions with its 95% confidence interval can be calculated using Excel.

In computing these statistics from the Crosstabulation table, the concordant cells are not used and only the information from the discordant cells is of interest as shown in Table 7.12. In Table 7.12, the two concordant cells (*a* and *d*) show the number of children who did or did not have appropriate knowledge at both the beginning and end of the camp. The two discordant cells (*b* and *c*) show the number of children who changed their knowledge status in either direction between the two occasions.

The counts in the discordant cells are used in calculating the change as a proportion and the SE of difference from the cell counts as follows:

Table 7.12 Presentation of data showing discordant cells

	No at end of camp			Yes at end of camp	Total
No at beginning of camp	27			29	56
		a	*b*		
		c	*d*		
Yes at beginning of camp	6			24	30
Total	33			53	*n* 86

Difference in proportions $= (b - c)/n$

$$\text{SE of difference} = 1/n \times \sqrt{(b + c - ((b - c)^2/n))}$$

For large sample sizes, the 95% confidence interval around the difference in proportions is calculated as $1.96 \times \text{SE}$. These statistics can be computed using the discordant cell counts in an Excel spreadsheet as shown in Table 7.13 and the proportions for appropriate knowledge at the beginning of the camp (Yes at Time 1) and end of the camp (Yes at Time 2). The table shows that the increase in knowledge converted back to a percentage is 26.7% (95% CI 14.5, 39.0). The 95% confidence interval does not cross the zero line of no difference which reflects the finding that the change in proportions is statistically significant.

Table 7.13 Excel spreadsheet to compute differences for paired data

	p2 Yes-Time2	p1 Yes-Time1	Total N	Difference	SE	95% CI width	CI lower	CI upper
Knowledge	0.616	0.349	86	0.267	0.062	0.122	0.145	0.390

A second outcome that was measured in the study was whether children knew when to use their rescue medication appropriately. The commands shown in Box 7.10 can be used to obtain a McNemar's test for this outcome by entering medication-time 1 into the rows and medication-time 2 into the columns of the crosstabulation. Again, only the total percentages are requested.

Crosstabs

Medication–Time1 * Medication–Time2 Crosstabulation

			Medication–Time2		Total
			No	Yes	
Medication–Time1	NO	Count	17	13	30
		% of total	19.8%	15.1%	34.9%
	Yes	Count	11	45	56
		% of total	12.8%	52.3%	65.1%
Total		Count	28	58	86
		% of total	32.6%	67.4%	100.0%

Chi-Square Tests

	Value	Exact sig. (two-sided)
McNemar test		0.839[a]
N of valid cases	86	

[a] Binomial distribution used.

The percentages in the discordant cells indicate a small increase in knowledge of 15.1% to 12.8%, or 2.3%. The Chi-Square Tests table shows that this difference is not significant with a *P* value of 0.839. The Excel spreadsheet shown in Table 7.13 can be used to obtain the paired difference and its 95% confidence interval as proportions as shown in Table 7.14. The increase in knowledge is 2.3% (95% CI −8.8%, 13.5%). The 95% confidence interval crosses the zero line of no difference reflecting the finding that the change in proportions is not statistically significant.

Table 7.14 Excel spreadsheet to compute differences for paired data

	p2 Yes-Time2	p1 Yes-Time1	Total N	Difference	SE	95% CI width	CI lower	CI upper
Medication	0.674	0.651	86	0.023	0.057	0.112	−0.088	0.135

Presenting the results

The analyses show that the number of children who knew how to manage their illness appropriately increased significantly and that the number of children who knew when to use their rescue medication increased slightly but not significantly on completion of the camp. These results could be presented as shown in Table 7.15. By reporting the per cent of children with knowledge on both occasions, the per cent increase and the *P* value, all information that is relevant to interpreting the findings is included.

Table 7.15 Changes in knowledge of management and medication use in 86 children following camp attendance

	Knowledge at entry	Knowledge on leaving	% increase and 95% CI	P value
Management	34.9%	61.6%	26.7% (14.5, 39.0)	<0.0001
Medication use	65.1%	67.4%	2.3% (−8.8, 13.5)	0.84

Notes for critical appraisal

There are many ways in which crosstabulations can be used and chi-square values can be computed. These values often depend on the sample size and can be biased by cells with only a small number of expected counts. When critically appraising an article that presents categorical data analysed using univariate statistics or crosstabulations, it is important to ask the questions shown in Box 7.11.

Box 7.11 Questions for critical appraisal

The following questions should be asked when appraising published results from analyses in which crosstabulations are used:
- Has any participant been included in an analysis more than once?
- Have the correct terms to describe rates or proportions been used?
- Is the correct chi-square value presented?
- Could any small cells have biased the *P* value?
- Are percentages reported so that the size of the difference is clear?
- Have 95% confidence intervals for percentages been reported?
- If two groups are being compared, is the difference between them shown?
- If the exposure variable is ordered, is a trend statistic reported?
- Is it clear how any 'missing data' have influenced the results?
- Are the most important findings reported as a figure?
- If the results of a trial to test an intervention are being reported, is NNT presented?
- If the data are paired, has a paired statistical test been used?

References

1. Bland M. An introduction to medical statistics (2nd edition). Oxford, UK: Oxford University Press, 1996; p. 3.
2. Altman DG. Confidence intervals for number needed to treat. BMJ 1998; 317: 1309–1312.

CHAPTER 8

Categorical variables: risk statistics

Clinicians have a good intuitive understanding of risk and even of a ratio of risks. Gamblers have a good intuitive understanding of odds. No one (with the possible exception of certain statisticians) intuitively understands a ratio of odds.[1]

Objectives

The objectives of this chapter are to explain how to:
- decide whether odds ratio or relative risk is the appropriate statistic to use
- use logistic regression to compute adjusted odds ratios
- report and plot unadjusted and adjusted odds ratios
- change risk estimates to protection and vice versa
- calculate 95% confidence intervals around estimates of risk
- critically appraise the literature in which estimates of risk are reported

---

Chi-square tests indicate whether two binary variables such as an exposure and an outcome measurement are independent or are significantly related to each other. However, apart from the *P* value, chi-square tests do not provide a statistic for describing the strength of the relationship. Two statistics that are useful for measuring the magnitude of the association between two binary variables measured in a 2 × 2 table are the odds ratio or a relative risk. Both of these statistics are estimates of risk and, as such, describe the probability that people who are exposed to a certain factor will have a disease compared to people who are not exposed to the same factor.

The choice of using an odds ratio or relative risk depends on both the study design and whether bivariate or multivariate analyses are required. Relative risk is an appropriate risk statistic to use when the sample has been selected randomly, such as in a cohort or cross-sectional study, and when only bivariate analyses are required. Odds ratios have the advantage that they can be used in any study design, including case–control studies in which the proportion of cases is unlikely to be representative of the proportion in the population, and they can be adjusted for the effects of other confounders in multivariate analyses.

Both odds ratio and relative risk are widely used in epidemiological and clinical research to describe the risk of people having a disease (or an outcome) in the presence of an exposure, which may be an environmental factor, a treatment or any other type of explanatory factor. In case–control studies, odds ratio is used to measure the odds that a case has been exposed compared to the odds that a control has had the same exposure.

The way in which tables to calculate risk statistics are classically set up in the clinical epidemiology textbooks is shown in Table 8.1.

Table 8.1 Table to measure the relation between a disease and an exposure

	Disease present	Disease absent	Total
Exposure present	a	b	$a+b$
Exposure absent	c	d	$c+d$
Total	$a+c$	$b+d$	N

The odds ratio and relative risk compare the likelihood of an event occurring between two groups. The odds is a ratio of the probability of an event occurring to the probability of an event not occurring[2]. The odds ratio is calculated by comparing the odds of an event in one group (e.g. exposure present) to the odds of the same event in another group (e.g. exposure absent). From Table 8.1, the odds of the disease in the exposed group compared to the odds of the disease in the non-exposed group can be calculated as follows:

Odds ratio (OR) $= (a/b)/(c/d) = (a \times d)/(b \times c)$

This calculation shows why an odds ratio is sometimes called a ratio of cross-products. On the other hand, relative risk compares the conditional probability of the event occurring in the exposed and non-exposed groups and is calculated as follows:

Relative risk (RR) $= \dfrac{a/(a+b)}{c/(c+d)}$

Coding

A problem arises in calculating odds ratio and relative risk using some statistical packages because the format of the table that is required to compute the correct statistics is different from the format used in clinical epidemiology textbooks. To use SPSS to compute these risk statistics, the variables need to be coded as shown in Table 8.2.

Table 8.2 Possible coding of variables to compute risk

Code	Alternate code	Condition	Interpretation
1	0	Disease absent	Outcome negative
2	1	Disease present	Outcome positive
1	0	Exposure absent	Risk factor negative
2	1	Exposure present	Risk factor positive

This will invert the table shown in Table 8.1 but as shown later in this chapter, this will allow the odds ratio to be read directly from the SPSS output generated in both the *Frequencies → Crosstabs* and the *Regression → Binary Logistic* menus.

If the reverse notation is used as in Table 8.1, the odds ratio and relative risk statistics printed by SPSS have to be inverted to obtain the correct direction of effect. The options are to either

- code the data as shown in Table 8.2 and in Table 7.3 in Chapter 7, which inverts the location of cells in Table 8.1 but not the statistics or
- code the data as shown in Table 8.1 which inverts the statistics but not the table.

In this chapter, the first option is used so that the layout of the tables is as shown in Table 7.3 in Chapter 7.

Odds ratio vs relative risk

Both odds ratio and relative risk are invaluable statistics for describing the magnitude of the relationship between the exposure and the outcome variables because they provide a size of effect that adds to the information provided by the chi-square value. A chi-square test indicates whether the difference in the proportion of participants with and without disease in the exposure present group and the exposure absent group is statistically significant, but an odds ratio quantifies the relative size of the difference between the groups.

The advantage of calculating the relative risk is that it has an intuitive interpretation. A relative risk of 2.0 indicates that the prevalence of disease in the exposed cases is twice as high as the prevalence in the non-exposed cases. Although a relative risk should not be calculated for some study designs, for example case–control designs, it is a useful statistic to describe risk in studies in which the participants are selected as a random sample of the population.

Odds ratio is a less valuable statistic because it represents the odds of disease, which is not as intuitive as the relative risk. Although the odds ratio is not the easiest of statistics to explain or understand, it is widely used for describing an association between an exposure and a disease because it can be calculated from studies of any design, including cross-sectional, cohort studies, case–control studies and experimental trials as shown in Table 8.3.

Table 8.3 Study type and statistics available

Type of study	Odds ratio	Relative risk
Cross-sectional	Yes	Yes
Cohort	Yes	Sometimes
Case–control	Yes	No
Clinical trial	Yes	Sometimes

Odds ratio has the advantage that it can be used to make direct comparisons of results from studies of different designs and, for this reason, odds ratios are often used in meta-analyses. The odds ratio and the relative risk are always in the same direction of risk or protection. However, the odds ratio does not give a good approximation of the relative risk when the exposure and/or the disease is relatively common[3]. The odds ratio is always larger than relative risk and therefore generally overestimates the true association between variables. For this reason, odds ratios are sometimes referred to as a poor man's relative risk.

The assumptions for using odds ratio and relative risk are exactly the same as the assumptions for using chi-square tests shown in Box 7.2 in Chapter 7.

Odds ratio

The odds ratio is the odds of a person having a disease if exposed to the risk factor divided by the odds of a person having a disease if not exposed to the risk factor. Conversely, an odds ratio can be interpreted as the odds of a person having been exposed to a factor when having the disease compared to the odds of a person not having been exposed to a factor when not having the disease. This converse interpretation is useful for case–control studies in which participants are selected on the basis of their disease status and their exposures are measured. In this type of study, the odds ratio is interpreted as the odds that a case has been exposed to the risk factor of interest compared to the odds that a control has been exposed.

Table 8.4 2 × 2 crosstabulation of disease and exposure

	Disease absent		Disease present	Total
Exposure absent	75		60	135
		d $\mid$ c		
		b $\mid$ a		
Exposure present	25		40	65
Total	100		100	200

The calculation of the odds ratio from the data shown in Table 8.4 is as follows:

$$
\begin{aligned}
\text{Odds ratio} &= (a/b)/(c/d) \\
&= (40/25)/(60/75) \\
&= (8/5)/(4/5) \\
&= 2.0
\end{aligned}
$$

Obviously, if an odds ratio is 1.0 then the odds that people with and without the disease have been exposed is equal and the exposure presents no difference in risk. An odds ratio of 2.0 can be interpreted as the odds that an exposed person has the disease present is twice that of the odds that a non-exposed person has the disease present. An odds ratio calculated in this way from a

2×2 table is called an unadjusted odds ratio because it is not adjusted for the effects of possible confounders. Odds ratios calculated using logistic regression are called adjusted odds ratios because they are adjusted for the effects of the other variables in the model.

Another way that an odds ratio of 2 can be interpreted is that if a person who is exposed to a risk factor and a person who is not exposed to the same risk factor are compared, a gambler would break even by betting 2:1 that the person who had been exposed would have the disease[1]. Naturally, these interpretations are not intuitive for most researchers and clinicians.

The size of odds ratio that is important is often debated and in considering this the clinical importance of the outcome and the number of people exposed need to be taken into account. An odds ratio above 2.0 is usually important. However, a smaller odds ratio between 1.0 and 2.0 can have public health importance if a large number of people are exposed to the factor of interest. For example, approximately 25% of the 5 million children aged between 1 and 14 years living in Australasia have a mother who smokes. The odds ratio for children to wheeze if exposed to environmental tobacco smoke is 1.3, which is close to 1.0. Based on this odds ratio and the high exposure rate, a conservative estimate is that 320 000 children wheeze as a result of being exposed, which amounts to an important public health problem[4]. If only 5% of children were exposed or if the outcome was more trivial, the public health impact would be less important.

Research question

The spreadsheet **asthma.sav** contains data from a random cross-sectional sample of 2464 children aged 8 to 10 years in which the exposure of allergy to housedust mites (HDM), the exposure to respiratory infection in early life, the characteristic gender and the presence of the disease, that is, asthma, were measured in all children.

Question:	Are HDM allergy, early infection or gender independent risk factors for asthma in this sample of children?
Null hypothesis:	That HDM allergy, respiratory infection in early life and gender are not independent risk factors for asthma.
Variables:	Outcome variable = Diagnosed asthma (categorical, two levels)
	Explanatory variables (risk factors) = allergy to HDM (categorical, two levels), early infection (categorical, two levels) and gender (categorical, two levels).

The SPSS commands shown in Box 8.1 can be used to obtain the crosstabulations for the three risk factors and their risk statistics. In calculating risk, the risk factors are entered in the rows, the outcome in the columns and the row percentages are requested. Each explanatory variable is crosstabulated separately with the outcome variable so three different crosstabulation tables are produced.

Box 8.1 SPSS commands to obtain risk statistics

SPSS Commands
asthma – SPSS Data Editor
       Analyze → Descriptive Statistics → Crosstabs
Crosstabs
       Highlight Allergy to HDM, Early infection, and Gender and click into
          Row(s)
       Highlight Diagnosed asthma and click into Column(s)
       Click Statistics
Crosstabs: Statistics
       Tick Chi-square, tick Risk, Click Continue
Crosstabs
       Click Cells
Crosstabs: Cell Display
       Tick Observed under Counts (default), tick Row under Percentages, click
          Continue
Crosstabs
       Click OK

*Allergy to HDM * Diagnosed asthma*

Crosstab

			Diagnosed asthma		Total
			No	Yes	
Allergy to HDM	No	Count	1414	125	1539
		% within allergy to HDM	91.9%	8.1%	100.0%
	Yes	Count	529	396	925
		% within allergy to HDM	57.2%	42.8%	100.0%
Total		Count	1943	521	2464
		% within allergy to HDM	78.9%	21.1%	100.0%

Chi-Square Tests

	Value	df	Asymp. sig. (two-sided)	Exact sig. (two-sided)	Exact sig. (one-sided)
Pearson chi-square	416.951[b]	1	0.000		
Continuity correction[a]	414.874	1	0.000		
Likelihood ratio	411.844	1	0.000		
Fisher's exact test				0.000	0.000
Linear-by-linear association	416.782	1	0.000		
N of valid cases	2464				

[a] Computed only for a 2 × 2 table.
[b] 0 cell (0.0%) has expected count less than 5. The minimum expected count is 195.59.

Risk Estimate

		95% confidence interval	
	Value	Lower	Upper
Odds ratio for allergy to HDM (no/yes)	8.468	6.765	10.600
For cohort diagnosed asthma = no	1.607	1.516	1.702
For cohort diagnosed asthma = yes	0.190	0.158	0.228
N of valid cases	2464		

The Crosstab table for HDM allergy shows that in the group of children who did not have HDM allergy 8.1% had been diagnosed with asthma and in the group of children who did have HDM allergy 42.8% had been diagnosed with asthma. The Pearson's chi-square value in the Chi-Square Tests table is used to assess significance because the sample size is in excess of 1000. The P value is highly significant at $P < 0.0001$ indicating that the frequency of HDM allergy is significantly different between the two groups. The odds ratio could be calculated from the crosstabulation as (396/529)/(125/1414), which is 8.468. This is shown in the Risk Estimate table, which also gives the 95% confidence interval. The odds ratio for the association between a diagnosis of asthma and HDM allergy is large at 8.468 (95% CI 6.765 to 10.60) reflecting the large difference in percentages of outcome given exposure and thus a strong relation between the two variables in this sample of children. The 95% confidence interval does not contain the value of 1.0, which represents no difference in risk, and therefore is consistent with an odds ratio that is statistically significant.

The cohort statistics below the odds ratio can also be used to generate relative risk, which is explained later in this chapter.

*Early infection * Diagnosed asthma*

Crosstab

			Diagnosed asthma		
			No	Yes	Total
Early infection	No	Count	1622	399	2021
		% within early infection	80.3%	19.7%	100.0%
	Yes	Count	321	122	443
		% within early infection	72.5%	27.5%	100.0%
Total		Count	1943	521	2464
		% within early infection	78.9%	21.1%	100.0%

Chi-Square Tests

	Value	df	Asymp. sig. (two-sided)	Exact sig. (two-sided)	Exact sig. (one-sided)
Pearson chi-square	13.247[b]	1	0.000		
Continuity correction[a]	12.784	1	0.000		
Likelihood ratio	12.599	1	0.000		
Fisher's exact test				0.000	0.000
Linear-by-linear association	13.242	1	0.000		
N of valid cases	2464				

[a] Computed only for a 2 × 2 table.
[b] 0 cell (0.0%) has expected count less than 5. The minimum expected count is 93.67.

Risk Estimate

	Value	95% confidence interval	
		Lower	Upper
Odds ratio for early infection (no/yes)	1.545	1.221	1.955
For cohort diagnosed asthma = no	1.108	1.042	1.178
For cohort diagnosed asthma = yes	0.717	0.602	0.854
N of valid cases	2464		

The second Crosstab table shows that 19.7% of children in the group who did not have an early respiratory infection had a diagnosis of asthma compared with 27.5% of the group who did have an early respiratory infection. Although the difference in percentages in this table (27.5% vs 19.7%) is not as large as for HDM allergy, the Pearson's chi-square value in the Chi-Square Tests table shows that this difference is similarly highly significant at $P < 0.0001$. However, the Risk Estimate table shows that the odds ratio for the association between a diagnosis of asthma and an early respiratory infection is much lower than for HDM allergy at 1.545 (95% CI 1.221 to 1.955). Again, the statistical significance of the odds ratio is reflected in the 95% confidence interval, which does not contain the value of 1.0, which represents no difference in risk.

*Gender * Diagnosed asthma*

Crosstab

			Diagnosed asthma		
			No	Yes	Total
Gender	Female	Count	965	223	1188
		% within gender	81.2%	18.8%	100.0%
	Male	Count	978	298	1276
		% within gender	76.6%	23.4%	100.0%
Total		Count	1943	521	2464
		% within gender	78.9%	21.1%	100.0%

Chi-Square Tests

	Value	df	Asymp. sig. (two-sided)	Exact sig. (two-sided)	Exact sig. (one-sided)
Pearson chi-square	7.751[b]	1	0.005		
Continuity correction[a]	7.478	1	0.006		
Likelihood ratio	7.778	1	0.005		
Fisher's exact test				0.006	0.003
Linear-by-linear association	7.747	1	0.005		
N of valid cases	2464				

[a] Computed only for a 2 × 2 table.
[b] 0 cell (0.0%) has expected count less than 5. The minimum expected count is 251.20.

Risk Estimate

		95% confidence interval	
	Value	Lower	Upper
Odds ratio for gender (female/male)	1.319	1.085	1.602
For cohort diagnosed asthma = no	1.060	1.017	1.104
For cohort diagnosed asthma = yes	0.804	0.689	0.938
N of valid cases	2464		

For gender, the Crosstab table shows that 18.8% of females had a diagnosis of asthma compared with 23.4% of males. At $P = 0.005$, the Pearson's chi-square value in the Chi-Square Tests table is less significant than for the other two variables and the odds ratio of 1.319 (95% CI 1.085 to 1.602) in the Risk Estimate table is also smaller, reflecting the smaller difference in proportions in diagnosed asthma between the two gender groups.

Reporting the results

The results from these tables can be presented as shown in Table 8.5. When reporting an odds ratio or relative risk, the per cent of cases with the outcome in the two comparison groups of interest are included. It is often useful to rank variables in order of the magnitude of risk.

Table 8.5 Unadjusted associations between risk factors and diagnosed asthma in a random sample of 2464 children aged 8 to 10 years

Risk factor (exposure)	%diagnosed asthma in exposed group	% diagnosed asthma in non-exposed group	Unadjusted odds ratio and 95% CI	Chi-square	P value
Allergy to HDM	42.8%	8.1%	8.5 (6.8, 10.6)	417.0	<0.0001
Early infection	27.5%	19.7%	1.5 (1.2, 2.0)	13.2	<0.0001
Gender	23.4%	18.8%	1.3 (1.1, 1.6)	7.8	0.005

Odds ratios larger than 1.0 are reported with only one decimal place because the precision of $1/100^{th}$ or $1/1000^{th}$ of an estimate of risk is not required. The decision of whether to include a column with the chi-square values is optional since the only interpretation of the chi-square value is the P value. From the table, it is easy to see how the odds ratio describes the strength of the associations between variables in a way that is not discriminated by the P values.

Protective odds ratios

An odds ratio greater than 1.0 indicates that the risk of disease in the exposed group is greater than the risk in the non-exposed group. If the odds ratio is less than 1.0, then the risk of disease in the exposed group is less than the risk in the non-exposed group.

Whether odds ratios represent risk or protection largely depends on the way in which the data are coded. For example, having HDM allergy is a strong risk factor for diagnosed asthma in the study sample but if the coding had been reversed with not having HDM allergy coded as 2, then not having HDM allergy would be a strong protective factor. For ease of interpretation, comparison and communication, it is usually better to present all odds ratios in the direction of risk rather than presenting some as risk and some as protection.

To illustrate this, the commands shown in Box 1.10 can be used to reverse the coding of HDM allergy from 2 = exposure to 1 = exposure and from 1 = no exposure to 2 = no exposure. In this example, the new variable is called hdm2 and its values have been added in Variable View before conducting any analyses. The SPSS commands shown in Box 8.1 can then be used with allergy to HDM re-coded as the row variable, diagnosed asthma as the column variable and the row percentages requested.

Allergy to HDM – Re-coded * Diagnosed Asthma Crosstabulation

| | | | Diagnosed asthma | | |
			No	Yes	Total
Allergy to HDM – re-coded	Allergy	Count	529	396	925
		% within allergy to HDM – re-coded	57.2%	42.8%	100.0%
	No Allergy	Count	1414	125	1539
		% within allergy to HDM – re-coded	91.9%	8.1%	100.0%
Total		Count	1943	521	2464
		% within allergy to HDM – re-coded	78.9%	21.1%	100.0%

Chi-Square Tests

	Value	df	Asymp. sig. (two-sided)	Exact sig. (two-sided)	Exact sig. (one-sided)
Pearson chi-square	416.951[b]	1	0.000		
Continuity correction[a]	414.874	1	0.000		
Likelihood ratio	411.844	1	0.000		
Fisher's exact test				0.000	0.000
Linear-by-linear association	416.782	1	0.000		
N of valid cases	2464				

[a] Computed only for a 2 × 2 table.
[b] 0 cell (0.0%) has expected count less than 5. The minimum expected count is 195.59.

Risk Estimate

		95% confidence interval	
	Value	Lower	Upper
Odds ratio for allergy to HDM – recoded (allergy/no allergy)	0.118	0.094	0.148
For cohort diagnosed asthma = no	0.622	0.588	0.659
For cohort diagnosed asthma = yes	5.271	4.386	6.334
N of valid cases	2464		

The per cent of children with diagnosed asthma in the exposed and un-exposed groups and the P value are obviously exactly the same as before. The only difference in the Crosstabulation table is that the rows have been interchanged. The odds ratio is now a protective factor of 0.118 (95% 0.094 to 0.148) rather than a risk factor of 8.468 (95% CI 6.765 to 10.60) as it was in the first analysis.

Summary statistics of odds ratio can easily be changed from protection to risk or vice versa by calculating the reciprocal value, that is

odds ratio (risk) = 1/odds ratio (protection)

$$= 1/0.118$$
$$= 8.474$$

When recalculated, the upper confidence interval becomes the lower confidence interval and vice versa.

Figure 8.1 shows an odds ratio expressed as a risk factor or as a protective factor. The x-axis is a logarithmic scale because odds ratios are derived from logarithmic values. In Figure 8.1, the dotted line passing through 1 indicates the line of no effect, that is, no difference in risk. When a factor is coded as risk or protection, the effect size is the same because on a logarithmic scale the odds ratios are symmetrical on either side of the line of unity.

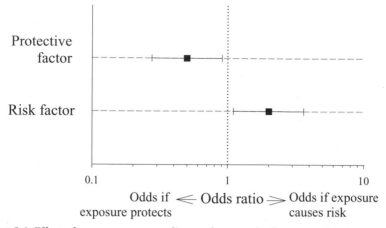

Figure 8.1 Effect of an exposure on a disease shown as both a protective factor and as a risk factor.

Adjusting for inter-relationships between risk factors

A problem with odds ratios calculated from 2 × 2 crosstabulations is that some explanatory factors may be related to one another. If cases with one factor present also tend to have another factor present, the effects of both factors in increasing the odds of disease will be included in each odds ratio. Thus, each odds ratio will be artificially inflated with the effect of the associated exposure, that is confounding will be present. Logistic regression is used to calculate the effects of risk factors as independent odds ratios with the effects of other confounders removed. These odds ratios are called adjusted odds ratios.

Figure 8.2 shows the percentage of cases with disease in each of three exposure groups. In group 1, participants had no exposure, in group 2 participants had exposure to factor I and in group 3 participants had exposure to factor I and factor II. If an unadjusted odds ratio were used to calculate the risk of disease in the presence of exposure to factor I, then in a bivariate analysis, groups 2 and 3 would be combined and compared with group 1. The effect of including cases also exposed to factor II would inflate the estimate of risk because their rate of disease is higher than for cases exposed to factor 1. Logistic regression is used to mathematically separate out the independent risk associated with exposure to factor I or to factor II.·

Binary logistic regression

Binary logistic regression is not really a regression analysis in the classic sense of the term but is a mathematical method to measure the effects of binary risk factors on a binary outcome variable whilst adjusting for inter-relationships.between them. In binary logistic regression, the variables that

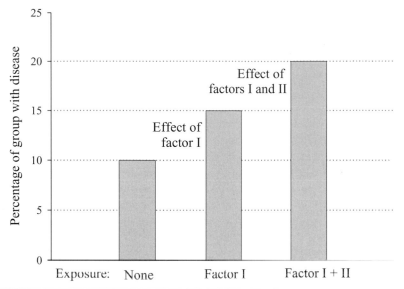

Figure 8.2 Rate of disease in group not exposed and in groups exposed to factor I or to both factors I and II.

affect the probability of the outcome are measured as odds ratios which are called adjusted odds ratios.

Logistic regression is primarily used to determine which binary explanatory variables independently predict the outcome, when the outcome is a binary variable[5]. The outcome variable normally reflects the presence or absence of a condition or a disease, for example, the presence or absence of asthma, or the occurrence or absence of a heart attack.

The assumptions for using logistic regression are shown in Box 8.2. In addition, the assumptions for the chi-square test as shown in Box 7.2 must also be met.

Box 8.2 Assumptions for using logistic regression

The assumptions that must be met when using logistic regression are as follows:
- the sample is representative of the population to which inference will be made
- the sample size is sufficient to support the model
- the data have been collected in a period when the relationship between the outcome and the explanatory variable/s remains constant
- all important explanatory variables are included
- the explanatory variables do not have a high degree of collinearity with one another

- if an ordered categorical variable or a continuous variable is included as an explanatory variable, the effect over levels of the factor must be linear
- alternate outcome and intervening variables are not included as explanatory variables

Although the explanatory variables or predictors in the model can be continuous or categorical variables, logistic regression is best suited to measure the effects of exposures or explanatory variables that are binary variables. Continuous variables can be included but logistic regression will produce an estimate of risk for each unit of measurement. Thus, the assumption that the risk effect is linear over each unit of the variable must be met and the relationship should not be curved or have a threshold value over which the effect occurs. In addition, interactions between explanatory variables can be included but these cause the same problems of collinearity as discussed for multiple regression in Chapter 6. Logistic regression is not suitable for matched or paired data or for repeated measures because the measurements are not independent – in these situations, conditional logistic regression is used. In addition, variables that are alternative outcome variables because they are on the same pathway of development as the outcome variable must not be included as independent risk factors.

A large sample size is usually required to support a reliable binary logistic regression model because a cell is generated for each unit of the variable. The data are divided into a multi-dimension array of cells in exactly the same way as for fuctorial ANOVA shown in Table 5.6 in Chapter 5 but the outcome variable is also included in the array. If three variables each with two levels are included in the analysis, for example an outcome and two explanatory variables, the number of cells in the model will be $2 \times 2 \times 2$, or eight cells. As with chi-square analyses, a general rule of thumb is that the number of cases in any one cell should be at least 10. When there are empty cells or cells with a small number of cases, estimates of risk can become unstable and unreliable. Thus, it is important to have an adequate sample size to support the analysis.

Although SPSS provides automatic forward and backward stepwise processes for building multivariate models, it is better to build a logistic regression model using the same sequential method described for multiple regression in Chapter 6. Using this method, variables are added to the model one at a time in order of the magnitude of the chi-square association, starting with the largest estimate. At each step, changes to the model can be examined to assess collinearity and instability in the model.

If an *a priori* decision is made to include known confounders, these can be entered first into the logistic regression and the model built up from there. Alternatively, confounders can be entered at the end of the model building sequence and only retained in the model if they change the size of the coefficients of the variables already in the model by more than 10%. It is important

to decide which is the most appropriate method of entering the variables before the analysis is conducted.

At each step of adding a variable to the model, it is important to compare the
P values, the standard errors and the odds ratios in the model from Block 1 of 1
with the values from the second model in Block 2 of 2. A standard error that
increases by an important amount, say 10%, is an indication that the model
has become less precise. In this situation, the model is less stable as a result
of two or more variables having some degree of collinearity and thus sharing
variation. The effect of shared variation is to inflate the standard errors. If
this occurs, then one of the variables must be removed. If the standard error
decreases, the model has become more precise. This indicates that the variable
added to the model is a good predictor of the outcome and explains some of
the variance. As with any multivariate model, the decision of which variable
to remove or maintain is based on biological plausibility for the effect and
decisions about the variables that can be measured with most accuracy.

Research question

The risk factors for asthma in the research question can now be examined in a
multivariate model by building a logistic regression using the SPSS commands
shown in Box 8.3. Based on the magnitude of the chi square values, the
variable allergy to HDM will be entered first, then early infection and finally
gender.

Box 8.3 SPSS commands to build a logistic regression model

SPSS Commands
asthma – SPSS Data Editor
       Analyze → Regression → Binary Logistic
Logistic Regression
       Highlight Diagnosed asthma and click into Dependent
       Highlight Allergy to HDM and click into Covariates
       Method = Enter (default)
       Under Block 1 of 1, click Next
       Highlight Early infection and click into Covariates under Block 2 of 2
       Method = Enter (default)
       Click OK

Logistic regression

Model Summary

Step	−2 Log likelihood	Cox & Snell R square	Nagelkerke R square
1	2130.337	0.154	0.239

Variables in the Equation

		B	S.E.	Wald	df	Sig.	Exp(B)
Step 1[a]	HDM	2.136	0.115	347.771	1	0.000	8.468
	Constant	−4.562	0.198	530.349	1	0.000	0.010

[a] Variable(s) entered on step 1: HDM.

In the Model Summary table, the Cox and Snell R square is similar to the multiple correlation coefficient in linear regression and measures the strength of the association. This coefficient which takes sample size into consideration is based on log likelihoods and cannot reach its maximum value of 1.[4] The Nagelkerke R square is a modification of the Cox and Snell so that a value of 1 can be obtained[6]. Consequently, the Nagelkerke R square is generally higher than Cox's and has values that range between 0 and 1. In this model, the Nagelkerke R square indicates that 23.9% of the variation in diagnosed asthma is explained by HDM allergy.

The Variables in the Equation table shows the model coefficients. The B estimate for HDM allergy of 2.136 is the odds ratio in units of natural logarithms, that is to the base e. The standard error of this estimate in log units is 0.115. When adding further variables to the model, it is important that this standard error does not inflate by more than 10%. The actual odds ratio of 8.468 is shown as the anti-log (or exponential) of the B estimate in the column $\exp(B)$.

The Wald statistic in the Variables in the Equation table has a chi-square distribution and is the result of dividing the B value by its standard error and then squaring the result. This value is used to calculate the significance (P) value for each factor in the model. In logistic regression, the constant is used in the prediction of probabilities but does not have a practical interpretation.

Block 2: Method = Enter

Model Summary

Step	−2 Log likelihood	Cox & Snell R square	Nagelkerke R square
1	2125.062	0.156	0.242

Variables in the Equation

		B	S.E.	Wald	df	Sig.	Exp(B)
Step 1[a]	HDM	2.123	0.115	342.608	1	0.000	8.360
	INFECT	0.307	0.133	5.369	1	0.020	1.360
	Constant	−4.911	0.252	380.375	1	0.000	0.007

[a] Variable(s) entered on step 1: INFECT.

The Model Summary table from Block 2 shows that the Nagelkerke R square has increased slightly from 0.239 to 0.242 and the odds ratio for HDM allergy has decreased slightly from 8.467 to 8.360. Importantly, the standard error for HDM allergy has remained unchanged at 0.115 indicating that the model is stable. The odds ratio for infection, which is the exponential of the beta coefficient (B) 0.307, that is 1.36, is significant at $P = 0.02$. This estimate of risk is reduced compared to the unadjusted odds ratio obtained from the 2×2 table.

The effect of gender can be added to the model using the commands shown in Box 8.3 by entering the variables allergy to HDM and early infection for the stable model in Block 1 of 1 and entering gender in Block 2 of 2.

Logistic regression

Model Summary

Step	−2 Log likelihood	Cox & Snell R square	Nagelkerke R square
1	2124.788	0.156	0.242

Variables in the Equation

		B	S.E.	Wald	df	Sig.	Exp(B)
Step	HDM	2.118	0.115	338.103	1	0.000	8.313
1[a]	INFECT	0.302	0.133	5.155	1	0.023	1.353
	GENDER	0.058	0.110	0.274	1	0.600	1.059
	Constant	−4.985	0.289	297.409	1	0.000	0.007

[a] Variable(s) entered on step 1: GENDER.

The addition of gender does not change the R square statistics in the Model Summary table and hardly changes the odds ratio for HDM allergy in the Variables in the Equation table. The odds ratio for HDM allergy falls slightly from 8.360 to 8.313 and there is no change in the standard error of 0.115. The odds ratio for infection falls slightly from 1.360 to 1.353, again with no change in the standard error of 0.133. However, gender which was a significant risk factor in the unadjusted analysis at $P = 0.005$ is no longer significant in the model with $P = 0.60$. The unadjusted odds ratio for gender was 1.319 in bivariate analyses compared to the adjusted value which is now 1.059.

The reduction in this odds ratio suggests that there is a degree of confounding between gender and HDM allergy or infection. The extent of the confounding can be investigated using the SPSS commands in Box 7.3 with allergy to HDM and early infection entered in the rows, gender entered in the columns and column percentages requested.

Allergy to HDM * Gender

Crosstab

				Gender		Total
				Female	Male	
Allergy to HDM	No	Count		805	734	1539
		% within gender		67.8%	57.5%	62.5%
	Yes	Count		383	542	925
		% within gender		32.2%	42.5%	37.5%
Total		Count		1188	1276	2464
		% within gender		100.0%	100.0%	100.0%

Chi-Square Tests

	Value	df	Asymp. sig. (two-sided)	Exact sig. (two-sided)	Exact sig. (one-sided)
Pearson chi-square	27.499[b]	1	0.000		
Continuity correction[a]	27.064	1	0.000		
Likelihood ratio	27.600	1	0.000		
Fisher's exact test				0.000	0.000
Linear-by-linear association	27.487	1	0.000		
N of valid cases	2464				

[a] Computed only for a 2 × 2 table.
[b] 0 cell (0.0%) has expected count less than 5. The minimum expected count is 445.98.

Early infection * Gender

Crosstab

				Gender		Total
				Female	Male	
Early infection	No	Count		1016	1005	2021
		% within gender		85.5%	78.8%	82.0%
	Yes	Count		172	271	443
		% within gender		14.5%	21.2%	18.0%
Total		Count		1188	1276	2464
		% within gender		100.0%	100.0%	100.0%

Chi-Square Tests

	Value	df	Asymp. sig. (two-sided)	Exact sig. (two-sided)	Exact sig. (one-sided)
Pearson chi-square	19.065[b]	1	0.000		
Continuity correction[a]	18.610	1	0.000		

Continued

	Value	df	Asymp. sig. (two-sided)	Exact sig. (two-sided)	Exact sig. (one-sided)
Likelihood ratio	19.228	1	0.000		
Fisher's exact test				0.000	0.000
Linear-by-linear association	19.058	1	0.000		
N of valid cases	2464				

[a] Computed only for a 2 × 2 table.
[b] 0 cell (0.0%) has expected count less than 5. The minimum expected count is 213.59.

The tables show that allergy to housedust mites and early respiratory infection are both related to gender, with males having a higher percentage of allergy and early respiratory infections. Thus, gender was a risk factor in the unadjusted estimates because of confounding between gender and the other two risk factors. The logistic regression shows that once the effects of confounding are removed, gender is no longer a significant independent risk factor for diagnosed asthma.

The interpretation of this model is that boys have a higher rate of diagnosed asthma because they have a higher rate of allergy to HDM and a higher rate of early respiratory infection than girls, and not because they are male per se. Separating out the confounding and identifying the independent effects of risk factors makes an invaluable contribution towards identifying pathways to disease.

Computing confidence intervals from logistic regression output

Odds ratios should be reported with their 95% confidence intervals although the intervals are not provided in the SPSS output. The calculation is simple but it needs to take account of the fact that the odds ratio (B) and the SE are in units of natural logarithms. Few people can think in logarithmic units. Thus, once the 95% confidence intervals are calculated, the anti-log of the units needs to be obtained for presenting summary statistics in a way that increases the transparency of the results and simplifies communicating the findings.

The 95% CI can be calculated in logarithmic units as follows:

95% CI = Beta ± (1.96 × SE)

and then the antilog of the two values can be calculated. This can be undertaken in an Excel spreadsheet as shown in Table 8.6. The beta coefficients and the standard errors (SE) are taken directly from the SPSS output. The formulae that are used to calculate the 95% confidence intervals around the odds ratios derived from SPSS are shown below, where exp indicates an exponential conversion. In Excel, clicking on Insert and then Function, the exponential function is listed as EXP under the Math and Trig Function Category.

Odds ratio = exp (beta)
  Lower CI = exp (beta − 1.96 × SE)
  Upper CI = exp (beta + 1.96 × SE)
Width down = odds ratio − lower CI
  Width up = upper CI − odds ratio

Table 8.6 Excel spreadsheet to compute confidence intervals around odds ratios derived from logistic regression

	Beta	SE	1.96 × SE	Odds ratio	Lower	Upper	Width down	Width up
HDM	2.118	0.115	0.225	8.313	6.637	10.417	1.678	2.102
Infection	0.302	0.133	0.261	1.353	1.042	1.755	0.310	0.403
Gender	0.058	0.11	0.216	1.059	0.854	1.315	0.206	0.255

Reporting the results

When reporting odds ratios from any type of study design, the percentages from which they are derived must also be reported so that the level of exposure can be used to interpret the findings. In this research question, the data were derived from a cross-sectional study and thus it is important to report the proportion of children who had asthma in the groups that were exposed or not exposed to the risk factors of interest as shown in Table 8.7. In a case–control study, it would be important to report the per cent of participants in the case and control groups who were exposed to the factors of interest. It is also important to report the unadjusted and adjusted values so that the importance of confounding factors is clear. The adjusted odds ratios from the binary logistic regression are smaller but provide an estimate that is not biased by confounding.

Table 8.7 Unadjusted and adjusted risk factors for children to have asthma

Risk factor	Exposed % with asthma	Non-exposed % with asthma	Unadjusted odds ratio (95% CI)	Adjusted odds ratio (95% CI)	P value
HDM allergy	42.8%	8.1%	8.5 (6.8, 10.6)	8.3 (6.6, 10.4)	<0.0001
Early infection	27.5%	19.7%	1.5 (1.2, 2.0)	1.4 (1.0, 1.8)	0.023
Gender	23.4%	18.8%	1.4 (1.1, 1.6)	1.1 (0.9, 1.3)	0.600

Odds ratios are multiplicative. Table 8.7 shows that the odds ratio for the association between childhood asthma and allergy to HDM is 8.3. However, the odds ratio for children to have diagnosed asthma is they are exposed to both allergy to HDM and to an early respiratory infection compared to the odds they are not exposed to either risk factor is 8.3 × 1.4, or 11.6.

Plotting the results in a figure

The lower and upper 95% confidence intervals have different widths as a result of being computed in logarithmic units, therefore they need to be overlaid as separate plots when using SigmaPlot as shown in Box 8.4. The estimates of odds ratios and confidence interval widths obtained in Excel can be entered into SigmaPlot worksheet with the odds ratio in column 1, the width down in column 2 and the width up in column 3 as follows:

Column 1	Column 2	Column 3
8.314	1.678	2.102
1.353	0.310	0.403
1.060	0.206	0.255

The graph can then be plotted using the commands shown in Box 8.4.

Box 8.4 SigmaPlot commands to plot odds ratios

SigmaPlot Commands
SigmaPlot – [Data 1*]
         Graph → Create Graph
Create Graph - Type
         Highlight Scatter Plot, click Next
Create Graph - Style
         Highlight Horizontal Error Bars, click Next
Create Graph – Error Bars
         Symbol Values = Worksheet Columns (default), click Next
Create Graph – Data Format
         Data Format — Highlight Many X, click Next
Create Graph – Select Data
         Data for Bar = use drop box and select Column 1
         Data for Error = use drop box and select Column 2
         Click Finish

The sequence is then repeated in *Graph → Add Plot* with column 1 again as the data for the bar and column 3 as the data for the error. Once this basic graph is obtained, the labels, symbols, axes, ticks and labels can be customised under the *Graph → Options* menus to obtain Figure 8.3. The x-axis needs to be a logarithmic base 10 scale, the first plot should have negative error bars only and the second plot should have positive error bars only.

Figure 8.3 shows the relative importance of the odds ratios. Early infection and allergy to HDM are significant risk factors which is reflected by their 95%

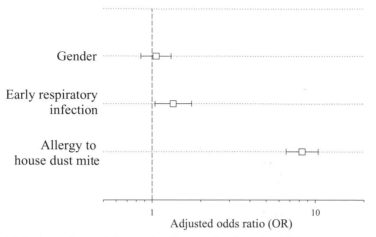

Figure 8.3 Independent risk factors for diagnosed asthma in children.

confidence intervals not crossing the line of no effect (unity). For gender, the odds ratio is close to unity and the confidence intervals lie on either side of the line of unity indicating an effect from protection to risk, which is therefore ambiguous.

Relative risk

Relative risk can only be used when the sample is randomly selected from the population and cannot be used in other studies, such as case–control studies or some clinical trials, in which the percentage of the sample with the disease is determined by the sampling method.

If the summary data shown in Table 8.4 had been collected from a random sample the relative risk would be calculated as follows:

$$\text{Relative risk} = a/(a+c)/b/(b+d)$$
$$= (40/100)/(25/100)$$
$$= 1.6$$

Thus the risk estimates are calculated by dividing the per cent of disease positive cases in one row by the per cent of disease positive cases in the other row. The calculation shows how the odds ratio of 2.0 calculated previously with the same data can overestimate the relative risk of 1.6.

In requesting risk statistics in conjunction with a 2 × 2 table in SPSS, three estimates are shown in the Risk Estimate table. The first set of statistics is the odds ratio and the next two sets of estimates are labelled 'For cohort = No' and 'For cohort = Yes'. If the 2 × 2 table is set up appropriately, one of these two statistics is the relative risk. If the 2 × 2 table is not set up appropriately, relative risk has to be computed from the risk estimates.

For obtaining relative risk in SPSS, the crosstabulation table needs to be set up with the outcome in the columns, the risk factor in the rows and the row percentages requested. If a table is constructed in this way, then either of the following two options can be used.

Option 1
The risk factor but not the outcome has to be re-coded with the exposure present (yes) coded as 1 and the exposure absent (no) coded as 2.

On the spreadsheet **asthma.sav**, allergy to HDM has been re-coded in this way into the variable HDM2. This coding is exactly opposite to the coding needed to easily interpret the output from logistic and linear regressions. This coding scheme will 'invert' the crosstabulation table so that the positive exposure is shown on the top row and no exposure is shown on the row below. This table with HDM allergy re-coded, which was shown previously, is shown again below. The relative risk can then be calculated as the row percentage for positive outcome divided by the row percentage for negative outcome, that is 42.8/8.1 or 5.28. This statistic is given in the line 'For cohort = Yes', with a negligible difference from the calculated value resulting from rounding of decimal places.

Crosstabs

Allergy to HDM – Re-coded * Diagnosed Asthma Crosstabulation

			Diagnosed asthma		
			No	Yes	Total
Allergy to HDM – recoded	Allergy	Count	529	396	925
		% within allergy to HDM – recoded	57.2%	42.8%	100.0%
	No allergy	Count	1414	125	1539
		% within allergy to HDM – recoded	91.9%	8.1%	100.0%
Total		Count	1943	521	2464
		% within allergy to HDM – recoded	78.9%	21.1%	100.0%

Risk Estimate

	Value	95% confidence interval	
		Lower	Upper
Odds ratio for HDM allergy – recoded (allergy/no allergy)	0.118	0.094	0.148
For cohort diagnosed asthma = no	0.622	0.588	0.659
For cohort diagnosed asthma = yes	5.271	4.386	6.334
N of valid cases	2464		

In the Risk Estimate table, 'For cohort diagnosed asthma = yes' shows the relative risk for children to have diagnosed asthma in the presence of HDM allergy is 5.271 (95% CI 4.386, 6.334). As with odds ratio, only the number of decimal places that infer a precision that can be interpreted is reported so the risk estimates from this table would be reported as a relative risk of 5.3 (95% CI 4.4, 6.3).

Option 2

If the risk factor for exposure is maintained as coded as 1 for exposure absent (no) and 2 for exposure present (yes), then the table that was obtained previously is shown again below.

Allergy to HDM * Diagnosed Asthma Crosstabulation

			Diagnosed asthma		
			No	Yes	Total
Allergy to HDM	No	Count	1414	125	1539
		% within allergy to HDM	91.9%	8.1%	100.0%
	Yes	Count	529	396	925
		% within allergy to HDM	57.2%	42.8%	100.0%
Total		Count	1943	521	2464
		% within allergy to HDM	78.9%	21.1%	100.0%

Risk Estimate

	Value	95% confidence interval	
		Lower	Upper
Odds ratio for allergy to HDM (no/yes)	8.468	6.765	10.600
For cohort diagnosed asthma = no	1.607	1.516	1.702
For cohort diagnosed asthma = yes	0.190	0.158	0.228
N of valid cases	2464		

In this case, the relative risk shown in the table is calculated as 8.1/42.8, or 0.190 and is in the direction of protection. The estimate in the direction of risk and the 95% confidence interval can be computed as the reciprocal of the estimates given for 'For cohort diagnosed asthma = yes' as follows:

$1/0.190 = 5.263$
$1/0.158 = 6.329$
$1/0.228 = 4.386$

Thus, the relative risk for children to have asthma in the presence of HDM allergy is 5.3 (95% CI 4.4, 6.3), which is identical to using the first option.

For both options, the estimate 'For cohort ... = no' is the relative risk of children having diagnosed asthma in the group that is not exposed to the risk factor of interest. This statistic is rarely used.

Number needed to be exposed for one additional person to be harmed

In epidemiological studies in which the influence of an exposure is described by an odds ratio, inclusion of the statistic number needed to be exposed for one additional person to be harmed (NNEH) can be a useful statistic that applies to a person rather than to a sample. As such, this statistic provides the number of people who need to be exposed to the risk factor of interest to cause harm to one additional person.

As with calculating NNT in Chapter 7, NNEH is calculated from a 2 × 2 table in which both the outcome and the exposure are coded as binary variables. The statistic NNEH can be easily calculated from a 2 × 2 crosstabulation in which the outcome is entered in the rows, the exposure is entered in the columns and the column percentages are requested. The statistic NNEH is then calculated from the absolute risk increase (ARI), which is simply the difference in the proportion of participants with the outcome of interest in the exposed and unexposed groups. From the tables for asthma and HDM allergy:

$$ARI = 0.43 - 0.08 = 0.35$$
$$NNEH = 1/ARI = 1/0.35 = 2.9$$

This indicates that for every three children with allergy to housedust mites, one additional child will be diagnosed with asthma. NNEH is only reported to whole numbers.

For early infection

$$ARI = 0.275 - 0.197 = 0.078$$
$$NNEH = 1/ARR = 1/0.078 = 12.8$$

This indicates that for every 13 children who have respiratory infection in early life, one additional child will be diagnosed with asthma. Obviously, the larger the odds ratio, the fewer the number of people who need to be exposed to cause harm.

Notes for critical appraisal

When critically appraising an article that reports risk statistics, it is important to ask the questions shown in Box 8.5.

Box 8.5 Questions to ask when critically appraising the literature in which risk statistics are presented

The following questions should be asked of studies that report risk statistics:
- If relative risk is reported, was the sample randomly selected?
- Have the proportions of disease in the exposed and non-exposed groups been reported in addition to the odds ratio or relative risk?
- Is it difficult to compare estimates if some of the factors are presented as risk factors and others as protective factors?
- Are confidence intervals presented for all estimates of odds ratio or relative risk?
- Can all of the variables in the model be classified as independent exposure factors or have alternative outcomes and intervening variables also been included?
- What type of method was used to build the logistic regression model and was collinearity between variables tested?

References

1. Guyatt G, Rennie D, Users guides to the medical literature—a manual for evidence based clinical practice by the Evidence-Based Medicine Working Group Chicago, USA: AMA Press, 2001; pp 356–357.
2. Bland JM, Altman DG. The odds ratio. BMJ 2000; 320: 1468.
3. Deeks J. When can odds ratios mislead. BMJ 1998; 317: 1155–1156.
4. Peat JK. Can asthma be prevented? Evidence from epidemiological studies in children in Australia and New Zealand in the last decade. Clin Exp Allergy 1998; 28: 261–265.
5. Wright RE. Logistic Regression. In: Reading and understanding multivariate statistics, Grimm LG, Yarnold PR (editors). Washington, USA: American Psychological Association, 1995; p. 217.
6. Tabachnick BG, Fidell LS. Testing hypotheses in multiple regression. In: Using multivariate statistics (4th edition). Boston, MA: Allyn and Bacon, 2001; pp 545–546.

CHAPTER 9

Categorical and continuous variables: tests of agreement

Truth cannot be defined or tested by agreement with 'the world'; for not only do truths differ for different worlds but the nature of agreement between a world apart from it is notoriously nebulous.

NELSON GOODMAN, PHILOSOPHER

Objectives

The objectives of the chapter are to explain how to:
- measure repeatability of categorical information collected by questionnaires
- measure the repeatability of continuous measurements
- critically appraise the literature that reports tests of agreement

Repeatability

Questionnaires are often tested for repeatability, which is an aspect of measuring agreement. Repeatability is an important issue especially when new instruments are being developed. In any type of research study, measurements that are accurate (repeatable) provide more reliable information. However, studies of repeatability must be conducted in a setting in which they do not produce a false impression of the accuracy of the measurement. Box 9.1 shows the

Box 9.1 Assumptions for measuring repeatability

The following methods must be used when measuring repeatability:
- the method of administration must be identical on each occasion
- at the second administration, both the participant and the rater (observer) must have no knowledge of the results of the first measurement
- the time to the second administration should be short enough so that the condition has not changed since the first administration
- if a questionnaire is being tested, the time between administrations must be long enough for participants to have forgotten their previous responses
- the setting in which repeatability is established must be the same as the setting in which the questionnaire or measurement will be used

assumptions under which the repeatability of categorical measurements and continuous measurements are tested. All of the assumptions relate to study design.

If a questionnaire is to be used in a community setting, then repeatability has to be established in a similar community setting and not for example in a clinic setting where the patients form a well-defined sub-sample of a population. Patients who frequently answer questions about their illness may have well rehearsed responses to questions and may provide an artificial estimate of repeatability when compared to people in the general population who rarely consider aspects of an illness that they do not have.

Repeatability of categorical data

Questionnaires are widely used in research studies to obtain information of personnel characteristics, illnesses and exposure to environmental factors. For a questionnaire to be a useful research tool, the responses must be repeatable, that is they must not have a substantial amount of measurement error. To test repeatability, the questionnaire is administered to the same people on two separate occasions. An important concept is that the condition that the questionnaire is designed to measure must not have changed in the period between administrations and the time period must be long enough for the participants to have little recollection of their previous responses. Repeatability is then measured as the proportion of responses in agreement on the two occasions using the statistic kappa.

Kappa is used to test the agreement between observers or between administrations for both binary and nominal scales. For data with three or more possible responses or for ordered categorical data, weighted kappa should be used. Kappa is an estimate of the proportion in agreement between two administrations or two observers in excess of the agreement that would occur by chance. A value of 1 indicates perfect agreement and a value of 0 indicates no agreement. In general, values less than 0.40 indicate poor agreement, values between 0.41 and 0.60 indicate moderate agreement, values between 0.61 and 0.80 indicate good agreement and above 0.81 indicate very good agreement[1].

Research question

The file **questionnaires. sav** contains the data of three questions which required a yes or no response. The questions were administered on two occasions to the same 50 people at an interval of 3 weeks. The research aim was to measure the repeatability of the questions. It is often important to establish how repeatable questions are because questions that are prone to a significant amount of random error or bias do not make good outcome or explanatory variables. The SPSS commands shown in Box 9.2 can be used to obtain repeatability statistics.

This command sequence can then be repeated to obtain the following tables and statistics for questions 2 and 3 of the questionnaire.

Box 9.2 SPSS commands to measure repeatability

SPSS Commands
questionnaires – SPSS Data Editor
    Analyze → Descriptive Statistics → Crosstabs
Crosstabs
    Highlight Question 1-time 1 and click into Row(s)
    Highlight Question1-time 2 and click into Column(s)
    Click on Statistics
Crosstabs: Statistics
    Tick Kappa, tick Continue
Crosstabs
    Click on Cells
Crosstabs: Cell Display
    Tick Observed under Counts (default), tick Total under Percentages
    Click Continue
Crosstabs
    Click OK

Crosstabs

Question 1 - Time 1 * Question 1 - Time 2 Crosstabulation

			Question 1 - time 2		
			No	Yes	Total
Question 1- time 1	No	Count	20	15	35
		% of total	40.0%	30.0%	70.0%
	Yes	Count	4	11	15
		% of total	8.0%	22.0%	30.0%
Total		Count	24	26	50
		% of total	48.0%	52.0%	100.0%

Symmetric Measures

	Value	Asymp. std. error[a]	Approx. T[b]	Approx. sig.
Measure of agreement Kappa	0.252	0.123	1.977	0.048
N of valid cases	50			

[a.] Not assuming the null hypothesis.
[b.] Using the asymptotic standard error assuming the null hypothesis.

From the Crosstabulation, the proportion in agreement is estimated from the per cent in the concordant No at Time 1-No at Time 2 and Yes at Time 1-Yes at Time 2 cells. Thus the proportion in agreement is 40% + 22%, or 0.62 as a proportion. The Symmetric Measures table shows that the kappa value is low at 0.252 indicating poor repeatability after agreement by chance is taken into account. Kappa is always lower than the proportion in agreement.

Although a *P* value is included in the Symmetric Measures table, it is not a good indication of agreement because its interpretation is that the kappa value is significantly different from zero. Measurements taken from the same people on two occasions in order to assess repeatability are highly related by nature and thus the *P* value is expected to indicate some degree of agreement. The standard error is also reported and can be used to calculate a confidence interval around kappa but this is also of little interest.

Crosstabs

Question 2 - Time 1* Question 2 - Time 2 Crosstabulation

| | | | Question 2 - time 2 | | Total |
			No	Yes	
Question 2 -time 1	No	Count	34	5	39
		% of total	68.0%	10.0%	78.0%
	Yes	Count	6	5	11
		% of total	12.0%	10.0%	22.0%
Total		Count	40	10	50
		% of total	80.0%	20.0%	100.0%

Symmetric Measures

	Value	Asymp. std. error[a]	Approx. T[b]	Approx. sig.
Measure of agreement Kappa	0.337	0.159	2.390	0.017
N of valid cases	50			

[a.] Not assuming the null hypothesis.
[b.] Using the asymptotic standard error assuming the null hypothesis.

Crosstabs

Question 3 - Time 1 * Question 3 - Time 2 Crosstabulation

| | | | Question 3 - time 2 | | Total |
			No	Yes	
Question 3 -time 1	No	Count	17	5	22
		% of total	34.0%	10.0%	44.0%
	Yes	Count	6	22	28
		% of total	12.0%	44.0%	56.0%
Total		Count	23	27	50
		% of total	46.0%	54.0%	100.0%

Symmetric Measures

	Value	Asymp. std. error[a]	Approx. T[b]	Approx. sig.
Measure of agreement Kappa	0.556	0.118	3.933	0.000
N of valid cases	50			

[a.] Not assuming the null hypothesis.
[b.] Using the asymptotic standard error assuming the null hypothesis.

In the second Crosstabulation table, the percentage in agreement is 68% + 10%, or 0.78 as a proportion, and kappa is higher than in the first table at 0.337. Although the percentage in agreement in the third table is 34% + 44%, also 0.78 as a proportion, kappa is higher than in the second table at 0.556 and the P value increases in significance from 0.017 to <0.001. Thus, kappa varies for the same proportion in agreement. With a higher proportion of Yes replies (56% for question 3 compared with 22% for question 2), kappa increases from poor to moderate range.

A feature of kappa is that the value increases as the proportion of 'No' and 'Yes' responses become more equal and when the proportion in agreement remains the same. This feature is a major barrier to comparing kappa values. For this reason, the value of kappa, the percentage of positive responses and the proportion in agreement must all be reported to help assess repeatability.

Reporting the results

Information about the repeatability of the three questions can be reported as shown in Table 9.1. It is difficult to say which question is the most repeatable and has the least non-systematic bias because all three questions have a different percentage of positive responses and therefore the kappa values cannot be compared. However, both questions 2 and 3 have a higher proportion in agreement than question 1. The differences in percentages suggest that the three questions are measuring different entities.

Table 9.1 Repeatability for three questions administered to 50 people at a 3-week interval

	Percentage of positive responses at time 1	Percentage of positive responses at time 2	Proportion in agreement	Kappa
Question 1	30%	52%	0.62	0.25
Question 2	22%	20%	0.78	0.34
Question 3	56%	54%	0.78	0.56

Repeatability of continuous measurements

Continuous measurements must also have a high degree of repeatability to be useful as a research tool. Variations in continuous measurements can result from inconsistent measurement practices, from equipment variation or from ways in which results are read or interpreted. These sources can be measured as within-observer (intra-observer) variation, between-observer (inter-observer) variation or within-subject variation. Variations that result from the ways in which researchers administer, read or interpret tests are within- or between-observer variations. Variations that arise from patient compliance factors or from biological changes are within-subject variations. To quantify these measurement errors, the same measurement is taken from the same participant on two occasions or from the same participant by two observers and the results are compared.

Research question

The file **observer-weights.sav** contains data from 32 babies who had their weight measured by two nurses who had no knowledge of each other's measurements. The weights measured by both nurses could be plotted against each other in a scatter plot. However, it is best that a Pearson's correlation coefficient is not used to describe repeatability because it does not make sense to test the hypothesis that two measurements taken from the same babies using the same equipment are related to one another[2]. In addition, a second measurement that is, for example, twice as large as the first measurement would have perfect correlation but poor agreement.

To estimate the measurement error, the *Transform → Compute* command is first used to calculate the mean of the two measurements for each baby using the *Mean* function and then the difference between the two measurements as a simple subtraction, that is measurement 1 – measurement 2 is calculated with this command. The subtraction can be in either direction but the direction must be indicated in the summary results and graphs. The two new variables are created at the end of the data sheet and should be labelled as mean and differences respectively.

The size of the measurement error can then be calculated from the standard deviation around the differences, which can be obtained using the *Analyze → Descriptive Statistics → Descriptives* commands with the differences variable entered as the *Variable(s)*.

Descriptives

Descriptive Statistics

	N	Minimum	Maximum	Mean	Std. deviation
Differences	32	−0.10	0.15	0.0125	0.06792
Valid *N* (listwise)	32				

The mean of the differences is 0.0125 and gives an estimate of the amount of bias between the two measurements. In this case, the measurements taken by nurse 1 are on average 0.0125 kg higher than nurse 2, which is a small difference. A problem with using the mean value is that large positive and large negative differences are balanced and therefore negated. However, the mean $\pm$ 1.96 SD can also be calculated from this table. This range is calculated as $0.0125 \pm (1.96 \times 0.0679)$, or -0.12 to 0.15 and is called the limits of agreement[3]. The limits of agreement indicate the interval in which 95% of the differences lie.

The mean and difference values can be plotted as a differences-vs-means plot to show whether the measurement error as estimated by the differences is related to the size of the measurement as estimated by the mean[4]. The shape of the scatter conveys important information about the repeatability of the measurements. A scatter that is evenly distributed above and below the zero line of no difference indicates that there is no systematic bias between the two observers. A scatter that is largely above or largely below the zero line of no difference or a scatter that increases or decreases with the mean value indicates a systematic bias between observers[5].

The values for the means and differences can be copied and pasted from SPSS to SigmaPlot and the figure can be created using the commands shown in Box 9.3. A recommendation for the axes of differences-vs-means plots is that the y-axis should be approximately one-third to one-half of the length of the x-axis[5].

Box 9.3 SigmaPlot commands to create a differences-vs-means plot

SigmaPlot Commands
SigmaPlot – [Data 1*]
Graph → Create Graph
Create Graph – Type
    Highlight Scatter Plot, click Next
Create Graph – Styles
    Highlight Simple Scatter, click Next
Create Graph – Data Format
    Under Data format, highlight XY pair, click Next
Create Graph – Select Data
    Highlight Column 1, click into Data for X
    Highlight Column 2, click into Data for Y
    Click Finish

The lines for the mean difference and limits of agreement can be added by typing the x coordinates in column 3 and y coordinates of the lines into columns 4 to 6 and adding three line plots by using the SigmaPlot commands *Graph → Add Plot → Line Plot → Simple Straight Line → XY Pair* options with x as column 3 each time and each y column. The columns for the coordinate data are as follows:

Column 3	Column 4	Column 5	Column 6
3.5	0.0125	−0.12	0.15
6.0	0.0125	−0.12	0.15

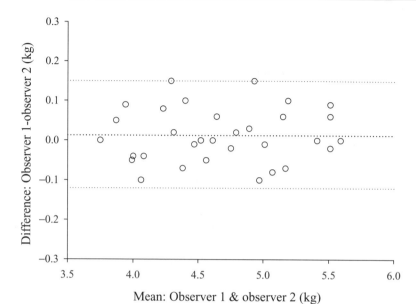

Figure 9.1 Differences-vs-means plot.

Figure 9.1 shows only a small amount of random error that is evenly scattered around the line of no difference and shows that most of the differences are within 0.1 kg. A wide scatter would indicate a large amount of measurement error. A Kendall's correlation coefficient between the means and the differences can be obtained using the commands shown in Box 6.3 in Chapter 6.

Non-parametric correlations

Correlations

			Differences	Mean
Kendall's tau_b	Differences	Correlation coefficient	1.000	0.045
		Sig. (two-tailed)	.	0.721
		N	32	32
	Mean	Correlation coefficient	0.045	1.000
		Sig. (two-tailed)	0.721	.
		N	32	32

The almost negligible correlation of 0.045 with a *P* value of 0.721 confirms the uniformity of variance in the repeated measurements. A systematic bias between the two measurements could be inspected using a paired t-test or a non-parametric rank sums test.

A more useful statistic to describe repeatability is to first calculate the measurement error from the standard deviation of the differences of observations in the same subject[3]. This is calculated as:

$$
\begin{aligned}
\text{Measurement error} &= \text{SD of differences}/\sqrt{2} \\
&= 0.06792/1.414 \\
&= 0.048 \text{ kg}
\end{aligned}
$$

This error can then be converted to a range by multiplying by a critical value of 1.96.

$$
\begin{aligned}
\text{Error range} &= \text{Measurement error} \times \text{Critical value} \\
&= 0.048 \times 1.96 \\
&= 0.09 \text{ kg}
\end{aligned}
$$

The error range indicates that the average of all possible measurements of a baby's weight is within the range of 0.09 kg above and 0.09 kg below the actual measurement taken. Thus for a baby with a measured weight of 4.01 kg, the average of all possible weights, which are expected to be close to the true weight, would be within the range 3.92 to 4.10 kg.

Intra-class correlation

The intra-class correlation coefficient (ICC) can be used to describe the relative extent to which two continuous measurements taken by different people or two measurements taken by the same person on different occasions are related. The advantage of ICC is that, unlike Pearson's correlation, a value of unity is only obtained when the two measurements are identical to one another. A high value of ICC of 0.95 indicates that 95% of the variance in the measurement is due to the true variance between the participants and 5% of the variance is due to measurement error or the variance within the participants or the observers. The SPSS commands to obtain ICC are shown in Box 9.4.

Box 9.4 SPSS commands to measure repeatability

SPSS Commands
observer-weights – SPSS Data Editor
  Analyze → Scale → Reliability Analysis
Reliability Analysis
  Highlight Weight–observer 1 and Weight–observer 2 and click into
   Items box
  Click Statistics

Reliability Analysis: Statistics
     Tick Intraclass correlation coefficient,
     Model: Two-Way Mixed (default)
     Type: Consistency (default)
     Test Value: 0 (default), click Continue
Reliability Analysis
     Click OK

Reliability

RELIABILITY ANALYSIS - SCALE (ALPHA)
              Intraclass Correlation Coefficients
        Two-Way Mixed Effects Model (Consistency Definition)

Measure	ICC Value	95% Confidence Interval Lower Bound	Upper Bound	F-Value	Sig.
Single Rater	.9922	.9841	.9962	255.4797	.0000
Average of Raters*	.9961	.9920	.9981	255.4797	.0000

Degrees of freedom for F-tests are 31 and 31. Test Value = 0.

* Assumes absence of People*Rater interaction.

Reliability Coefficients

N of Cases =   32.0   N of Items = 2
Alpha =   .9961

In this example, there are two raters (observers) and the ICC is 0.9961, that is less than 1% of the variance is explained by within-subject differences. The 95% confidence interval around an ICC is rarely used and the significance of the ICC is of no importance because it is expected that two measurements taken from the same person are highly related.

When reporting the results, the differences-vs-means plot gives the most informative description of agreement or repeatability. Additional information of the mean difference, the limits of agreement and the 95% range are direct measures of agreement between two continuous measurements whereas the intra-class correlation coefficient is a relative measure of agreement. All of these statistics should be included when reporting information of the agreement or repeatability between two measurements because they all convey relevant information.

Notes for critical appraisal

Paired measurements to estimate agreement must be treated appropriately when analysing the data. When critically appraising an article that presents these types of statistics, it is important to ask the questions shown in Box 9.5.

Box 9.5 Questions for critical appraisal

The following questions should be asked when appraising published results from paired categorical follow-up data or data collected to estimate the repeatability of questionnaire responses or continuous measurements:
- Is the sample size large enough to have confidence in the summary estimates?

For repeatability of categorical data:
- Is the percentage of positive or negative responses and proportion in agreement included in addition to kappa?
- Are kappa values inappropriately compared?

For repeatability of continuous measurements:
- Have a differences-vs-means plot, the limits of agreement, a 95% range and the intra-class correlation been reported?
- Is Pearson's correlation used inappropriately?

References

1. Altman DG. Inter-rater agreement in practical statistics for medical research. London, UK: Chapman and Hall 1996; pp 403–409.
2. Bland JM, Altman DG. Measurement error and correlation coefficients. BMJ 1996; 313: 41–42.
3. Bland JM, Altman DG. Measurement error. BMJ 1996; 313: 744.
4. Bland JM, Altman DG. Statistical methods for assessing agreement between two methods of clinical measurement. Lancet 1986; 1: 307–310.
5. Peat JK, Mellis CM, Williams K, Xuan W. Health science research: a handbook of quantitative methods. Crows Nest, Australia: Allen and Unwin, 2002; pp 205–229.

CHAPTER 10

Categorical and continuous variables: diagnostic statistics

Like dreams, statistics are a form of wish fulfilment.
JEAN BAUDRILLARD (b. 1929), FRENCH SEMIOLOGIST

Objectives

The objectives of the chapter are to explain how to:
• compute sensitivity, specificity and likelihood ratios
• understand the limitations of positive and negative predictive values
• select cut-off points for screening and diagnostic tests
• critically appraise studies that use or evaluate diagnostic tests

In clinical practice it is important to know how well diagnostic tests, such as x-rays, biopsies or blood and urine tests, can predict that a patient has a certain condition or disease. The statistics positive predictive value (PPV), negative predictive value (NPV), sensitivity and specificity are all used to estimate the utility of a test in predicting the presence of a condition or a disease. A statistic that combines the utility of sensitivity and specificity is the likelihood ratio (LR). If the outcome of the diagnostic test is binary, a likelihood ratio can be calculated directly. If the test result is on a continuous scale, a receiver operating characteristic (ROC) curve is used to determine the point that maximises the LR.

Diagnostic statistics are part of a group of statistics used to describe agreement between two measurements. However, these statistics should only be calculated when there is a 'gold standard' to measure the presence or absence of disease against which the test can be compared. If a gold diagnostic standard does not exist, a proxy gold standard may need to be justified[1]. In this situation, the test being evaluated must not be included in the definition of the gold standard[1]. In measuring the diagnostic utility of a test, the person interpreting the test measurement must have no knowledge of the disease status of each patient.

Coding

For diagnostic statistics, it is best to code the variable indicating disease status as 1 for disease present as measured by the gold standard or test positive and

2 for disease absent or test negative. This coding will produce a table with the rows and columns in the order shown in Table 10.1. In this table, the row and column order is the reverse of that used to calculate an odds ratio from a 2 × 2 crosstabulation but is identical to the coding shown in Table 8.1 in Chapter 8 which is frequently used in clinical epidemiology textbooks.

Table 10.1 Coding for diagnostic statistics

	Disease present	Disease absent	Total
Test positive	*a*	*b*	*a + b*
Test negative	*c*	*d*	*c + d*
Total	*a + c*	*b + d*	*N*

Positive and negative predictive values

In estimating the utility of a test, PPV is the proportion of patients who are test positive and in whom the disease is present and NPV is the proportion of patients who are test negative and in whom the disease is absent. These statistics indicate the probability that the test will make a correct diagnosis[2]. Both PPV and NPV are statistics that predict from the test to the disease and indicate the probability that patients will or will not have a disease if they have a positive or negative diagnostic test. Intuitively, it would seem that PPV and NPV would be the most useful statistics; however, they have serious limitations in their interpretations[2].

The statistics PPV and NPV should only be calculated if the study sample is from a population and not if groups of patients and healthy people are recruited independently, which is often the case. From Table 10.1, the PPV and NPV can be calculated as follows:

$$PPV = a/(a + b)$$
$$NPV = d/(c + d)$$

Research question

The file **xray.sav** contains the data from 150 patients who had an x-ray for a bone fracture. A positive x-ray means that a fracture appears to be present on the x-ray, and a negative x-ray means that there is no indication of a fracture on the x-ray. The presence or absence of a fracture was later confirmed during surgery. Thus surgery is the 'gold standard' for deciding whether or not a fracture was present. The research question is how accurate are x-rays in predicting fractures in people. In computing diagnostic statistics, a hypothesis is not being tested so that the P value for the crosstabulation has little meaning.

Diagnostic statistics of PPV and NPV are computed using the SPSS commands shown in Box 10.1 with row percentages requested because PPV and NPV are calculated as proportions of the test positive patients and test negative patients who have the disease. In SPSS, PPV and NPV are not produced directly or labelled as such but can be simply derived from the row percentages. Although the figures are given in percentages, diagnostic statistics are more commonly reported as proportions, that is, in decimal form.

Box 10.1 SPSS commands to compute diagnostic statistics

SPSS Commands
xray - SPSS Data Editor
Analyze → Descriptive Statistics → Crosstabs
Crosstabs
       Highlight Xray results (test) and click into Row(s)
       Highlight Fracture detected by surgery (disease) and click into Column(s)
       Click on Statistics
Crosstabs: Statistics
       Check all boxes are empty, click Continue
Crosstabs
       Click on Cells
Crosstabs: Cell Display
       Under Percentages tick Row, tick Continue
       Click OK

Crosstab

X-ray Results * Fracture Detected by Surgery Crosstabulation

			Fracture detected by surgery (disease)		
			Present	Absent	Total
X-ray results (test)	Positive	Count	36	24	60
		% within x-ray results	60.0%	40.0%	100.0%
	Negative	Count	8	82	90
		% within x-ray results	8.9%	91.1%	100.0%
Total		Count	44	106	150
		% within x-ray results	29.3%	70.7%	100.0%

From the crosstabulation the row percentages are used and are simply converted to a proportion by dividing by 100.

Positive predictive value = 0.60 (i.e. 36/60)

Negative predictive value = 0.91 (i.e. 82/90)

This indicates that 0.60 of patients who had a positive x-ray had a fracture and 0.91 who had a negative x-ray did not have a fracture.

To measure the certainty of diagnostic statistics, confidence intervals for PPV and NPV can be calculated as for any proportion. If the confidence interval around a proportion contains a value less than zero, exact confidence intervals based on the binomial distribution should be used rather than asymptotic statistics based on a normal distribution[3]. The formula for calculating the standard error around a proportion was shown in Chapter 7. The Excel spreadsheet shown in Table 10.2 can be used to calculate 95% confidence intervals for PPV and NPV. The confidence interval for PPV is based on the total number of patients who have a positive test result and the confidence interval for NPV is based on the total number of patients who have a negative test result.

Table 10.2 Excel spreadsheet to calculate 95% confidence intervals

	Proportion	*N*	SE	Width	CI lower	CI upper
PPV	0.6	60	0.063	0.124	0.476	0.724
NPV	0.91	90	0.030	0.059	0.851	0.969

The interpretation of the 95% confidence interval for PPV is that with 95% confidence, 47.6% to 72.4% of patients with a positive x-ray will have a fracture. The interpretation of the 95% confidence interval for NPV is that with 95% confidence, 85.1% to 96.9% of patients with a negative x-ray will not have a fracture. Confidence intervals should be interpreted taking the sample size into account. The larger the sample size, the narrower the confidence intervals will be.

Although PPV and NPV seem intuitive to interpret, both statistics vary with changes in the proportion of patients in the sample who are disease positive. Thus, these statistics can only be applied to the study sample or to a sample with the same proportion of disease positive and disease negative patients. For this reason, PPV and NPV are not commonly used in clinical practice. Box 10.2 shows why these statistics are limited in their interpretation.

Box 10.2 Limitations in the interpretation of positive and negative predictive values

Positive and negative predictive values:
- are strongly influenced by the proportion of patients who are disease positive
- increase when the per cent of patients who have the disease in the sample is high and decrease when the per cent who have the disease is small
- cannot be applied or generalised to other clinical settings with different patient profiles
- cannot be compared between different diagnostic tests

In practice, the statistics PPV and NPV are only useful in settings in which the per cent of patients who have the disease present is the same as the prevalence of the disease in the population. This naturally rules out most clinical settings.

Sensitivity and specificity

The statistics that are most often used to describe the utility of diagnostic tests in clinical applications are sensitivity, specificity[4] and likelihood ratio[5]. These diagnostic statistics can be computed from Table 10.1 as follows:

Sensitivity $= a/(a+c)$
Specificity $= d/(b+d)$
Likelihood ratio $=$ Sensitivity$/(1 -$ specificity$)$

Sensitivity indicates how likely patients are to have a positive test if they have the disease and specificity indicates how likely the patients are to have a negative test if they do not have the disease. In this sense, these two statistics describe the proportion of patients in each disease category who are test positive or negative. Although the usefulness of these statistics is not as intuitive, sensitivity and specificity have advantages over PPV and NPV as shown in Box 10.3.

Box 10.3 Advantages of using sensitivity and specificity to describe the application of diagnostic tests

The advantages of using sensitivity and specificity to describe diagnostic tests are that these statistics:
• do not alter if the prevalence of disease is different between clinical populations
• can be applied in different clinical populations and settings
• can be compared between studies with different inclusion criteria
• can be used to compare the diagnostic potential of different tests

---

The interpretation of sensitivity and specificity is not intuitive and therefore to calculate these statistics it is recommended that the notations of true positives (TP), false positives (FP), true negatives (TN) and false negatives (FN) are written in each quadrant of crosstabulation as shown in Table 10.3. The false negative group is the proportion of patients who have the disease and who have a negative test result. The false positive group is the proportion of patients who do not have the disease and who have a positive test result.

Thus, sensitivity is the rate of true positives in the disease-present group $(a/a+c)$ and specificity is the rate of true negatives in the disease-absent group $(d/b+d)$. The 'opposites' rule applies to remembering the meaning of the terms sensitivity and specificity because: sensitivity has a 'n' in it and this

Table 10.3 Terms used in diagnostic statistics

	Disease present	Disease absent	Total
Test positive	a TP (sensitivity) (true +ve)	b FP (false +ve)	
Test negative	c FN (false −ve)	d TN (specificity) (true −ve)	
Total	a + c	b + d	N

applies to the true positives, which begin with 'p' and specificity has a 'p' in it and this applies to the true negatives, which begin with 'n'.

Is this logical? Well no, but the terminology is well established and this reverse code helps in remembering which term indicates the true negatives or true positives. From Table 10.3 it can be seen that the rate of false negatives is the complement of the true positives for patients who have the disease. Similarly, the rate of false positives is the complement of the true negatives for patients who do not have the disease.

SpPin and SnNout

SpPin and SnNout are two clinical epidemiology terms that are commonly used to aid in the interpretation of sensitivity and specificity in clinical settings[6].

SpPin stands for **Sp**ecificity-**P**ositive-**in,** which means that if a test has a high specificity (TN) and therefore a low 1 – specificity (FP), a positive result rules the disease in. A test that is used to diagnose an illness in patients with symptoms of the illness needs to have a low false positive rate because it will then identify most of the people who do not have the disease. Although specificity needs to be high for a diagnostic test to rule the disease in, it is calculated solely from patients without the disease.

SnNout stands for **Sn**ensitivity-**N**egative-**out**, which means that if the test has a high sensitivity (TP) and a low 1 – sensitivity (FN), a negative test result rules the disease out. A test that is used to screen a population in which many people will not have the disease needs to have high sensitivity because it will then identify all of the people with the disease. Although sensitivity needs to be high in a screening test to rule the disease out, it is calculated solely from patients with the disease.

The SPSS commands shown in Box 10.1 can be used to compute sensitivity and specificity but the column percentages rather than the row percentages are requested because sensitivity is a proportion of the disease positive group and specificity is a proportion of the disease negative group.

Crosstab

X-ray Results * Fracture Detected by Surgery Crosstabulation

| | | | Fracture detected by surgery (disease) | | |
			Present	Absent	Total
X-ray results (test)	Positive	Count	36	24	60
		% within fracture detected by surgery	81.8%	22.6%	40.0%
	Negative	Count	8	82	90
		% within fracture detected by surgery	18.2%	77.4%	60.0%
Total		Count	44	106	150
		% within fracture detected by surgery	100.0%	100.0%	100.0%

The column percentages can be simply changed into proportions by dividing by 100. Thus, from the above table:

Sensitivity $\quad = TP = 0.82$
$1 - \text{sensitivity} = FN = 0.18$
Specificity $\quad = TN = 0.77$
$1 - \text{specificity} = FP = 0.23$

The sensitivity of the test indicates that 82% of patients with a fracture will have a positive x-ray and the specificity of the test indicates that 77.4% of patients with no fracture will have a negative x-ray.

Confidence intervals

The confidence intervals for sensitivity and specificity can be calculated using the spreadsheet shown in Table 10.2. This produces the intervals shown in Table 10.4. Again, if the confidence interval of a proportion contains a value less than zero, exact confidence intervals should be used[3].

Table 10.4 Excel spreadsheet for calculating confidence intervals around a proportion

Proportion	*N*	SE	Width	CI lower	CI upper
0.82	44	0.058	0.114	0.706	0.934
0.18	44	0.058	0.114	0.066	0.294
0.77	106	0.041	0.080	0.690	0.850
0.23	106	0.041	0.080	0.150	0.310

These 95% confidence intervals are based on the number of patients with the disease present for sensitivity and the number of patients with the disease absent for specificity. Because each 95% confidence interval is based on only a subset of the sample rather than on the total sample size, the confidence intervals can be surprisingly wide if the number in the group is quite small.

The interpretation of the intervals for sensitivity is that with 95% confidence between 70.6% and 93.4% of patients with a fracture will have a positive x-ray. Similarly, the interpretation for specificity is that with 95% confidence between 69.0% and 85% of patients without a fracture will have a negative x-ray.

Study design

In calculating the required sample size to estimate sensitivity and specificity, it is important to have an adequate number of people with and without the disease. A high sensitivity rules the disease out, therefore it is essential to enrol a large number of people with disease present to calculate the proportion of true positives with precision. A high specificity rules the disease in, so it is essential to enrol a large number of people with the disease absent to calculate the proportion of true negatives with precision.

It is not always understood that to show that a test can rule a disease out, a large number of people with the disease present must be enrolled and that to show that a test is useful in ruling a disease in, a large number of people without the disease must be enrolled. For most tests, a large number of people with the disease present and with the disease absent must be enrolled to provide tighter confidence intervals around both sensitivity and specificity.

Likelihood ratio

Both sensitivity and specificity can be thought of as statistics that 'look backwards' in that they show the probability that a person with a disease will have a positive test rather than looking 'forwards' and showing the probability that the person who tests positive has the disease. Also, sensitivity and specificity should not be used in isolation because each is calculated from separate parts of the data. To be useful in clinical practice, these statistics need to be converted to a likelihood ratio that uses data from the total sample to estimate the relative predictive value of the test. The LR is calculated as follows:

$$LR = \frac{\text{Likelihood of a positive result in people with disease}}{\text{Likelihood of a positive result in people without disease}}$$

$$= \text{Sensitivity}/(1 - \text{specificity})$$

$$= TP/FP$$

The LR is simply the ratio of true positives to the false positives and indicates how likely a positive result will be found in a person with the disease than in a person without the disease[1]. From the previous calculation:

$$LR = 0.82/(1 - 0.77) = 3.56$$

Confidence intervals around LR are best generated using dedicated programs (see useful websites). The LR indicates how much a positive test will alter the pre-test probability that a patient will have the illness. The pre-test probability is the probability of the disease in the clinic setting where the test is being used. The post-test probability is the probability that the disease is present when the test is positive. To interpret the LR, a likelihood ratio nomogram can be used to convert pre-test probability of disease into post-test probability[3, 7]. Alternatively, the following formula can be used to convert the pre-test probability (Pre-TP) into a post-test probability (Post-TP):

$$Post-TP = (Pre-TP \times LR)/(1 + Pre-TP \times (LR - 1))$$

The size of the LR indicates the utility of the test in diagnosing an illness. As a rule, a LR greater than 10 is large and means a conclusive change from pre-test to post-test probability. On the other hand a LR between 5 and 10 results in only a moderate shift between pre- and post-test probability, a LR between 2 and 5 results in a small shift but sometimes reflects an important shift, and a LR below 2 is small and rarely important[4].

The advantages of using a likelihood ratio to interpret the results of diagnostic tests are shown in Box 10.4.

Box 10.4 Advantages of using likelihood ratio as a predictive statistic for diagnostic tests

The advantages of likelihood ratio are that this predictive statistic:
• allows valid comparisons of diagnostic statistics between studies
• the diagnostic value can be applied in different clinical settings
• provides the certainty of a positive diagnosis

ROC curves

Receiver operating characteristic (ROC) curves are an invaluable tool for finding the cut-off point in a continuously distributed measurement that best predicts whether a condition is present, for example whether patients are disease positive or disease negative[8]. ROC curves are used to find a cut-off value that delineates a 'normal' from an 'abnormal' test result when the test result is a continuously distributed measurement. ROC curves are plotted by calculating the sensitivity and specificity of the test in predicting the diagnosis for each value of the measurement. The curve makes it possible to determine a cut-off point for the measurement that maximises the rate of true positives (sensitivity) and minimises the rate of false positives (1 – specificity), and thus maximises the likelihood ratio.

Research question

The file **xray.sav**, which was used in the previous research question, also contains data for the results of three different biochemical tests and a variable that indicates whether the disease was later confirmed by surgery. ROC curves are used to assess which test is most useful in predicting that patients will be disease positive.

Before constructing a ROC curve, the amount of overlap in the distribution of the continuous biochemical test measurement in both the disease positive and disease negative groups can be explored using the SPSS commands shown in Box 10.5.

Box 10.5 SPSS commands to obtain scatter plots

SPSS Commands
xray - SPSS Data Editor
         Graphs → Scatter
Scatterplot
         Click on Simple, click on Define
Simple Scatterplots
         Highlight BiochemA and click into the Y Axis
         Highlight Disease positive and click into the X Axis
         Click OK

These SPSS commands can be repeated to obtain scatter plots for the test BiochemB and BiochemC as shown in Figure 10.1. In the plots, the values and labels on the *x*- and *y*-axes are automatically assigned by SPSS and are not selected labels. For example, in Figure 10.1 the tests are never negative as suggested by the negative values on the *y*-axis and the group labels of 1 for disease present and 2 for disease absent on the *x* axis are not displayed. Although the scatter plots are useful for understanding the discriminatory value of each continuous variable, they would not be reported in a journal article.

In the first plot shown in Figure 10.1, it is clear that the values for BiochemA in the disease positive group (coded 1) overlap almost completely with the values for BiochemA in the disease negative group (coded 2). With complete overlap such as this, there will never be a cut-off point that effectively delineates between the two groups.

In the plots for BiochemB and BiochemC as shown in Figure 10.1, there is more separation of the test measurements between the groups, particularly for BiochemC. The value of the tests in distinguishing between the disease positive and disease negative groups can be quantified by plotting ROC curves using the commands shown in Box 10.6. In the data set, disease positive is coded as 1 and this value is entered into the State Variable box.

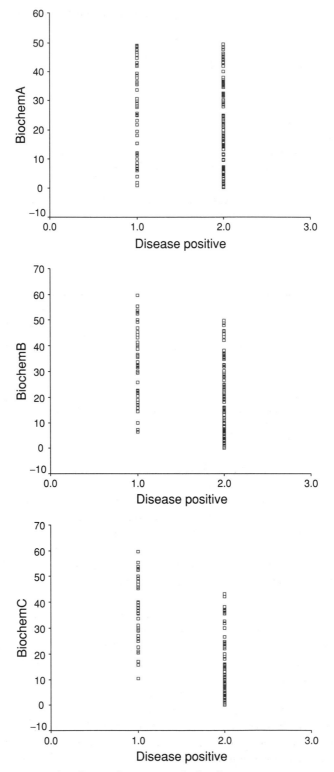

Figure 10.1 Scatter plots for BiochemA, B and C by disease status.

Box 10.6 SPSS commands to plot a ROC curve

SPSS Commands
xray - SPSS Data Editor
Graphs → ROC Curve
ROC Curve
    Highlight BiochemA, BiochemB and BiochemC and click into Test Variable
    Highlight Disease positive and click into State Variable
    Type in 1 as Value of State Variable
    Under Display tick ROC Curve (default), With diagonal reference line,
       and Standard error and confidence interval
    Click OK

Area Under the Curve

Test result varible(s)	Area	Std. error[a]	Asymptotic sig.[b]	Asymptotic 95% confidence interval	
				Lower bound	Upper bound
BiochemA	0.580	0.051	0.114	0.479	0.681
BoichemB	0.755	0.042	0.000	0.673	0.837
BiochemC	0.886	0.028	0.000	0.832	0.940

[a] Under the non-parametric assumption.
[b] Null hypothesis: true area = 0.5.

In a ROC curve, sensitivity is calculated using every value of BiochemA in the data set as a cut-off point and is plotted against the corresponding 1 – specificity at that point, as shown in Figure 10.2. Thus the curve is the true positives plotted against the false positives calculated using each value of the test as a cut-off point. In Figure 10.2, the diagonal line indicates where the test would fall if the results were no better than chance at predicting the presence of a disease, that is no better than tossing a coin. BiochemA lies close to this line confirming that the test is poor at discriminating between disease positive and disease negative patients.

The area under the diagonal line is 0.5 of the total area. The greater the area under the ROC curve, the more useful the measurement is in predicting the patients who have the disease. A curve that falls substantially below the diagonal line indicates that the test is useful for predicting patients who do not have the disease.

The Area Under the Curve table indicates that the area under the curve for BiochemA is 0.580 with a non-significant P value (asymptotic significance) of 0.114, which shows that the area is not significantly different from 0.5. The 95% confidence intervals contain the value 0.5 confirming the P value that shows that this test is not a significant predictor of disease status.

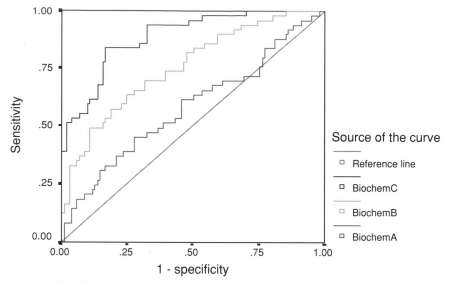

Figure 10.2 ROC curves for Biochem A, B and C.

The ROC curves in Figure 10.2 show that, as expected from the previous scatter plots, the tests BiochemB and BiochemC detect the disease positive patients more effectively than BiochemA. In the Area under the Curve table, BiochemC is the superior test because the area under its ROC curve is the largest at 0.886. Both BiochemB and BiochemC have an area under the curve that is significantly greater than 0.5 and in both cases, the P value is <0.0001. The very small amount of overlap of confidence intervals between BiochemB and BiochemC suggests that BiochemC is a significantly better diagnostic test than BiochemB, even though the P values are identical.

The choice of the cut-off point that optimises the utility of the test is often an expert decision taking factors such as the sensitivity, specificity, cost and purpose of the test into account. In diagnosing a disease, the gold standard test may be a biopsy or surgery, which is invasive, expensive and carries a degree of risk, for example the risk of undergoing an anaesthetic. Tests that are markers of the presence or absence of disease are often used to reduce the number of patients who require such invasive interventions. The exact points on the curve that are selected as cut-off points will vary according to each situation and are best selected using expert opinion.

Three different cut-off points on the curve are used for a diagnostic test, a general optimal test and a screening test. The cut-off point for a screening test is chosen to maximise the sensitivity of the test and for a diagnostic test is chosen to maximise the specificity of the test. The cut-off point for a general optimal test is chosen to optimise the rate of true positives whilst minimising the rate of false positives. All three points can be identified from the coordinates of the ROC curve. By entering only BiochemC into the Test Variable box of *Graphs → ROC* and ticking the box 'Coordinate Points of the ROC Curve' the

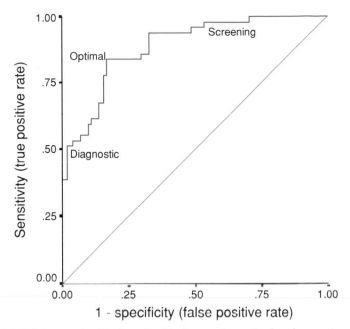

Figure 10.3 ROC curve for BiochemC with diagnostic, optimal and screening cut-off points.

ROC curve and a list of the points on the graph are printed as shown in Figure 10.3.

The cut-off point for a *general optimal test*, which is sometimes called the optimal diagnostic point, is the point on the curve that is closest to the top of the left hand *y*-axis. This point is shown in Figure 10.3 and the test cut-off value can be identified from the coordinate points of the curve. The coordinate points from the central section of the SPSS output have been copied to an Excel spreadsheet and are shown in Table 10.5. In the table, the Excel function option has been used to also calculate Specificity and 1 – sensitivity for each point.

To find the coordinates of the optimal diagnostic point, a simple method is to use a ruler to calculate the coordinate value for 1 – specificity of the optimal cut-off point. Once the point is identified on the graph as being the closest point to the top of the *y*-axis on the ROC curve, a line can be drawn vertically down to the *x*-axis. The value for 1 – specificity is then calculated as the ratio of the distance of the point from the *y*-axis to the total length of the *x*-axis. Using this method, this value is estimated to be 0.167. In the '1 – specificity' column of Table 10.5, there are three values of 0.168, which are closest to 0.167. For the first value of 0.168, sensitivity equals 0.837 after which it begins to fall to 0.796 and 0.776. Thus, of the three points, the first point optimises sensitivity while 1 – specificity remains constant at 0.168. At this value, specificity is 1 – 0.168, or 0.832. The value of BiochemC at this coordinate is 24.8, which is the cut-off point for an optimal general test or is the optimal diagnostic point.

Table 10.5 Excel spreadsheet to identify clinical cut-off points

Cut-off point	Sensitivity True positives	1 – specificity False positives	Specificity True negatives	1 – sensitivity False negatives	Distance
14.950	0.980	0.584	0.416	0.020	0.342
15.150	0.980	0.564	0.436	0.020	0.319
15.350	0.980	0.554	0.446	0.020	0.308
15.550	0.980	0.545	0.455	0.020	0.297
15.750	**0.980**	**0.535**	**0.465**	**0.020**	**0.286**
15.900	0.959	0.535	0.465	0.041	0.288
16.500	0.959	0.485	0.515	0.041	0.237
17.500	0.939	0.485	0.515	0.061	0.239
18.450	0.939	0.406	0.594	0.061	0.169
19.450	0.939	0.396	0.604	0.061	0.161
20.200	0.939	0.327	0.673	0.061	0.111
20.700	0.918	0.327	0.673	0.082	0.113
21.500	0.857	0.327	0.673	0.143	0.127
22.300	0.857	0.297	0.703	0.143	0.109
22.650	0.837	0.297	0.703	0.163	0.115
22.850	0.837	0.287	0.713	0.163	0.109
23.500	0.837	0.228	0.772	0.163	0.079
24.050	0.837	0.188	0.812	0.163	0.062
24.350	0.837	0.178	0.822	0.163	0.058
24.800	**0.837**	**0.168**	**0.832**	**0.163**	**0.055**
25.400	0.796	0.168	0.832	0.204	0.070
26.150	0.776	0.168	0.832	0.224	0.079
26.750	0.776	0.158	0.842	0.224	0.075
28.000	0.735	0.158	0.842	0.265	0.095
29.200	0.714	0.158	0.842	0.286	0.107
29.650	0.694	0.158	0.842	0.306	0.119
29.950	0.673	0.158	0.842	0.327	0.132
30.500	0.673	0.139	0.861	0.327	0.126
31.400	0.612	0.139	0.861	0.388	0.170
31.850	0.612	0.129	0.871	0.388	0.167
32.300	0.612	0.119	0.881	0.388	0.164
33.200	0.612	0.109	0.891	0.388	0.162
34.600	0.592	0.109	0.891	0.408	0.178
35.550	0.592	0.099	0.901	0.408	0.176
35.650	0.571	0.099	0.901	0.429	0.193
35.900	0.551	0.099	0.901	0.449	0.211
36.350	0.551	0.079	0.921	0.449	0.208
36.650	0.551	0.069	0.931	0.449	0.206
36.800	0.531	0.069	0.931	0.469	0.225
37.050	0.531	0.050	0.950	0.469	0.223
37.600	0.531	0.040	0.960	0.469	0.222
38.100	0.510	0.040	0.960	0.490	0.241

Continued

Table 10.5 *(Conitnued)*

Cut-off point	Sensitivity True positives	1 – specificity False positives	Specificity True negatives	1 – sensitivity False negatives	Distance
38.500	0.510	0.020	0.980	0.490	0.240
38.250	0.510	0.030	0.970	0.490	0.241
39.200	0.490	0.020	0.980	0.510	0.261
39.850	0.469	0.020	0.980	0.531	0.282
41.100	0.388	0.020	0.980	0.612	0.375
42.700	0.388	0.010	0.990	0.612	0.375
44.250	0.388	0.000	1.000	0.612	0.375

An alternative method to identify the cut-off point from the Excel spreadsheet is to use the following arithmetic expression, which uses Pythagoras' theorem, to identify the distance of each point from the top of the y-axis. In this calculation, the 'distance' has no units but is a relative measure:

$$\text{Distance} = (1 - \text{Sensitivity})^2 + (1 - \text{Specificity})^2$$

This value was calculated for all points in Table 10.5 using the function option in Excel. The minimum distance value is 0.055 for the cut-off point 24.8. Above and below this value the distance increases indicating that the points are further from the optimal diagnostic point. When the point closest to the top of the y-axis is not readily identified from the ROC curve, this method is useful for identifying the cut-off value.

The cut-off points that would be used for diagnostic and screening tests can also be read from the ROC curve coordinates. For a diagnostic test, it is important to maximise specificity while optimising sensitivity. From the ROC curve figure, the value that would be used for a *diagnostic test* is where the curve is close to the left hand axis, that is where the rate of false positives (1 – specificity) is low and thus the rate of true negatives (specificity) is high. At the cut-off point where the test value is 38.5, there is a sensitivity of 0.510 and a low 1 – specificity of 0.02. At this test value, specificity is high at 0.98 which is a requirement for a diagnostic test. Ideally, specificity should be 1.0 but this has to be balanced against the rate of true positives. At the three test values that have the same sensitivity of 0.510, the rate of false positive is higher for the cut-off points of 38.1 and 38.25 than for the cut-off point of 38.5, which maximises specificity while optimising sensitivity. At the cut-off points below 38.5 where specificity is also 0.98, a significant reduction in true positives would occur if the cut-off point of 41.10 with a sensitivity of 0.388 was selected.

The value that would be used for a *screening test* is where the curve is close to the top axis where the rate of true positives (sensitivity) is maximised. For a screening test, it is important to maximise sensitivity while optimising specificity. At the cut-off point where the test value is 15.75, a high sensitivity of 0.98 is attained for a specificity of 0.465 (Table 10.5). At this point the false negative rate (1 – sensitivity) is low at 0.02 which is a requirement of a screening test. Ideally, sensitivity should be 1.0 but this has to be balanced against the rate of false positives. The original SPSS output (not shown here) indicates that there are 13 test values below 15.75 at which sensitivity remains constant at 0.980 but there is a large gain in the rate of false positives across these cut-off points from 0.535 to 0.703. Thus, at several cut-off values below 15.75, specificity decreases for no change in sensitivity.

For all three cut-off points, the choice of a cut-off value needs to be made using expert opinion in addition to the ROC curve. In this, the decision needs to be made about how important it is to minimise the occurrence of false negative or false positive results.

Reporting the results

The results from the above analyses could be reported as shown in Table 10.6. The positive likelihood ratio is computed for each cut-off point as sensitivity/1 – specificity. A high positive likelihood ratio is more important for a diagnostic test than for a screening test. The 95% confidence intervals for sensitivity and specificity are calculated using the Excel spreadsheet in Table 10.2 with the numbers of disease positive (49) and disease negative (101) patients respectively used as the sample sizes.

Table 10.6 Cut-off points and diagnostic utility of test BiochemC for identifying disease positive patients

Purpose	Cut-off value	Sensitivity (95% CI)	Specificity (95% CI)	Positive likelihood ratio
Screening	15.8	0.98 (0.94, 1.02)	0.47 (0.37, 0.57)	1.8
Optimal	24.8	0.84 (0.74, 0.94)	0.83 (0.76 to 0.90)	4.9
Diagnostic	38.5	0.51 (0.37, 0.65)	0.98 (0.95, 1.0)	25.5

Notes for critical appraisal

When critically appraising an article that presents information about diagnostic tests, it is important to ask the questions shown in Box 10.7. In diagnostic tests, 95% confidence intervals are rarely reported but knowledge of the precision around measurements of sensitivity and specificity is important for applying the test in clinical practice. In addition, estimating sample size in the disease positive and negative groups is of paramount importance in designing studies to measure diagnostic statistics with accuracy.

Box 10.7 Questions for critical appraisal

The following questions should be asked when appraising studies from which diagnostic statistics are reported:

- Was a standard protocol used for deciding whether the diagnosis and the test were classified as positive or negative?
- Was a gold standard used to classify the diagnosis?
- Was knowledge of the results of the test witheld from the people who classified patients as having a disease and vice versa?
- How long was the time interval between the test and the diagnosis? Could the condition have changed through medication use, natural progression, etc. during this time?
- Are there sufficient disease positive and disease negative people in the sample to calculate both sensitivity and specificity accurately?
- Have confidence intervals been calculated for sensitivity and specificity?

References

1. Greenhalgh T. How to read a paper: papers that report diagnostic or screening tests BMJ 1997; 315: 540–543.
2. Altman DG, Bland JM. Diagnostic tests 2: predictive values. BMJ 1994; 309: 102.
3. Deeks JJ, Altman DG. Sensitivity and specificity and their confidence intervals cannot exceed 100%. BMJ 1999; 318: 193.
4. Altman DG, Bland JM. Diagnostic tests 1: sensitivity and specificity. BMJ 1994; 308: 1552.
5. Sackett DL, Richardson WS, Rosenberg W, Haynes RB. How to practice and teach evidence-based medicine. New York: Churchill Livingstone, 1997; pp 118–128.
6. Sackett DL. On some clinically useful measures of the effects of treatment. Evidence-based Medicine 1996; 1: 37–38.
7. Fagan TJ. Nomogram for Bayes' theorem. New Engl J Med 1975; 293:257.
8. Altman DG, Bland JM. Diagnostic tests 3: receiver operating characteristics plots. BMJ 1994; 309: 188.

CHAPTER 11

Categorical and continuous variables: survival analyses

The individual source of the statistics may easily be the weakest link. Harold Cox tells a story of his life as a young man in India. He quoted some statistics to a judge who was an Englishman. The judge said, Cox, when you are a bit older, you will not quote Indian statistics with that assurance. The Government are very keen on amassing statistics—they collect them, add them, raise them to the nth power, take the cube root and prepare wonderful diagrams. But what you must never forget is that every one of those figures comes in the first instance from the chowkidar (village watchman), who just puts down whatever he pleases.

JOSIAH CHARLES STAMP (1880 – 1941)

Objectives

The objectives of the chapter are to explain how to:
- decide when survival analyses are appropriate
- obtain and interpret the results of survival analyses
- ensure that the assumptions for survival analyses are met
- report results in a graph or a table
- critically appraise the survival analyses reported in the literature

Survival analyses are used to investigate the time between entry into a study and the subsequent occurrence of an event. Although survival analyses were designed to measure differences between time to death in study groups, they are frequently used for time to other events including discharge from hospital; disease onset; disease relapse or treatment failure; or cessation of an activity such as breastfeeding or use of contraception.

With data relating to time, a number of problems occur. The time to an event is rarely normally distributed and follow-up times for patients enrolled in cohort studies vary, especially when it is impractical to wait until the event has occurred in all patients. In addition, patients who leave the study early or who have had less opportunity for the event to occur need to be taken into account. Survival analyses circumvent these problems by taking advantage of the longitudinal nature of the data to compare event rates over the study period and not at an arbitrary time point[1].

Survival analyses are ideal for analysing event data from prospective cohort studies and from randomised controlled trials in which patients are enrolled in the study over long time periods. The advantages of using survival analyses rather than logistic regression for measuring the risk of the event occurring are that the time to the event is used in the analysis and that the different length of follow-up for each patient is taken into account. This is important because a patient in one group who has been enrolled for only 12 months does not have an equal chance for the event to occur as a patient in another group who has been enrolled for 24 months. Survival analyses also have an advantage over regression in that the event rate over time does not have to be constant.

Censored observations

Patients who leave the study or do not experience the event are called 'censored' observations. The term censoring is used because, in addition to patients who survive, the censored group includes patients who are lost to follow-up, who withdraw from the study or who die without the investigators' knowledge. Classifying patients who do not experience the event for whatever reason as 'censored' allows them to be included in the analysis.

Assumptions

The assumptions for using Kaplan–Meier survival analyses are shown in Box 11.1. These analyses are non-parametric tests and thus no assumptions about the distributions of variables need to be met.

Box 11.1 Assumptions for using Kaplan–Meier survival analysis

The assumptions for using Kaplan–Meier survival analysis are that:
- the participants must be independent, that is each participant appears only once in their group
- the groups must be independent, that is each participant is in one group only
- the measurement of time to the event must be precise
- the start point and the event must be clearly defined
- participants' survival prospects remain constant, that is participants enrolled early or late in the study have the same survival prospects
- the probability of censoring is not related to the probability of the event

---

In survival analyses, it is essential that the time to the event be measured accurately. For this, regular observations need to be conducted rather than, for example, surmising that the event occurred between two routine examinations[2]. When it is only known that an event occurred between two points in time, for example if observations are only taken every 6 months, the data are said to be interval censored[3]. If time to the event is not measured precisely, the survival probabilities will be biased.

Both the start point, that is entry into the study, the inclusion criteria and the event must be well defined to avoid bias in the analyses. This is especially important when using survival analyses to describe the natural history of a condition[4]. Using start points that are prone to bias, such as patient recall of a diagnosis or attendance at a doctor surgery to define the presence of an illness, will result in unreliable survival probabilities.

The reason for the event must also be clearly defined. When an event occurs that is not due to the condition being investigated, careful consideration needs to be given to whether it is treated as an event or as a withdrawal. In clinical trials, combined events for example an event that combines death, acute myocardial infarction or cardiac arrest are often used to test the effectiveness of interventions[5].

In addition, patients who are censored must have the same survival prospects as patients who continue in the study, that is the risk of the event should not be related to the reasons for censoring or loss to follow-up[2]. Thus factors that influence patients' survival prospects, such as different treatment options, should not change over the study period and patients who experience more sickness in one treatment group should not be preferentially lost to follow-up compared with patients who experience less sickness in another treatment group. Secular trends in survival can also occur if patients enrolled early have a different underlying prognosis from those enrolled towards the end of the study. This would bias estimates of risk of survival in a cohort study but is not so important in clinical trials in which randomisation balances important prognostic factors between the groups.

As with all analyses, if the total number of patients in any group is small, say less than 30 participants in each group, the standard errors around the summary statistics will be large and therefore the survival estimates will be imprecise.

When conducting a survival analysis, the data need to be entered with one binary variable indicating whether or not the event occurred and a continuous variable indicating the time to the event or the time to follow-up. The event is usually coded as '1' and censored cases coded as '0', although other coding such as '1' and '2' could be used.

Research question

The file **survival.sav** contains the data from 56 patients enrolled in a trial of two treatments in which 30 patients received the new treatment and 26 patients received the standard treatment. A total of 39 patients died.

Question:	Is the survival rate in the new treatment group higher than in the standard treatment group?
Null hypothesis:	That there is no difference in survival rates between treatment groups.

Variables: Outcome variable = death (binary event)
Explanatory variables = time of follow-up (continuous),
treatment group (categorical, two levels)

The commands shown in Box 11.2 can be used to obtain a Kaplan–Meier statistic to assess whether the differences in survival times between the two treatment groups are significantly different.

Box 11.2 SPSS commands to obtain survival curves

SPSS Commands
survival – SPSS Data Editor
        Analyze → Survival→ Kaplan-Meier
Kaplan-Meier
        Highlight days and click into Time
        Highlight event and click into Status
        Click on Define Event
Kaplan-Meier: Define Event for Status Variable
        Type 1 in Single value box, click Continue
Kaplan-Meier
        Highlight Treatment group and click into Factor
        Click Compare Factor
Kaplan-Meier: Compare factor levels
        Under Test Statistics tick Log rank, Breslow, Tarone Ware, click Continue
Kaplan-Meier
        Click Options
Kaplan-Meier: Options
        Under Statistics tick Survival table(s) (default) and tick Mean and median survival (default)
        Under Plots, tick Survival
        Click Continue
Kaplan-Meier
        Click OK

Kaplan–Meier

```
Survival Analysis for DAYS
Factor GROUP = New treatment
```

Time	Status	Cumulative Survival	Standard Error	Cumulative Events	Number Remaining
5	0			0	29
7	0			0	28
8	0			0	27
9	1	.9630	.0363	1	26
9	0			1	25
12	1	.9244	.0514	2	24

Time	Status	Cumulative Survival	Standard Error	Cumulative Events	Number Remaining
15	1	.8859	.0620	3	23
16	1	.8474	.0703	4	22
16	0			4	21
16	0			4	20
19	0			4	19
20	0			4	18
23	0			4	17
24	0			4	16
25	0			4	15
29	0			4	14
31	0			4	13
32	1	.7822	.0902	5	12
32	0			5	11
36	1	.7111	.1064	6	10
38	0			6	9
40	0			6	8
41	0			6	7
41	0			6	6
42	0			6	5
43	0			6	4
48	0			6	3
49	0			6	2
58	0			6	1
59	0			6	0

Number of Cases: 30   Censored: 24 (80.00%)   Events: 6

	Survival Time	Standard Error	95% Confidence Interval
Mean:	49	4	(41, 56)(Limited to 59)

Survival Analysis for DAYS
Factor GROUP = Standard treatment

Time	Status	Cumulative Survival	Standard Error	Cumulative Events	Number Remaining
1	1			1	25
1	1			2	24
1	1	.8846	.0627	3	23
2	1	.8462	.0708	4	22
3	1	.8077	.0773	5	21
4	1			6	20
4	1	.7308	.0870	7	19
6	0			7	18
7	1	.6902	.0911	8	17
17	1	.6496	.0944	9	16
20	0			9	15
21	1			10	14
21	1	.5630	.0997	11	13
31	0			11	12
31	0			11	11
32	0			11	10
33	0			11	9
33	0			11	8
36	0			11	7

39	0		11	6
40	0		11	5
40	0		11	4
41	0		11	3
43	0		11	2
50	0		11	1
65	0		11	0

```
Number of Cases:   26      Censored:   15   ( 57.69%)   Events:11
           Survival Time   Standard Error   95% Confidence Interval
  Mean:         40                    6 ( 29, 51 )(Limited to 65 )
```

The Survival Analysis for Days tables show the cumulative survival rate at each follow-up time point which is calculated each time an event occurs. The column labelled 'Time' indicates the day the event occurred. From the Cumulative Survival column, the cumulative survival is 0.7111 at 36 days in group 1 (new treatment) and 0.5630 at 21 days in group 2 (standard treatment). The Kaplan–Meier method produces a single summary statistic of survival time, that is the mean[6]. Mean survival is calculated as the summation of time divided by the number of patients who remain uncensored. The mean survival time shown at the foot of each table is higher in the new treatment group at 49 days than in the standard treatment group at 40 days.

Survival Analysis for DAYS

		Total	Number Events	Number Censored	Per cent Censored
GROUP	New treatment	30	6	24	80.00
GROUP	Standard treatment	26	11	15	57.69
Overall		56	17	39	69.64

The final Survival Analysis for Days table also shows summary statistics of the number in each group, the number of events and the number and per cent censored. These statistics show that there were fewer events but more patients who were censored in the new treatment group.

Test Statistics for Equality of Survival Distributions for GROUP

	Statistic	**df**	**Significance**
Log Rank	3.27	1	.0705
Breslow	5.32	1	.0211
Tarone-Ware	4.39	1	.0362

The Test Statistics for Equality of Survival Distributions table shows the three tests that can be used to test the null hypothesis that there is an equal risk of death in both groups, that is the Log Rank, Breslow and Tarone-Ware tests. These tests are similar to chi-square tests in that the number of observed events is compared with the number of expected events. All three tests have low power for detecting differences when survival curves cross one another.

The Log Rank statistic, which is derived from a whole pattern test in which the entire survival curve is used, is the most commonly reported survival statistic[7]. The Log Rank test is appropriate when the survival curves continue to diverge over time but this test becomes unreliable if one or more groups have small numbers and is not recommended if the survival curves from two groups cross one another.

The Breslow and Tarone-Ware tests are both weighted variants of the Log Rank test because in these tests different weightings are given to particular points of the survival curve[7]. The Breslow test gives greater weight to early observations when the sample size is larger and is less sensitive to later observations when the sample size is smaller. This test is appropriate when there are few ties in the data, that is patients with equal survival times. The Tarone-Ware test provides a compromise between the Log Rank and the Breslow tests but is rarely used.

The SPSS output shows how the three tests can lead to different conclusions about whether there is a significant difference in the survival rate between groups. The Log Rank test is not significant at $P = 0.0705$. However, this test is not appropriate in this situation in which the number of patients remaining after 33 to 36 days is small with less than 10 patients in each group.

The Breslow test is significant at $P = 0.0211$ and is the most appropriate test to report here because more weight is placed on earlier observations when group sizes are larger. In this example, the Breslow P value is more significant than the Log Rank P value because more weight has been placed on the early observations when survival rates between the groups are different than on later observations when survival rates between the groups are more similar as shown in the Survival Functions plot in the next section. If early observations were more similar between groups and later observations more different, the Log Rank P value would have been more significant than the Breslow P value.

Reporting the results

When reporting data from survival analyses, the P values from the statistical analyses do not convey information about the size of the effect. In addition to P values, summary statistics such as the follow-up time of each group, the total number of events and the number of patients who remain event free are important for interpreting the data. This information can be reported as shown in Table 11.1.

Table 11.1 Survival characteristics of study sample

Group	Number of cases	Number of events	Number censored	Mean survival time in days (95% CI)
New treatment	30	6	24 (80.0%)	49 (41, 56)
Standard treatment	26	11	15 (57.7%)	40 (29, 51)

Survival plots

Survival plots, which are called Kaplan–Meier curves, are widely used with 40% of publications from randomised controlled trials including a survival plot[5]. In plotting Kaplan–Meier curves, the data are first ranked in ascending order according to time. A curve is then plotted for each group by calculating the proportion of patients who remain in the study and who are censored each time an event occurs. Thus, the curves do not change at the time of censoring but only when the next event occurs.

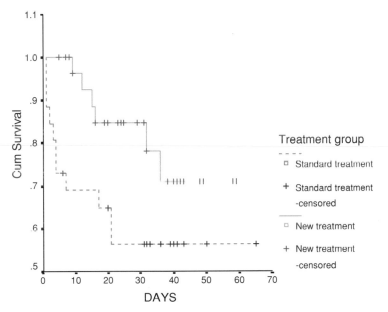

Figure 11.1 Plot showing survival functions of treatment group.

The survival plot shows the proportion of patients who are free of the event at each time point. The steps in the curves occur each time an event occurs and the bars on the curves indicate the times at which patients are censored. The plots show the survival time for a typical patient. In the survival plot shown in Figure 11.1 the standard treatment group, which is the lower curve, has a poorer survival time than the new treatment group, which is the upper curve. The sections of the curves where the slope is steep, in this case the earlier parts, indicate the periods when patients are most at risk for experiencing the event. It is always advisable to plot survival curves before conducting the tests of significance.

Plotting survival curves

There are several ways to plot survival curves and the debate about whether they should go up or down and how the y-axis should be scaled continues[5].

In SPSS, different presentations of the survival curve can be obtained in the *Plot → Options* commands.

Plotting survival curves is not problematic when the study sample is large and the follow-up time is short. However, when the number of patients who remain at the end is small, survival estimates are poor. Thus, it is important to end plots when the number in follow-up has not become too small. In the above example, the curves should be truncated to 31 days when the number in each group is 10 or more and should not be continued to 65 days when all patients in the standard treatment group have experienced the event or are censored.

The scaling of the *y*-axis is important because differences between groups can be visually magnified or reduced by shortening or lengthening the axis. In practice, a scale only slightly larger than the event rate is generally recommended to provide visual discrimination between groups rather than the full scale of 0 to 1.[5] However, this can tend to make the differences between the curves seem larger than they actually are, as in the SPSS plot in which the *y*-axis scale ranges from 0.5 to 1.0.

Questions for critical appraisal

The questions that should be asked when critically appraising a journal article that reports a survival analysis are shown in Box 11.3.

Box 11.3 Questions to ask when critically appraising the literature

The following questions can be asked when critically appraising the literature:
- Is the start point and event clearly defined and free of recall or other bias?
- Has time been measured accurately?
- Have any factors preferentially changed the patient's survival prospects over the course of the study?
- Is a figure reported appropriately?
- Is the sample size in each group sufficient?

References

1. Altman DG, Bland M. Time to event (survival) data. BMJ 1998; 317:468–469.
2. Bland JM, Altman DG. Survival probabilities (the Kaplan–Meier method). BMJ 1998; 317:1572.
3. Collett D. Modelling survival data in medical research London, UK. Chapman and Hall, 1994, pp 2–3.
4. Norman GR, Streiner DL. Biostatistics. The bare essentials. Missourie, USA: Mosby Year Book Inc., 1994, pp 182–195.

5. Pocock SJ, Clayton TC, Altman DG. Survival plots of time-to-event outcomes in clinical trials: good practice and pitfalls. Lancet 2002; 359:1686–1689.
6. Tabachnick BG, Fidell LS. Using multivariate statistics (4th edition). Boston, USA: Allyn and Bacon, 2001; pp 791–796.
7. Wright RE. Survival analysis. In: Reading and understanding more multivariate statistics, Grimm LG, Yarnold PR (editors). Washington, USA, pp 363–406.

Glossary

Adjusted *R* square *R* square is the coefficient of determination that is adjusted for the number of explanatory variables included in the regression model. This value can be used to compare regression models that have a different number of explanatory variables.

Asymptotic methods Commonly used statistical tests based on assumptions that the sample size is large and the data are normally distributed or, if the data are categorical, that the condition of interest occurs frequently, say in more than 5% of the sample.

Balanced design Studies with a balanced design have an equal number of observations in each cell. This can only be achieved in experimental studies or by data selection. Most observational studies have an unbalanced design with unequal number of observations in the cells.

Bivariate tests Tests in which the relation between two variables is estimated, for example an outcome and an explanatory variable.

Case–control study A study design in which individuals with the disease of interest (cases) are selected and compared to a control or reference group of individuals without the disease.

Censoring A term used to indicate that an event did not occur in a survival analysis. The reasons for censoring could be that the participant withdrew, was lost to follow-up or did not experience the event.

Chi-square A statistic used to test whether the frequency of an outcome in two or more groups is significantly different, or that the rows and columns of a crosstabulation table are independent.

Collinearity A term used when two variables are strongly related to one another. Collinearity between explanatory variables inflates the standard errors and causes imprecision because the variation is shared. Thus, the model becomes unstable (i.e. unreliable).

Complete design A study design is complete when there are one or more observations in each cell and is incomplete when some cells are empty.

Confidence interval The 95% confidence interval is the interval in which there is 95% certainty that the true population value lies. Confidence intervals are calculated around summary statistics such as mean values or proportions. For samples with more than 30 cases, a 95% confidence is calculated as the summary statistic $\pm$ (SE $\times$ 1.96), where SE equals standard error. The confidence limits are the values at the ends of the confidence interval.

Confounder Confounders are nuisance variables that are related to the outcome and to the explanatory variables and whose effect needs to be minimised in the study design or analyses so that the results are not biased.

Cook's distances Measure of influence used in multivariate models. Values greater than $4/(n - k - 1)$ are considered influential ($n =$ sample size, $k =$ number of variables in model).

Discrepancy A measure of how much a case is in line with other cases in a multivariate model.

Dummy variables A series of binary variables that have been derived from a multi-level ordinal variable.

Effect size The distance between two mean values described in units of their standard deviations.

Error term See Residual.

Eta squared A measure of the strength of association between the outcome and the explanatory factors. As such, eta^2 is an approximation to R squared.

Exact statistics Statistics calculated using exact factorial or binomial methods rather than asymptotic methods. Exact statistics are used when the numbers in a cell or group are small and the assumptions for asymptotic statistical tests are violated.

Explanatory variable A variable that is a measured characteristic or an exposure and that is hypothesised to influence an event or a disease status (i.e. outcome variable). In cross-sectional and cohort studies, explanatory variables are often exposure variables.

F value An F value is a ratio of variances. For one-way ANOVA, F is the between-group MS/within MS where MS equals mean sum of squares. For factorial ANOVA, F is the MS for factor/residual MS. For regression, F is the MS regression/residual MS.

Factorial ANOVA A factorial ANOVA is used to examine the effects of two or more factors, or explanatory variables, on a single outcome variable. When there are two explanatory factors, the model is described as a two-way ANOVA, when there are three factors as a three-way ANOVA, etc.

Heteroscedasticity Heteroscedasticity indicates that the variances in cells in a multivariate model are unequal or the variance across a model is not constant.

Homoscedasticity Homoscedasticity indicates that the variances in cells in a multivariate model are not different or that there is constant variance over the length of a model.

Incidence Rate of new cases in a random population sample in a specified time, for example, 1 year.

Influence Influence is calculated as leverage multiplied by discrepancy and is used to assess the change in a regression coefficient when a case is deleted.

Inter-quartile range A measure of spread that is the width of the band that contains the middle half of the data that lies between the 25th and 75th percentiles.

Interval scale variable A variable with values where differences in intervals or points along the scale can be made e.g. the difference between 5 and 10 is the same as the difference between 85 and 90.

Intervening variable A variable that acts on the pathway between an outcome and an exposure variable.

Kurtosis A measure of whether the distribution of a variable is peaked or flat. Measures of kurtosis between −1 and 1 indicate that the distribution has an approximately normal bell shape curve and values around −2 to +2 are a warning of some degree of kurtosis. Values below −3 or above +3 indicate that there is significant peakedness or flatness and therefore that the data are not normally distributed.

Leverage A measure of the influence of a point on the fit of a regression. Leverage can range from 0 (no influence) to $n - 1/n$ where n equals the sample size. Leverage values close to 1 indicate total influence.

Likelihood ratio A statistic used to combine sensitivity and specificity into a single estimate that indicates how a positive test result will change the odds that a patient has the disease.

Linear-by-linear association A statistic used to test whether a binary outcome increases or decreases over an ordered categorical exposure variable. Although this is printed by SPSS when chi-square is requested, the trend is computed using a Pearson correlation coefficient.

Mahalanobis distance This is the distance between a case and the centroid of the remaining cases, where the centroid is the point where the means of the explanatory variables intersect. Mahalanobis distance is used to identify multivariate outliers in regression analyses. A case with a Mahalanobis distance above the chi-squared critical value at $P < 0.001$ with degrees of freedom equal to the number of explanatory variables in the model is a multivariate outlier.

Maximum value The largest numerical value of a variable.

Mean A measure of the centre or the average value of the data.

Mean square A term used to describe variance in a regression model. This term is the sum of the squares divided by their degrees of freedom.

Median The point at which half the measurements lie above and below this value, that is the point that marks the centre of the data.

Minimum value The smallest numerical value of a variable.

Multivariate tests Tests with more than one explanatory variable in the model.

Negative predictive value The proportion of individuals who have a negative diagnostic test result and who do not have the disease.

Nominal variable A variable with values that do not have any ordering or meaningful ranking and are generally categories e.g. values to indicate retired, employed or unemployed.

Normal score See z score.

Null hypothesis A null hypothesis states that there is no difference between the means of the populations from which the samples were drawn, that is population means are equal or that there is no relationship between two or more variables. If the null hypothesis is accepted, this does not necessarily mean that the null hypothesis is true but can suggest that there is not sufficient or strong enough evidence to reject it.

Odds ratio An estimate of risk of disease given exposure, or vice versa, that can be calculated from any type of study design.

One-tailed tests When the direction of the effect is specified by the alternate hypothesis e.g. $\mu > 50$ a one-tailed test is used. The tail refers to the end of the probability curve. The critical region for a one sided test is located in only one tail of the probability distribution. One-tailed tests are more powerful than two-tailed tests for showing a significant difference because the critical value for significance is lower and are rarely used in health care research.

Ordinal variable A variable with values that indicate a logical order such as codes to indicate socioeconomic or educational status.

Outcome variable The outcome of interest in a study, that is the variable that is dependent on or is influenced by other variables (explanatory variables) such as exposures, risk factors, etc.

Outliers There are two types of outliers: univariate and multivariate. Univariate outliers are defined as data points that have an absolute z score greater than 3. This term is used to describe values that are at the extremities of the range of data points or are separated from the normal range of the data. For small sample sizes, data points that have an absolute z score greater than 2.5 are considered to be univariate outliers. Multivariate outliers are data values that have an extreme value on a combination of explanatory variables and exert too much leverage and/or discrepancy.

***P* value** A P value is the probability of a test statistic occurring if the null hypothesis is true. P values that are large are consistent with the null hypothesis. On the other hand, P values that are small, say less than 0.05, lead to rejection of the null hypothesis because there is a small probability that the null hypothesis is true. P values are also called significance levels. In SPSS output, P value columns are often labelled 'Sig.'

Partial correlation The correlation between two variables after the effects of a third or confounding variable have been removed.

Population A collection of individuals to whom the researcher is interested in making an inference, for example all people residing in a specific region or in an entire country, or all people with a specific disease.

Positive predictive value The proportion of individuals with a positive diagnostic test result who have the disease.

Power The ability of the study to demonstrate an effect or association if one exists, that is to avoid type II errors. Power can be influenced by many factors including the frequency of the outcome, the size of the effect, the sample size and the statistical tests used.

Prevalence Rate of total cases in a random population sample in a specified time, for example 1 year.

Quartiles Obtained by placing observations in an increasing order and then dividing into four groups so that 25% of the observations are in each group.

The cut-off points are called quartiles. The four groups formed by the three quartiles are called 'fourths' or 'quarters'

Quintiles Obtained by placing observations in an increasing order and then dividing into five groups so that 20% of the observations are in each group. The cut-off points are called quintiles.

R square The R square value (coefficient of determination) is the squared multiple correlation coefficient and indicates the per cent of the variance in the outcome variable that can be explained or accounted for by the explanatory variables.

r value Pearson's correlation coefficient that measures the linear relationship between two continuous normally distributed variables.

R Multiple correlation coefficient that is the correlation between the observed and predicted values of the outcome variable.

Range The difference between the lowest and the highest numerical values of a variable, that is the maximum value subtracted from the minimum value. The term range is also often used to describe the values that are the limits of the range, that is the minimum and the maximum values e.g. range 0 to 100.

Ratio scale variable An interval scale variable with a true zero value so that the ratio between two values on the scale can be calculated, e.g. age in years is a ratio scale variable but calendar year of birth is not.

Relative risk The risk of disease given exposure divided by the risk of disease given no exposure, which can only be calculated directly from a random population sample. In case–control studies, relative risk is estimated by an odds ratio.

Residual The difference between a participant's value and the predicted value, or mean value, for the group. This term is often called the error term.

Risk The probability that any individual will develop a disease. Risk is calculated as the number of individuals who have the disease divided by the total number of individuals in the sample or population.

Risk factor An aspect of behaviour or lifestyle or an environmental exposure that is associated with a health related condition.

Sample Selected and representative part of a population that is used to make inferences about the total population from which it is drawn.

Sensitivity Proportion of disease positive individuals who are correctly diagnosed by a positive diagnostic test result.

Significance level See P value.

Skewness A measure of whether the distribution of a variable has a tail to the left or right hand side. Skewness values between −1 and +1 indicate slight skewness and values around −2 and +2 are a warning of a reasonable degree of skewness but possibly still acceptable. Values below −3 or above +3 indicate that there is significant skewness and that the data are not normally distributed.

Specificity The proportion of disease negative individuals who are correctly identified as disease free by a negative diagnostic test result.

Standard deviation A measure of spread such that it is expected that 95% of the measurements lie within 1.96 standard deviations above and below the mean. This value is the square root of the variance.

Standardised coefficients Partial regression coefficients that indicate the relative importance of each variable in the regression equation. These coefficients are in standardised units similar to z scores and their dimension allows them to be compared with one another.

Standard error A measure of precision that is the size of the error around a mean value or proportion, etc. For continuous variables, the standard error around a mean value is calculated $SD/\sqrt{n}$. For other statistics such as proportions and regression estimates, different formulae are used. For all statistics, the SE will become smaller as the sample size increases for data with the same spread or characteristics.

SE of the estimate This is the approximate standard deviation of the residuals around a regression line. This statistic is a measure of the variation that is not accounted for by the regression line. In general, the better the fit, the smaller the standard error of the estimate.

String variable A variable that generally consists of words or characters but may include some numbers. This type of variable is also known as an alphanumeric variable.

t-value A t-distribution is closely related to a normal distribution but depends on the number of cases in a sample. A t-value, which is calculated by dividing a mean value by its standard error, gives a number from which the probability of an event occurring is estimated from a t-table.

Trimmed mean The 5% trimmed mean is the mean calculated after 5% of the data (i.e. outliers) are removed. This method is sometimes used in sports competitions, for example skating, when several judges rate performance on a scale.

Two-tailed tests When the direction of the effect is not specified by the alternate hypothesis e.g. $\mu \neq 50$ a two-tailed test is used. The tail refers to the end of the probability curve. The critical region for a two sided test is located in both tails of the probability distribution. Two-tailed tests are used in most research studies.

Type I error A term used when a statistically significant difference between two study groups is found although the null hypothesis is true. Thus, the null hypothesis is rejected in error.

Type II error A term used when a clinically important difference between two study groups does not reach statistical significance. Thus, the null hypothesis is not rejected when it is false. Type II errors typically occur when the sample size is small.

Type sum of squares (SS) Type III SS are used in ANOVA for unbalanced study designs when all cells have equal importance but no cells are empty. This is the most common type of study design in health research. Type I SS are used when all cell numbers are equal, type II is used when some cells have equal importance and type IV is used when some cells are empty.

Univariate tests Descriptive tests in which the distribution or summary statistics for only one variable are reported.

Unstandardised coefficients These are the regression estimates such as y and x in the equation $y = a + bx$ where 'a' is the constant and 'b' is the coefficient for explanatory variable.

Variance A measure of spread that is calculated from the sum of the deviations from the mean, which have been squared to remove negative values.

Z score This is the number of standard deviations of a value from the mean. Z scores, which are also known as normal scores, have a mean of zero and a standard deviation of one unit. Values can be converted to z scores for variables with a normal or non-normal distribution; however, conversion to z scores does not transform the shape of the distribution.

Useful Web sites

A New View of Statistics
http://www.sportsci.org/resource/stats/index.html
A peer-reviewed website that includes comprehensive explanations and discussion of many statistical techniques including confidence intervals, chi-squared and ANOVA, plus some Excel spreadsheets to calculate summary statistics that are not available from commonly used statistical packages.

Diagnostic test calculator
http://araw.mede.uic.edu/cgi-alansz/testcalc.pl
Online program for calculating statistics related to diagnostic tests such as sensitivity, specificity and likelihood ratio.

Epi Info
http://www.cdc.gov/epiinfo/downloads.htm
With Epi Info, a questionnaire or form can be developed, the data entry process can be customised and data can be entered and analysed. Epidemiologic statistics, tables, graphs, maps, and sample size calculations confidence intervals around a proportion can be produced. Epi Info can be downloaded free.

Graphpad Quickcalcs Free Online calculators for scientists
http://www.graphpad.com/quickcalcs/index.cfm
Online program for calculating many statistical tests from summary data including McNemars, NNT, etc.

HyperStat Online Textbook
http://davidmlane.com/hyperstat/
Provides information on a variety of statistical procedures, with links to other related Web sites, recommended books and statistician jokes.

Martin Bland Web page
http://www.mbland.sghms.ac.uk
Web page with links to talks on agreement, cluster designs, etc. and statistics advice and access to free statistical software. Also includes an index to all BMJ statistical notes that are online.

Multivariate Statistics: Concepts, Models and Applications

http://www.psychstat.smsu.edu/multibook2/mlt.htm

A Web site that includes graphs to illustrate multivariate concepts and detailed examples of multiple regression, two-way ANOVA and other multivariate tests. Includes examples of how to interpret SPSS output.

PA 765 Statnotes: An Online Textbook by G David Garson

http://www2.chass.ncsu.edu/garson/pa765/statnote.htm

Notes on a range of statistical tests including t-tests, chi-squared, ANOVA, ANCOVA, correlations, regression and logistic regression are presented in detail. Also, assumptions for each statistical test, definition of terms and links to other statistical Web sites are given.

Public Health Archives

http://www.jiscmail.ac.uk/archives/public-health.html

Mailbase to search for information or post queries about statistics, study design issues, etc. This site also has details of international courses, etc.

Raynald's SPSS Tools

http://pages.infinit.net/rlevesqu/index.htm

Web site with syntax, macros and online tutorials on how to use SPSS and with links to other statistical Web sites.

Russ Lenth's power and sample size page

http://www.stat.uiowa.edu/~rlenth/Power/

A graphical interface for studying the power of one or more tests including the comparison of two proportions, t-tests and balanced ANOVA.

Simple Interactive Statistical Analysis (SISA)

http://home.clara.net/sisa

Simple interactive program that provides tables to conduct statistical analysis such as chi-square and t tests from summary data.

Statistics on the Web

http://www.execpc.com/~helberg/statistics.html

Links to statistics resources including online education courses, statistics books and programs and professional organisations.

StatPages.net

http://members.aol.com/johnp71/javastat.html

A conveniently accessible statistical software package with links to online statistics books, tutorials, downloadable software, and related resources.

StatSoft – Electronic Statistics Textbook

http://www.statsoft.com/textbook/stathome.html

Provides an overview of elementary concepts and continues with a more indepth exploration of specific areas of statistics including ANOVA, regression and survival analysis. A glossary of statistical terms and a list of references for further study are included.

Stat/Transfer

http://www.stattransfer.com.

Stat/Transfer is designed to simplify the transfer of statistical data between different programs. Stat/Transfer automatically reads statistical data in the internal format of one of the supported programs such as Microsoft Access, FoxPro, Minitab, SAS and Epi Info and will then transfer as much of the information as is present and appropriate to the internal format of another.

UCLA Academic Technology Services

http://www.ats.ucla.edu/stat/spss/

Helpful Web site with online SPSS textbook and examples and frequently asked questions, with detailed information about regression and ANOVA.

Index

Note: Page numbers in *italic* refer to figures, those in **bold** refer to tables.

Contents

Preface

This book is the first textbook of rural medicine in the UK. It should prove invaluable for anyone with an interest in rural health matters. Its publication is timely: rural life is misunderstood and under threat but there is now more political and media attention on rural issues than there has been for many years.

Although 20% of UK residents (11 million people) live in rural areas, little attention has been paid to their health needs or to the needs of the people who provide them with healthcare. This book is aimed particularly at doctors and nurses in practice or in training. It should also be of interest and value to other rural primary healthcare workers, including community physiotherapists, occupational therapists, psychologists, dicticians and chiropodists. Practice managers and others responsible for managing our health services in health authorities and trusts will find that the book helps them to understand rural healthcare. And as undergraduate medical education moves from medical schools out into the community, the book should be of value to medical students and their teachers.

We hope you find this book both useful and enjoyable. We would welcome your comments, corrections and suggestions.

Jim Cox
Iain Mungall
September 1998

List of contributors

Jim Cox, MD, FRCP Edin, FRCGP, General Practitioner, Caldbeck, Cumbria

Iain Mungall, FRCGP, General Practitioner, Bellingham, Northumberland

Gordon Baird, FRCGP, MRCOG, General Practitioner, Sandhead, Wigtownshire

David Baker, MB, BS, MRCS, LRCP, Retired General Practitioner, Bassingham, Lincoln

Neil Frame, BVM&S, MRCVS, Veterinary Surgeon, Penrith, Cumbria

Laura Marshall, MRCGP, General Practitioner, Isle of Lewis

Eleri Roderick, FRCGP, General Practitioner, Caldbeck, Cumbria

Philip Spencer, PhD, MRCGP, General Practitioner, Caldbeck, Cumbria

Antoinette Ward, RGN, RM, RHV, Practice Nurse, Caldbeck, Cumbria

Professor Ian Watt, MPH, MFPHM, Centre for Reviews and Dissemination, York University

John Wynn-Jones, FRCGP, General Practitioner, Montgomery, Powys

Acknowledgements

We thank our families and members of the Rural Practice Group of the Royal College of General Practitioners for their help and support.
  We are extremely grateful to Dr Michael Cox for the illustrations.

Colour plate section produced with the aid of an educational grant from Glaxo Wellcome.

1
Introduction

What is different about rural practice?

Rural communities are extraordinarily diverse. Some are commuter areas, others consist of a predominantly elderly and retired population, the young having migrated to study or work elsewhere. Tourist areas have their own characteristics and visitors bring their own health needs. Much employment in tourist areas is low paid and seasonal.

Although most of the work of rural practitioners is common to colleagues working in non-rural areas, there is sufficient that is different to merit description and study. Rural doctors and nurses find that rurality affects the way they work, but that these aspects are poorly understood by their urban colleagues.

In general, rural people are healthier than their urban counterparts but there is wide variation across the country, with some rural populations being less healthy than some urban populations. Certain rural occupations have their own health risks. Country dwellers are often seen as more stoical and there is evidence to support this view.

Certain diseases, for example zoonoses, are peculiar to the countryside and its occupations. Trauma is common, often associated with farming, and the local surgery is often the first port of call for casualty services. Health, social and voluntary services tend to be less accessible than they are in more densely populated areas.

Rural deprivation affects health, but it is often hidden. Existing indices of deprivation do not adequately define rural deprivation, so there is poor targeting of scarce resources. Twenty per cent of the rural population of England and 25% of rural households live in 'absolute poverty' (on an income of less than 140% of supplementary benefit entitlement), and elderly people are worst affected. Transport is of vital concern in the countryside. Lack of public transport means that many of the poorest members of society must run their own vehicle, thus compounding their poverty.

With constant pressure to find 'efficiency savings', and 'value for money', there is a clear trend towards centralisation of health services at all levels. As we write, the government has promised equitable access to healthcare, but it is unclear how commissioning groups and health authorities will achieve equity in all geographical areas.

There are major concerns about recruitment of both doctors and nurses to rural areas, particularly where arrangements for the provision of out-of-hours care remain unresolved.

What is it like to be a rural health worker in the UK?

Living in the countryside has its own special joy. Most of us who live and work in rural areas have chosen to do so and consider ourselves lucky. However, the perfect setting on a fine spring morning can be hideous during a foul winter.

Practices tend to be small, and isolated from neighbouring colleagues. List sizes are likely to be low, allowing longer patient contact time but more time spent in travel. Practice populations tend to be stable with relatively slow turnover, so the patients are well known. The professionals may well be seen as 'community property'. Some find the lack of anonymity difficult, especially if they are diffident about taking on a wider role within the community. Travelling is also a major feature for health professionals in isolated areas, sometimes with long drives for schooling, entertainment, etc.

Practice staff may well be patients, with consequent problems of confidentiality and multilayered relationships. Meeting and learning with colleagues and managers can be difficult, engendering a feeling of professional isolation. Information technology (IT) offers the prospect of exciting solutions.

The last decade has seen an explosion of interest in rural health issues.

The Montgomeryshire Medical Society

Since 1979 the society has organised a successful annual conference for rural GPs at Gregynog Hall in Powys, Wales. The event has been influential in developing links between rural health professionals within the UK and internationally.

Rural Practice Group

In 1993 the Royal College of General Practitioners formed a Rural Practice Group to define and address some of the issues concerning rural health. The group has stimulated research, organised conferences and helped to raise the profile of rural practice, publishing an Occasional Paper on Rural Practice in the UK in 1995.[1] It has an Internet forum at: http://www.rcgp.org.uk/forums/rural/wwwboard.htm

The Institute of Rural Health

Formed in 1996 and based at Gregynog Hall in Wales, the Institute is helping to establish a multidisciplinary academic foundation for rural practice. Current initiatives include:

* young persons' health needs
* a project on suicide
* a series of briefing papers on relevant topics such as zoonoses, farming accidents, etc.

The Centre for Health Services Research at Newcastle University

In 1994 the Centre published a comprehensive and useful literature review[2] and in 1997 it completed important research on equity and access in rural primary care.[3] The work has highlighted areas for future research.

EURIPA

Founded in 1997, the European Rural and Isolated Practitioners Association aims to address the health needs of rural communities in Europe and the professional needs of those serving them. It has established a moderated newsgroup (euripa@dial.pipex.com) on the Internet and produced a Charter for Rural Practice, which is accessible on the website.

WONCA

In 1995 the World Organisation of Family Doctors (WONCA) published a seminal report on training for rural general practice.[4] It held its second international conference of rural practice in Durban, South Africa, in September 1997.

The contributors

All the contributors to this book have been chosen as experienced rural practitioners with a track record of involvement in developments within rural practice, often with previous research and publication within their particular fields.

Many of the contributors are members of the RCGP Rural Practice Group, which has been at the forefront in pursuing the rural health agenda. Antoinette Ward has worked as a rural district nurse, midwife, health visitor, practice nurse and educator. She is particularly well qualified to provide a rural nurse's perspective. Neil Frame is a veterinary surgeon. His chapter on animal diseases is essential reading for health workers in agricultural areas who want to know what their patients are talking about.

The future

The enormous upsurge in interest in rural issues, the commitment by government to promote equitable access to healthcare for all and the rapid development of IT suggest an exciting future. However, provision of services in country areas is inevitably more expensive than it is in towns and cities. It remains to be seen how primary care groups respond to the challenge.

There is a compelling need for more research into rural healthcare. This should be easier once the new infrastructure for primary care research in the UK is established.

References

1   Cox J (ed) (1995) *Rural Practice in the United Kingdom*. Occasional paper 71. Royal College of General Practitioners, London.

2 Rousseau N, McColl E and Eccles M (1994) *Primary Health Care in Rural Areas: issues of equity and resource management – a literature review.* (Report no. 66). Centre for Health Services Research, University of Newcastle upon Tyne.
3 Rousseau N and McColl E (1997) *Equity and Access in Rural Primary Care: an exploratory study in Northumberland and Cumbria.* (Report no. 83). Centre for Health Services Research, University of Newcastle upon Tyne.
4 Working Party on Training for Rural Practice (1995) *Policy on Training for Rural Practice.* World Organisation of Family Doctors (WONCA), Victoria, Australia.

2
Rural diseases

Iain Mungall

Most diseases seen in rural areas of the UK are similar to those seen by our non-rural colleagues. Others are more common and important in rural areas, and some are seen only rarely in urban areas.

The conditions described in this chapter are selected because they are more common in rural than urban areas and because they are clinically important. There remains a great deal of uncertainty about the incidence and prevalence of many rural diseases. Symptoms can be non-specific and infections subclinical. There are few published studies that systematically record the incidence and prevalence of rural diseases, so we must recognise that reported incidence may not reflect true incidence. There is a great need for both national and regional studies to define and describe illnesses presenting in rural areas.

Musculoskeletal

Farming is associated with an increased incidence of osteoarthritis, especially of the hips and knees. Other rural occupations are associated with industrial diseases; for example, the use of chain saws in forestry work is associated with vibration disease.

Mental health

Farmers are at greater risk of suicide than average. It is not clear whether there is an increase in depression in the farming population or whether farming is an unduly stressful occupation. It could be related to farmers spending considerable lengths of time alone. It could also be because they have ready access to efficient means of suicide, e.g. shotguns and poisons. Whatever the reasons, we need to maintain a high level of awareness of the possibility of depression and suicide in the farming population.

Insect stings

Wasp and bee stings are common and cause local and occasionally systemic effects. The local effects are caused by injection of amines and peptides, including enzymes and locally active substances such as histamine, dopamine, noradrenaline and GABA. Reactions, which normally last only a few hours, are characterised by pain, swelling, erythema and pruritus. Treatment is by oral antihistamines and local application of ice or 1% hydrocortisone cream. Antihistamine ointments can themselves be allergenic and should be avoided.

Systemic reactions to stings are because of hypersensitivity and can include urticaria, faintness, shortness of breath, nausea, vomiting and palpitations. In severe cases, anaphylaxis with bronchospasm, oedema and shock can be fatal. Normally these reactions begin within a few minutes of the sting. Sensitisation is the result of a previous sting, although there may have been no adverse effects on that occasion.

Wasp stings are retained by the wasp, but bee stings are left in the victim's skin. Bee stings should be removed as quickly as possible by gentle scraping to prevent continuing envenomation.

Hypersensitivity reactions are caused by a variety of allergenic proteins, and should be treated by subcutaneous or intramuscular injection of 0.5–1 ml epinephrine (adrenaline) 1:1000 given as early as possible. Although it only contains 0.3 ml, the EpiPen is a convenient form of epinephrine and may be prescribed to at-risk patients for them to carry at all times. Hypersensitive patients should avoid exposure as best they can. Desensitisation can be very successful.

Horse fly bites ('clegs')

Horse fly bites cause painful, itchy, local skin reactions, often with oedema and urticaria. Oral antihistamines and possibly local hydrocortisone cream may be helpful. Secondary bacterial infection can occur, requiring antibiotics.

Ticks

Rural doctors and nurses are frequently asked to remove ticks from patients. One method of removing a tick is to grasp it firmly, but not too tightly, with tweezers and, with a steady pull, remove it whole. Occasionally the tick's head will be left behind, in which case this can be removed by scraping with a needle. Removal may be easier if the tick is first painted with nail varnish or Tipp-Ex.

There is some suggestion that squeezing the tick's body may cause regurgitation of parasitic organisms into the host, so it is better not to grasp the bloated abdomen directly, but rather grasp it between the belly and the victim's skin. Special tick-removal forceps are available.

Alternative remedies include killing the tick by applying spirit or a tiny amount of fly spray, suffocating it with Vaseline, or burning it with a lighted cigarette then leaving it to die and drop off. The same principles apply to removal of ticks from dogs and other animals.

In areas where tick-borne diseases are prevalent, people should inspect themselves or each other 4-hourly and remove ticks early, before they become engorged.

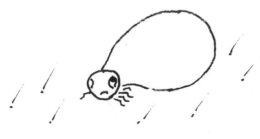

Adder bites

Adders or common vipers (*Vipera berus*) are the only indigenous venomous snakes in the UK. They are distributed unevenly. At birth, which is usually in late summer, adders are 16–17 cm long with fully developed fangs and venom glands, although the volume of venom that a juvenile can inject when biting is considerably less than that delivered by an adult. Fully grown adults often reach a length of 65 cm. They are dark with a clearly defined zigzag stripe along the centre of the back. Adders are cold-blooded and are usually encountered on sunny days in quiet moorland areas, often lying on dead grass or rocks, absorbing warmth. They are usually easy to spot.

Adders hibernate in the winter and are usually not seen between mid-October and February, although in the south of England they may emerge from hibernation as early as January. They are usually most active between May and September. Most adder bites occur during June, July and August.

Venom

Viper venom is produced by modified salivary glands and stored in venom sacs under and beneath the orbit. It is injected 2–3 mm subcutaneously into the victim through two hollow retractable fangs situated at the front of the mouth. A variable volume of venom is delivered. Venom consists of a complex mixture of high molecular weight proteins, proteases, peptide hydrolases, hyaluronidase and phospholipases.

Site of adder bites

In a study of 834 cases of adder bite in the UK and Europe, the site of the bite was hand in 51.6% and foot in 32.8% of cases. Bites on the hand were usually the result of the victim attempting to pick up the snake. Most victims are young males. In my practice I saw one teenager who successfully put five adders in a jar but was less successful with the sixth. There are, however, more bizarre sites. For example, a 14-month-old baby boy was bitten on the ear as he lay in some grass, and in Sweden an 8-year-old boy was bitten on the neck while swimming.[1] I have heard a report of a family of adders swimming through an outdoor swimming pool in the north of England.

Effects of adder bites

Most adder bites result in trivial symptoms and there may be bites without envenomation. (Seventy per cent of reported adder bites result in either no or very mild effects.) However, death can occur between 6 and 60 hours after a bite. The critical period is usually the first 12 hours after being bitten. Children and the elderly are most at risk.

Adder bites engender great alarm, but they are rarely fatal.[2] The last death recorded in Britain was of a 5-year-old boy in Scotland in 1975, so one can generally offer a very optimistic prognosis. Estimates of frequency may not be accurate, but between 1982 and 1990, 72 people attended hospitals in Scotland following adder bites.

In the 1980s a retired GP knelt in rough grass beside his caravan and immediately experienced severe pain in his knee. In the subsequent 12 hours the entire leg became grossly swollen and painful and he felt unwell. The following day, while driving, he blacked out, overturning his car, fortunately without serious injury. It was only some two days later that the diagnosis of adder bite was made.

Local effects

The principal local effect is oedema, sometimes massive, which may occur within minutes but is nearly always present within 2 hours. Bruising may also occur. The site of the bite is usually but not always painful. Bruising and tissue tenderness increase during the first 1–3 days then slowly subside.

Systemic effects

Hypotension is the most important sign of systemic envenomation, usually developing within 2 hours. The victim may feel faint or drowsy and become semi-conscious. Nausea and vomiting are common and diarrhoea may also occur. Other systemic symptoms include abdominal colic, incontinence of urine and faeces, sweating, vasoconstriction, tachycardia, oedema of the face, lips, gums, tongue and throat, urticaria and bronchospasm. There may be some cardiotoxic component in the venom that can cause T wave inversion, myocardial damage and second-degree heart block. A blood sample may show neutrophil leucocytosis, thrombocytopenia and sometimes late anaemia.

Treatment

The effects of adder bites are unpredictable and victims should therefore be monitored closely, usually in hospital.

First aid

Immobilise the affected part to delay spread of venom. Do not manipulate, incise or suck the area, or apply a tourniquet. Local treatments, such as potassium permanganate soaks and ice packs, should not be used because they increase the risk of local tissue necrosis. Strong reassurance of the victim is important and may help to delay systemic envenomation.

Monitor the patient closely for at least 2 hours by recording pulse rate, blood pressure, respiratory rate, progression of local swelling and any new symptoms. Asymptomatic victims with no local swelling within 2 hours can be discharged from care.

Most cases require no treatment other than symptomatic therapy, e.g. analgesia and antiemetics. Systemic steroids, such as intravenous hydrocortisone or oral prednisolone, have been used extensively and may be of value when there are systemic symptoms, but they have not been evaluated critically. There is no indication for prescribing antibiotics.

Antivenom

Antivenom may reduce morbidity, prevent death and reduce convales-cent time in moderate or severe cases. Indications for treatment include systemic symptoms or within 4 hours of a bite on the hand or foot with swelling extending beyond the wrist or ankle.

Antivenom is produced in Zagreb and widely available. It should only be given in hospital. Reactions to antivenom are rare, but a history of allergy or hypersensitivity to equine antiserum carries an increased risk of adverse reactions.

Summary

All adder bite victims should be admitted to hospital for observation for a minimum of 2 hours. Victims, particularly children and the elderly, showing evidence of local or systemic envenomation should be observed for a minimum of 24 hours. Monitoring should include pulse, blood pressure, respiratory rate, progression of local swelling and appearance of new symptoms. Consider giving intravenous hydrocortisone. Antivenom should be given if there is any evidence of systemic envenomation or if local symptoms are severe. Adrenaline should be immediately available for the treatment of anaphylactic reactions to antivenom. Reassurance of the victim is a most important aspect of treatment.

> During a First Aid class for forestry workers in Northumberland I was asked 'Is it true that if two adders are tied together by their tail they will fight each other to the death?'. Naturally, being dedicated to evidence-based medicine, I did not immediately find a reply, but the following week I was advised by the same class that 'No, it isn't true, the two adders just go to sleep'.

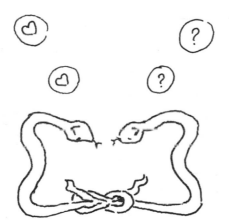

Organophosphate poisoning

Organophosphate insecticides inhibit the enzyme acetyl cholinesterase in insects, but they also inhibit the enzyme in mammals, including humans. Introduced around the time of the Second World War, they have become the principal means of agricultural pest control throughout the world.

Acute, severe poisoning can occur following skin contact, ingestion or inhalation. Inability to break down acetylcholine causes cholinergic effects, including nausea, vomiting, light-headedness, abdominal pain, excessive salivation, blurred vision, headache and subsequent neuropathy. There can be lasting damage to the nervous system, with persistent EEG changes, and reduced performance in neuropsychological testing.[3] Acute poisoning is unusual in the UK.

Treatment is by injection of both atropine sulphate (2 mg intramuscularly or intravenously) and pralidoxime mesylate (30 mg/kg intravenously, slowly), and hospital admission.

Sheep dipping

The widespread use of organophosphates in sheep dip is of particular concern in rural areas. Guidelines exist for the safe use of sheep dips, but these are often impracticable and ignored. As dipping is a long hot hard job, farm workers often have considerable skin contact with the sheep dip solution. However, there is little conclusive evidence of significant illness as a result of exposure.

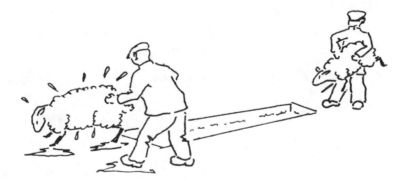

Several studies have detected no difference in symptomatology and CNS function between sheep dippers and controls, but some other studies have shown that exposed sheep farmers are less able to sustain attention or process information and that they may have peripheral sensory loss.[3] Other studies have suggested that sheep farmers are more vulnerable to psychiatric disorder than controls, but it is unclear how far this is related to organophosphates or to other economic and social factors.

More long-term studies are required to determine adverse effects, particularly psychological ones.[4,5] Investigations into 'Gulf War syndrome' may furnish more information.

Diagnosis

Enquire about sheep dipping in farmers with non-specific illness. The diagnosis can be confirmed by a blood test, demonstrating reduced erythrocyte cholinesterase activity. In subclinical poisoning activity may be reduced to 50% and in severe poisoning to 10% of normal.

Dust diseases

Farmers are often exposed to dust, which may contain grain dust, bacteria and metabolites, fungi and metabolites, endotoxins and mites. Two syndromes have been described: allergic alveolitis or hypersensitivity pneumonitis (HP) and organic dust toxic syndrome (ODTS). These two illnesses may represent parts of a spectrum of response to complex organic dusts and not distinct clinical entities.

Farmer's lung

Farmer's lung is a hypersensitivity pneumonitis or extrinsic allergic alveolitis following exposure to mouldy hay on which thermophilic actinomycetes (e.g. *Micropolyspora faeni*) have grown. For the purposes of compensation, it is recognised as an industrial disease. When disturbed, mouldy hay releases clouds of millions of spores. A recent report from Canada has identified further possible antigens, *Penicillium brevicompactum* and *Penicillium alevicolor*, which are responsible for a farmer's lung-like condition that can progress to fatal pulmonary fibrosis.

Prevalence

In the UK the prevalence ranges from 10 to 50 per 100 000 farmers. The higher the rainfall, and therefore the more likely the hay to be mouldy, the greater the prevalence of the disease.

Symptoms

Fever, chills, general malaise and flu-like symptoms, including cough and dyspnoea without wheezing, arise 4–8 hours following exposure. Repeated exposure can cause irreversible lung damage.

Management

Management of the condition is largely to do with early diagnosis and prevention. It demands a careful history to discover the source of occupational exposure. Once diagnosed, patients must be counselled about the importance of avoiding exposure to mouldy hay, working with hay in the open air, staying upwind of it and using a face mask. Change of working practices, e.g. making silage instead of hay, or even a change of occupation should be discussed.

Diagnosis

Serology can be useful to help confirm a diagnosis. Chest X-ray can be helpful but is not as specific as CT scanning. Pulmonary function tests show loss of vital capacity and exercise-induced hypoxaemia.

Treatment

Removal from the source is imperative. A course of oral steroids, e.g. prednisolone 1 mg/kg daily for 1–2 weeks, gradually withdrawing over the subsequent 6 weeks, is often helpful, particularly if symptoms are severe.

Prognosis

Smoking adversely affects farmer's lung disease, reducing the 10-year survival rate from over 90% to 70%.[6] Farmer's lung is potentially very serious. Death can occur following heavy exposure to mould. Mortality has been estimated at 0.7%, occurring on average 8 years following diagnosis.

Other causes of hypersensitivity pneumonitis

There are many other causes of hypersensitivity pneumonitis, including mushroom worker's lung (*Micropolyspora faeni*), bird fancier's lung, sauna taker's lung, paprika splitter's lung (*Mucor stolonifer*), dog house disease (*Aspergillus versicolor*), cheese washer's lung (*Penicillium casii*) and sewage worker's lung (*Cephalosporium*). The principles of diagnosis and management are similar to farmer's lung.

Organic dust toxic syndrome

ODTS is characterised by a febrile reaction to inhaled mould dust. Unlike hypersensitivity pneumonitis, which is associated with heavy exposure over days or weeks, ODTS is associated with extreme exposure occurring on a single day. There is evidence that dust masks protect against dust inhalation and that they can be practicable in the farming environment.[7]

Creutzfeldt-Jakob disease (CJD)

CJD is caused by an infectious, proteinaceous particle, which is devoid of nucleic acid (a prion). There are two forms. Both are difficult to diagnose in the early stages.

Classic CJD typically presents in late middle age with rapidly progressive dementia, usually fatal within 6 months. The annual incidence worldwide is 0.5–1 per million per annum.

New-variant CJD, which was first described in 1996, presents in younger people (aged under 42), and is characterised by behavioural change, ataxia, progressive cognitive impairment and a longer duration of illness (up to 23 months). Both types are invariably fatal and there is no specific treatment. The brains of victims with new-variant CJD have a different appearance to those with classic CJD, with similar lesions to those found in scrapie.[8]

Brain biopsy, the only certain way to diagnose the condition, shows spongiform changes in both types.

CJD and BSE

A report from the National CJD Surveillance Unit in Edinburgh in 1996 suggested that bovine spongiform encephalopathy (BSE) in cattle was a likely cause of new-variant CJD. This link was confirmed in 1997 by studies showing identical incubation periods and pathological brain lesions when material from new-variant CJD patients and animals with BSE were innoculated into susceptible mice. The Advisory Committee on Dangerous Pathogens has now classified BSE as a disease of humans.[8]

This link has had a major impact on farmers, as the government has introduced restrictions in an attempt to eradicate BSE from herds and to bring confidence back to consumers.

Zoonoses

Zoonoses are infections passed to man from animals. There are many illnesses in this category, but not all are seen in the UK. Many zoonotic infections produce non-specific symptoms or only subclinical illness in man. Many remain undiagnosed by GPs. Others are only diagnosed in retrospect by antibody tests. Information about incidence and geographic distribution within the UK is hard to come by. There is a need for more research.

Box 2.1: Notifiable zoonoses in England and Wales

- Anthrax
- Food poisoning, e.g. due to *Salmonella, Campylobacter, E. coli, Cryptosporidium*, etc.
- Lassa fever
- Leptospirosis
- Marburg disease
- Viral haemorrhagic disease
- Plague
- Rabies
- Relapsing fever (louse-borne *Borrelia* infection)
- Tuberculosis
- Murine typhus
- Yellow fever
- Brucellosis

The Public Health Laboratory Service Communicable Disease Surveil-lance Centre in Cardiff, commissioned by the Health and Safety Executive (HSE), has published research which gives valuable insight into the prevalence and incidence of zoonoses in UK farm workers.[9] The key messages from the study of three different farm types and geographic areas are:

- infections with ringworm, orf, cowpox, *Coxiella*, *Chlamydia* and *Toxoplasma* are common in UK farm workers

- Lyme disease, leptospirosis and brucellosis are uncommon in UK farm workers

- Hantavirus and *Bartonella* infections occur in rural UK populations

- *Coxiella* and *Toxoplasma* infections occur more frequently in livestock farmers than people in other occupations

- ringworm infection is associated with exposure to cattle. Hantavirus and cowpox infections are associated with exposure to rats. Orf is associated with sheep. *Coxiella* is associated with total farm contact and exposure to cattle. *Chlamydia* is associated with sheep, specifically with lambing

- *Helicobacter pylori* and *Neospora caninum* may be acquired by zoonotic transmission.

They showed that antibodies to Q fever (27.3%), *Chlamydia* (79.6%) and *Toxoplasma* (50.2%) are common in UK farm workers, but antibodies to Lyme disease (0.3%), leptospirosis (0.2%) and brucellosis (0.7%) are uncommon (but the study did not include areas known to be associated with Lyme disease). Also, 4.7% of farm workers had antibodies to Hantavirus, 0.7% to orthopox virus, 4.5% to parapox virus, 2% to *Bartonella* spp. and 1.5% to *Echinococcus granulosis*. Orf occurs in 2% of farmers each year and ringworm occurs in farmers at a rate of 4% per year.

Table 2.1. Relationship between animal exposure and disease antibodies

Antibody	Animal
Hantavirus and cowpox	Rats
Coxiella (Q fever)	Cattle
Chlamydia	Sheep (specifically with lambing)
Orf	Sheep
Ringworm	Cattle

The relationship between animal exposure and particular disease antibodies is shown in Table 2.1.

Lyme disease

This was first described in 1977 after an outbreak of juvenile rheumatoid arthritis in the Lyme area of Connecticut, USA. However, there is retrospective evidence that the first European case was in the late 19th century and the first American case over 80 years later. It is important because it is a serious disease, which is eminently treatable if diagnosed. In the UK, Lyme disease is most commonly found in East Anglia, Scotland, Northern Ireland and the New Forest.[10]

Organism and route of transmission

The tick *Ixodes ricinus* acts as a vector for the spirochaete *Borrelia burgdorferi*, which causes the disease. There is a reservoir of infection in mammals, particularly deer. *B. burgdorferi* has recently been divided into three groups, each associated with different disease patterns:

- *B. burgdorferi* sensu stricto, associated with arthritis
- *B. garinii*, associated with neurological manifestations
- *B. afzelius*, associated with late or persistent Lyme disease.

The incubation period is 3–32 days following the tick bite.

Clinical

Lyme disease is a systemic inflammatory disease with three stages typical of spirochaetal diseases (such as syphilis). The first stage consists of an area of expanding erythema around the site of a tick bite. The lesion may grow to as large as 15 cm in diameter and have red borders and central pallor. They are sometimes called target lesions because of the central red macule, surrounding pallor and red border. Similar lesions may develop at other sites forming the syndrome of erythema chronicum migrans. There is frequently a flu-like illness, which may include fatigue, headache, fever, meningism and musculoskeletal aches and pains. The first stage is most likely to occur during summer, when people and ticks are more active in the countryside.

The second stage occurs several weeks or months later and may include cardiac effects (such as A–V block or myopericarditis) and neurological manifestations (including meningitis and cranial nerve involvement, especially of the 7th nerve). There are increased numbers of lymphocytes in the cerebrospinal fluid. Neurological problems may last for many months, but usually resolve completely.

As in syphilis, the third stage may begin many years later. Intermittent arthritis is present in about 80% of patients. There are asymmetrically migratory joint pains, usually of large joints, with polymorphonuclear synovial fluid. Fatigue is common but fever is uncommon. Ten per cent of patients develop persistent arthritis and some develop persistent neurological disease, which can mimic multiple sclerosis, psychiatric illness or transverse myelitis.

Diagnosis

With a history of tick bite in a geographical area where Lyme disease is known to exist, erythema chronicum migrans is the most important sign.

Tests

It is not possible to culture the spirochaete, but there are three useful immunological tests: immunofluorescence assays (IFA), enzyme-linked immunosorbent assays (ELISA) and immuno blots. These serological tests are not always helpful, particularly in the early stages, and treatment on purely clinical grounds is reasonable.[11] Antibiotic treatment may alter the humoral response. Serology tests are most useful for late Lyme disease (third stage). Low-titre positive or borderline results are usually suggestive of early Lyme disease, and high-titre positives are likely to be associated with late infection. Antibodies to B. burgdorferi alone do not confirm active Lyme disease, but merely that the patient has been exposed to the organism. (A study in rural Wigtownshire showed that approximately 10% of asymptomatic patients had antibodies.[12])

Prevention

Vaccination for Lyme disease is currently in development.

Prevalence

Lyme disease is most common in East Anglia, Scotland, Northern Ireland and the New Forest.

Treatment

Erythema chronicum migrans is treated with tetracycline 250 mg four times daily for 10 days, amoxycillin or, in children, penicillin V. These effectively shorten the illness and prevent subsequent stages of the disease.

Treatment of the second and third stages with intravenous penicillin has been shown to reduce the duration of meningitis from 30 weeks to 10 days and to cure arthritis in 55% of cases. Oral doxycycline is equally effective in the second and third stages.

Morbidity

Much remains unknown about Lyme disease. It is not possible to predict which patient exposed to the organism will go on to develop the disease. It is not clear whether antibiotics should be given prophylactically to patients following tick bites in areas where Lyme disease is prevalent. Nor is it clear whether antibiotics should be given to patients who develop non-specific symptoms such as fatigue, headache and fever following tick bites. Serological tests may help our understanding of the epidemiology and management of Lyme disease. In the meantime, many doctors use antibiotics even if there is only a small possibility of Lyme disease.

The ACP journal club reviewed the results of a controlled trial of antibiotics prescribed for 387 people within 7 days of deer tick bites.[13] Fifteen per cent of people were infected with the spirochaete but only two developed symptomatic Lyme disease. They concluded that the risk of infection without treatment was 1.2% and that giving amoxycillin could eliminate the risk. They also concluded that routine antibiotic treatment after most tick bites is not indicated, but may be worth considering in pregnant women and in those patients who present with highly engorged ticks. Because the spirochaete is most likely to be regurgitated into the host towards the end of feeding, the risk of infection increases with the duration of feeding.

Orf (contagious pustular dermatitis or ecthyma)

Most patients are aware of the diagnosis and come to the doctor for confirmation and management advice.

Organism

Orf is caused by a parapox virus that normally affects lambs, but can affect cattle and goats. Lambs' lips, which are the principal source of infection in humans, are the usual part involved, but it can infect any part of the skin. The virus is resistant and may survive in dust, on walls and on the wood of sheep pens. Another parapox virus occurs on cows teats causing milker's nodule, distinguishable from cowpox by the absence of vesicles and pustules.

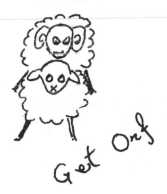

Route of transmission

The virus is transmitted through the skin. Human orf is an occupational hazard for farmers and shepherds and those who handle sheep carcasses, including abattoir workers and vets. Person-to-person transmission is uncommon. The incubation period is thought to be 3–4 days.

Clinical

The orf lesion develops as a single, macular then papular rash, usually on the hand or lower arm. Subsequently a vesicle forms, which evolves into a soft, solid lesion, usually up to 2 cm in diameter. The mature lesion looks rather like a pustule, but incision shows only a solid, soft keratosis. The whole lesion disappears within 5–6 weeks. Several lesions can occur in the same patient. Generally the patient remains well, but there may be some fever. Generalised viraemia is rare, although a severe infection known as giant orf has been reported in a patient with lymphoma.

Erythema multiforme is a recognised complication.

Treatment

Some patients develop a secondary cellulitis and benefit from treatment with antibiotics, e.g. flucloxacillin 250 mg 6-hourly for 7 days. Otherwise no treatment is necessary and the patient can be assured of complete recovery. Immunity develops so that subsequent infections are less likely. Buchan, in an unpublished study from Powys, suggests that shave biopsy may shorten the duration of the lesion. There is no evidence that antiviral drugs are effective or indicated, but local idoxuridine paint or cryotherapy are sometimes used.

Little is known about the behaviour of the orf virus during pregnancy. However, a case was reported in 1993 from South Dakota where a lady developed orf at 33 weeks gestation. There were no pathological findings in the baby, which was born at term, or in the placenta.

Prevalence

The HSE study suggested prevalence among farmers of around 4% in a year.

Cowpox

Organism and route of transmission

Cowpox is caused by an orthopox virus and is transmitted by hand contact with an infected ulcer on a cow's teat. It affects 0.7% of farmers per year.

Clinical

There may be one or more vesicular or pustular lesions on the hand, which scab. There may also be a lymphangitis and lymphadenopathy.

Diagnosis and treatment

Diagnosis is by virus culture from a lesion. There is no treatment.

Ringworm

Organism

The most common ringworm organisms in rural areas are *Trichophyton mentagrophytes* and *Trichophyton verrucosum*, which affect cattle and horses. A variant is caused by *Microsporum canis*, which affects dogs and cats. *Microsporum* fluoresces under Wood's lamp, but *Trichophyton* species do not.

The incubation period is 4–10 days. Although ringworm has low infectivity, it is communicable as long as lesions persist, so patients should be advised to use personal facecloths and towels. Secondary infection may occur and require systemic antibiotics.

Incidence

The HSE study (see above) showed that 29.5% of farmers had a history of ringworm at some time, and that 1.6% had had it during the preceding year. There was a strong association between infection and exposure to cattle.

Clinical

Generally the skin disease starts as a small papule, which slowly extends with central healing, causing an enlarging ring with an active raised edge and normal central skin. A variant, called a kerion, causes a boggy, raised, suppurative lesion. Reinfection is rare.

Diagnosis and treatment

Diagnosis can be confirmed by examining skin scrapings taken with a razor blade on to black paper. Placing the skin scrapings on to a glass slide and adding potassium hydroxide reveals hyphae under microscopy.

Treatment with a topical imidazole cream, such as clotrimazole or miconazole, is normally adequate. Occasionally a keratolytic such as Whitfield's ointment can be effective. Improvement can be expected within one week and a cure within one month. For severe cases griseofulvin (500 mg daily by mouth for at least a month) may be necessary. For griseofulvin-resistant cases, oral terbinafine is effective.

Anthrax

Organism

Anthrax is a serious disease caused by the bacterium *Bacillus anthracis*, a spore-forming organism.

Route of transmission

Anthrax most commonly infects the skin, through direct contact with infected animals and animal products, but can affect the gastrointestinal (GI) tract and the respiratory system, following ingestion or inhalation of spores. Workers in wool and bone processing, and tanning may be at risk. The incubation period is usually within 48 hours.

Incidence

The incidence of anthrax has declined enormously since 1965, probably because of improved animal infection control, with better occupational control over the handling of animal products. Vaccination is available, but is seldom required and can cause significant side effects. Since 1975 only 28 cases have been recorded, nearly all of them occupational.

Clinical

Anthrax usually presents as a skin lesion with itching, followed by the development of a papule which progressively becomes vesicular, then a depressed black 'eschar' surrounded by considerable oedema.

Inhalation anthrax presents with a mild upper respiratory tract infection, developing fever and severe shock and death within 3–5 days. Meningitis can develop.

Mortality

Untreated, anthrax of the skin has a mortality rate of 5–20%, but with antibiotic treatment death is rare. Treatment is by IM penicillin G, 2 million units 6-hourly initially, for 5–7 days. GI and inhalation anthrax have a high mortality.

Helicobacter

Organism and route of transmission

The causative organism is *Helicobacter pylori*. Transmission is largely person to person, but there is some evidence that the bacterium is present in cats, and that other species of *Helicobacter* are found in other animals. There is no evidence of an increased occupational risk associated with farming, but it may be acquired from animals. It is not known whether human infection is more common in rural areas. Incubation is 5–10 days.

Prevalence

Between 20% and 50% of adults in developed countries have the infection, usually acquired during childhood.

Clinical

It is associated with chronic gastritis, peptic ulceration and gastric adenocarcinoma.

Treatment

'Triple therapy', for example a one-week course of:

- metronidazole 400 mg twice daily
- amoxycillin 500 mg twice daily
- omeprazole 20 mg twice daily.

Brucellosis ('undulant fever')

Organism and route of transmission

The causative organism is *Brucella abortus* or *B. mellitensis*. Transmission is usually through handling infected animals, placentas or aborted foetuses (through breaks in the skin), or through ingestion of unpasteurised milk and dairy products from infected animals. Incubation is usually 5–60 days.

Prevalence

Brucellosis has been eradicated from cattle in the UK, and so new cases are extremely unusual. However, relapses can occur after many years.

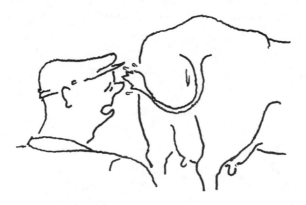

Clinical

The rather non-specific symptomatology, e.g. insidious onset of intermittent or irregular fever, headache, weakness, sweating, chills, arthralgia, depression, generalised aching and weight loss, may make diagnosis difficult. Neurotic symptoms are sometimes misdiagnosed as chronic brucellosis. Serological tests can be helpful. However, interpretation of tests in chronic and recurring cases can be especially difficult because titres are usually low.

Treatment

Treatment is with rifampicin 600–900 mg daily and doxycycline 200 mg daily for at least 6 weeks.

Psittacosis

Organism and route of transmission

The causative organism is *Chlamydia psittaci*, which is inhaled from pet birds, but may be associated with turkey or duck farming and processing. The incubation period is 1–4 weeks.

Clinical

Psittacosis is an acute systemic illness often with fever, myalgia, headaches and respiratory symptoms. The latter are often relatively mild in comparison to X-ray findings of pneumonia.

The diagnosis is confirmed by isolation of the organism from infected material after culture in mice, egg or cell culture.

Treatment is with tetracyclines, e.g oxytetracycline or erythromycin 250 mg 6-hourly, taken for 2 weeks after fever subsides.

Ovine chlamydiosis

Organism and route of transmission

The causative organism is the strain of *Chlamydia psittaci* that causes enzoootic abortion of ewes (EAE). It is responsible for approximately 30% of sheep abortions and many stillborn, weak and premature lambs. Pregnant women in contact with sheep during pregnancy, particularly during the second and third trimesters, can become infected.

Clinical

Infection during pregnancy can have serious consequences, including foetal death. Severe multisystem disease in the woman can result in hepatic and renal dysfunction and disseminated intravascular coagulation.

The diagnosis is made by complement fixation test or immunofluorescence. The platelet count may be low. Prognosis improves with early diagnosis and treatment with erythromycin and metronidazole. Close observation of the pregnancy is mandatory and early induction of labour may be indicated. Erythromycin has been used to treat neonates for 2 weeks after birth.

Prevention

The most important measure is to educate farming communities about the problem, encouraging pregnant women to maintain scrupulous personal hygiene and avoid contact with lambs, placentas, amniotic fluid and contaminated clothing during lambing.

Streptobacillosis (rat bite fever)

Organism and route of transmission

The causative organism is *Streptobacillus moniliformis*. Infection is usually through a rat bite, but can occur without a bite in rat-infested buildings. Contaminated milk or water has been suspected as the route of transmission in outbreaks. Incubation is 3–10 days.

Clinical

There is acute onset of chills and fever, headaches and muscle pains, followed within 1–3 days by a maculopapular rash, mainly on the extremities. One or more large joints may become inflamed. Serious complications include bacterial endocarditis, pericarditis, parotitis, tenosynovitis and soft tissue and brain abscesses.

Morbidity

Untreated, fatality rates can be 7–10%. Relapses occur commonly. Treatment is with penicillin 250 mg or tetracycline 250 mg 6-hourly for 7–10 days.

Prevention

Penicillin or doxycycline can be used prophylactically following a rat bite.

Leptospirosis (Weil's disease) (haemorrhagic jaundice)

Organism

In the UK the commonest organisms are *Leptospira icterohaemorrhagica* (from rats) and *L. hardjo* (from cattle). Others include *L. hebdomidis.*

Route of transmission

The organism can be transmitted through the skin, especially if abraded, or mucous membranes. It can also be ingested in food or drink contaminated by infected urine from domestic or wild animals, particularly rats and cattle. Leptospirosis is a recreational hazard for bathers, campers and sportsmen, as well as for water bailiffs, fish processors and sewerage workers. Person-to-person transmission is rare. Incubation period is usually 10 days (4–19).

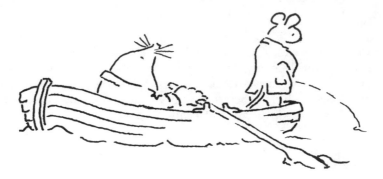

Prevalence

The HSE study showed 0.2% of farm workers had antibodies.

Clinical

Leptospirosis can be a serious illness with fever, sudden-onset headache, severe myalgia, conjunctivitis, meningitis, palatal rash, haemolytic anaemia, skin haemorrhages, hepatorenal failure, jaundice, mental confusion/depression, myocarditis and pulmonary involvement. However, many cases are very mild and undiagnosed.

Serological evidence of leptospirosis is found in 10% of cases initially diagnosed as meningitis and encephalitis. Resistance to the specific strain of leptospirosis follows infection, but this may not protect against infection with a different serovar.

Prevention

Doxycycline 200 mg weekly has been shown to prevent leptospirosis in people exposed to contaminated water.

Treatment

Prompt treatment is most important. Doxycycline 100 mg twice daily, penicillin G 1.5 megaunits 6-hourly and amoxycillin for 7 days have all been shown to be effective if commenced before the onset of jaundice.

Q fever

Organism

Q fever is caused by *Coxiella burnetii*, a rickettsia highly resistant to physical and chemical agents.

Route of transmission

Transmission is principally from sheep. The organism can be tick borne or transmitted by inhalation of infected dust from premises containing placental tissue, birth fluids or excreta of infected animals. There seems to be no evidence of person-to-person transmission. The incubation period is usually 2–3 weeks.

Prevalence

A recent study of farming communities in England and Wales showed little reported disease, but high prevalence of antibodies (27.3%). Evidence of previous exposure was higher in those in direct contact with animals, particularly those involved with calving and handling the products of cattle conception.

Clinical

Symptoms include acute febrile illness, retrobulbar headache, weakness, malaise and severe sweats. A pneumonitis may be shown on chest X-ray and there may be liver involvement and chronic endocarditis.

Diagnosis is made by antibody tests. The rickettsia may also be identified by electron microscopy or immunofluorescent testing in tissues and blood. Immunity follows recovery, preventing further infections. Immunisation is available, but is still experimental; it may be recommended for laboratory, abattoir or veterinary workers at risk.

Treatment

Oral tetracycline (250 mg 6-hourly) or chloramphenicol should be continued for several days after the fever subsides. Tetracycline combined with rifampicin or ciprofloxacin may also be effective. If endocarditis occurs, surgical replacement of an abnormal or prosthetic heart valve may be necessary. Mortality is negligible in treated cases, but as high as 1% if untreated.

Toxoplasmosis

Organism and route of transmission

Toxoplasmosis is caused by the organism *Toxoplasma gondii*. The normal host for *Toxoplasma gondii* is cats, but intermediate hosts include sheep, goats, rodents, swine, cattle and chickens. Infection may also be acquired from raw or undercooked meat, particularly pork or mutton containing *Toxoplasma* cysts, or from food or water contaminated with cat faeces. There is no evidence of person-to-person transmission, except from pregnant mother to foetus. Antibodies persist for many years. The incubation period varies from 5 to 23 days.

Prevalence

Systematic surveys show that it is greatly underdiagnosed. Antibodies are found in approximately 30% of the asymptomatic population and as many as 50% of UK farm workers. Approximately 660 cases are confirmed every year. There is some suggestion that most infection takes place in childhood.

Clinical

Toxoplasmosis may be asymptomatic or undiagnosed because it is similar to infectious mononucleosis, presenting as an acute disease with only lymphadenopathy, fever and lymphocytosis which may persist for days or weeks. As the illness subsides, *Toxoplasma* cysts containing viable organisms may remain in the tissues, reactivating later if the immune system becomes compromised. Diagnosis is by detection of blood antibodies.

Treatment

Treatment is not routinely indicated for a healthy person. For severe cases, pyrimethamine 50–75 mg per day, with sulphadiazine 2–6 g per day and folinic acid 10–15 mg daily for 4 weeks is the treatment of choice. Clindamycin can be added for patients with ocular toxoplasmosis.

Echinococcus (hydatid disease)

Organism

The tapeworm *Echinococcus granulosus* is a small worm found in dogs, especially when they have consumed uncooked viscera, e.g. from sheep.

Route of transmission

Human infection, 'cystic hydatid disease', occurs through hand-to-mouth transfer of eggs from dogs' faeces. Children in contact with dogs or dog faeces are at particular risk because of their generally poor personal hygiene.

Incubation and clinical

Cysts slowly enlarge in varying parts of the body, taking several years to develop and eventually mimicking tumours.

Diagnosis is by serology, with X-ray, CAT scans or ultrasound scan evidence of cysts.

Prevention involves avoidance of animal viscera, worming dogs and advice about the dangers of contact with dog faeces.

Treatment

Patients may require surgical excision of cysts, but albendazole 400 mg twice daily for 28 days alone may be successful.

Toxocariasis

This is also known as visceral larva migrans, and is rather similar to the cutaneous larva migrans occasionally seen in travellers from abroad.

Organism

The larval forms of a roundworm present in both dog (*Toxocara canis*) and cat (*T. catis*) faeces cause it. Infection from dogs is much the commonest cause of the illness, which is particularly common in young children.

Route of transmission

The eggs are present in contaminated soil and are then ingested. Up to 30% of soil samples from certain parks in the UK contain *T. canis* eggs, which can remain viable in soil for many months.

Incubation period is weeks or months.

Incidence

In recent years an average of 29 cases per year have been recorded by the Public Health Laboratory Service.

Clinical

Once eaten, eggs hatch out in the bowel and larvae penetrate the systemic circulation affecting organs such as the liver, lungs, spleen, lymph glands and eyes. The illness may take weeks or months to become apparent and eye involvement may develop as long as 10 years after infection.

The illness is characterised by eosinophilia, hepatomegaly, hyperglobulinaemia, fever and lung symptoms. WBC counts may be as high as 100 000 with 80–90% eosinophilia. There can be chronic abdominal pain, generalised rash and, sometimes, focal neurological signs.

Diagnosis and treatment

ELISA serology is sensitive in up to 90% of cases.

Mebendazole 100–200 mg twice daily for five doses is the treatment of choice.

Prevention

Parents should be made aware of the risks associated with pets. They should discourage children from contact with dog or cat faeces or contaminated soil, for example in play areas. Cats and dogs should be 'wormed' regularly.

Hantavirus

Organism and morbidity

Hantaviruses cause haemorrhagic fever with renal complications. One form found in the USA causes severe respiratory failure and cardiogenic shock with a mortality rate of up to 50%. The predominant European form is caused by the Puumala virus which causes a less severe illness, 'nephropathia epidemica', with a fatality rate of under 1%.

Route of transmission

Rats are the usual source of infection; the virus is present in their urine, faeces and saliva. The disease is not transmissible from person to person. The incubation period is 1–8 weeks.

Prevalence

The HSE study showed that the seroprevalence of Hantavirus antibodies is 4.7%, increasing to 9.4% over the age of 60.

Clinical

Classically there are five clinical phases: afebrile, hypotensive, oliguric, diuretic and convalescent. Fever, headache, malaise and anorexia are followed by severe abdominal or back pain, often with nausea and vomiting, skin petechiae and conjunctival injection, persisting for 3–7 days. The hypotensive phase begins abruptly and may progress to shock and haemorrhages. During the oliguric phase blood pressure returns to normal or may be elevated. During the recovery diuretic phase there may be polyuria of 3–6 litres per day. Full recovery takes months.

It is of note that the HSE showed that a significant number of farmers seroconverted during the study year, but without associated severe illness. Presumably many infections occur subclinically and without obvious or direct contact with rats.

Diagnosis is made by serology using ELISA or IPHA.

Treatment

Appropriate inpatient treatment for shock and renal failure is required. Early IV antiviral treatment has been found to improve the management.

Infectious diarrhoeas

Salmonella

Organism and route of transmission

Many strains of Salmonella cause diarrhoea. The organism is normally passed through contaminated food. Epidemics have been reported arising from non-chlorinated water supplies, but this is very uncommon in the UK. The infective dose may be as little as 1000 organisms, so person-to-person transmission is often seen in families. Larger epidemics are usually due to mishandling of food, together with poor temperature control, which enables multiplication of the Salmonella.

The organism is found in a wide range of animals, including poultry, pigs, cattle, rodents, cats and dogs, as well as human carriers. The importance of avoiding raw and undercooked eggs and poultry has been appreciated in recent years and cannot be overstated.

The incubation period is normally 12–36 hours. A small proportion of infected people may become carriers, excreting the organism for over one year.

Prevalence

The Public Health Laboratory Service noted an increase in salmonellosis starting in the mid-1980s and peaking in 1993 with over 30 000 reported cases. During this time an increasing proportion of the organisms were *Salmonella enteritidis*. Over recent years a rise in antibiotic resistance has been noted and frequently *Salmonella typhimurium* is now multiply resistant.

Clinical

Salmonella causes a diarrhoeal illness with systemic effects, including headache, nausea and vomiting and dehydration which may be severe.

Diagnosis of Salmonella is by culture of faeces. Serological tests are not useful.

Treatment is normally merely rehydration but antibiotics may be indicated in infants of under 2 months, the elderly and those with immune deficiency. Ciprofloxacin or amoxycillin may be effective.

Campylobacteriosis

Organism and route of transmission

Campylobacter jejuni and *C. coli* are the causative organisms. Sporadic cases, for which no source is found, are common but outbreaks are often associated with undercooked chicken, unpasteurised milk and non-chlorinated water supplies. The organism is known to affect many animals, particularly poultry and cattle, but also young cats and dogs, pigs, sheep and rodents.

Incubation is usually 2–5 days.

Prevalence

This is now the most commonly isolated GI pathogen in England and Wales. Over 44 000 cases were recorded in 1994.

Clinical

The illness is of varying severity. Many infections are asymptomatic. There can be severe diarrhoea with abdominal pain and fever, usually lasting 2–5 days, but prolonged illness may occur.

Diagnosis is by isolation of the organism from faeces.

Treatment

Some Campylobacter organisms are susceptible to erythromycin 250 mg 6-hourly for 7 days or tetracyclines, but antibiotics are generally only of value if taken early in the illness.

Cryptosporidiosis

Organism and route of transmission

The parasite *Cryptosporidium parvum* is the causative organism. It can be found in humans, cattle and other domestic animals. Infection may follow faecal ingestion from contaminated water supplies or food.

Incubation is probably 1–12 days.

Prevalence

Prevalence is unknown, but in developed countries the organism has been found in between 1% and 4.5% of stool samples sent to laboratories from patients with diarrhoea.

Clinical

Cryptosporidium causes profuse, watery diarrhoea, abdominal pains and fever, normally settling spontaneously within one month. Immunocompromised people, e.g. those with AIDS, may be unable to overcome the infection, which may then contribute to death.

Diagnosis is by demonstrating small oocysts of *Cryptosporidium parvum* in stool samples.

The only treatment is rehydration. Antibiotics have not been shown to be effective.

Entero-haemorrhagic *E. coli* (0157)

Organism

E. coli are the most frequent normal flora of the human gut. Some serotypes (verotoxic *E. coli*, VTEC) produce verocytotoxin, an entero-toxin like that from Shigella. The 0157 strain is the most common toxin-producing, entero-haemorrhagic strain of *E. coli*. Other strains of VTEC are widely encountered as travellers' diarrhoea.

Route of transmission

Epidemics have been associated with inadequately cooked beef, unpasteurised milk and infected water supplies.

Incubation is usually 3–4 days but up to 8 days. Only very small doses of infected material are required to cause the disease.

Clinical

E. coli 0157 causes diarrhoea. This may be mild or it may be extremely severe with major haemorrhage, especially in the elderly, and, in children, haemolytic uraemic syndrome (the most common cause of acquired renal failure in children). Normally there is no fever. Death may ensue.

Diagnosis is by stool culture. Treatment is by fluid and electrolyte replacement. It is not clear whether or not antibiotics have a role to play.

Tetanus

Organism and route of transmission

Tetanus is caused by *Clostridium tetani*. The spores are introduced through wounds in the skin from contaminated soil, dust, animal (especially horse) or human faeces. Infection occasionally occurs through trivial wounds. Neonatal tetanus, due to infection of the umbilical stump, is an important cause of death in Asia and Africa. It is not spread from person to person.

Incubation is usually 3–31 days. The shorter the incubation, the worse the disease.

Prevalence

Although tetanus is entirely preventable by immunisation, some 800 000 neonates worldwide die annually. In Western society adults are more likely than children to be infected. The USA has fewer than 100 cases reported yearly. Between 1984 and 1995 there were 145 reported cases in England and Wales, 53% in people over 65 years.[14]

Clinical

The organism grows anaerobically, producing an exotoxin that causes painful muscular contractions, often beginning in the jaw and neck ('lockjaw' or trismus), trunk and abdominal wall. Opisthotonus and risus sardonicus are characteristic. Mortality varies from 10% to 90%, depending on the age of the patient (it is higher in the young and the elderly), the incubation period and the availability of intensive care facilities.

Diagnosis and treatment

The organism is rarely cultured and antibodies rarely rise. Diagnosis is clinical, with a high index of suspicion in the presence of a recent wound.

Respiratory support must be available, in hospital. The wound is cleaned and debrided. Intramuscular penicillin and tetanus antitoxin should be given promptly. Diazepam helps to relieve muscle spasms or, for severe cases, the patient is paralysed and ventilated. Tetanus immunisation needs to be started.[14]

Prevention

In the UK, all children should be immunised routinely in the first year of life. A primary course of three injections of tetanus vaccine over one year followed by two booster vaccines at 10-year intervals should be completely protective. Because of the risk of reactions, a total of five immunisations in a lifetime is probably sufficient, other than at the time of a tetanus-prone injury. The following are considered to be tetanus-prone wounds:[14]

- any wound or burn sustained more than 6 hours before surgical treatment of the wound or burn

- any wound or burn at any interval after an injury that shows one or more of the following characteristics:
  - a significant degree of devitalised tissue
  - puncture-type wound
  - contact with soil or manure likely to harbour tetanus organisms clinical evidence of sepsis.

Liver flukes

Organism and route of transmission

The trematode (flatworm) *Fasciola hepatica* can infect humans. It is found particularly in marshy, sheep-bearing areas. Sheep are the main primary host, but other animals, e.g. cattle, may also host the worm. A semi-aquatic snail, *Lymnaea* spp., is the intermediate host. Egg cysts remain just under the water surface, attached to grass (or watercress). When swallowed by man or other animals, flukes penetrate the duodenum and reside in the gall bladder, bile duct or liver parenchyma.

Incubation is 8–16 weeks.

Clinical

Many patients have no symptoms. There may be dull pain in the right hypochondrium, particularly in the afternoon. As the disease progresses, pain becomes more persistent, with lassitude, anorexia, fever and hepatomegaly. Cholangitis, cholangiocarcinoma, cirrhosis or portal hypertension may develop.

Diagnosis and treatment

Ova are found on microscopy of faeces or bile. Treatment with albendazole, mebendazole or praziquantel is usually effective.

Prevention

Awareness of the dangers of ingesting water or watercress in sheep areas.

References

1   Persson H and Irestedt B (1981) A study of 136 cases of adder bite treated in Swedish hospitals during one year. *Acta Medica Scandinavica.* **210**:433–9.

2   Reading CJ (1996) Incidence, pathology and treatment of adder (*Vipera berus* L) bites in man. *Journal of Accident & Emergency Medicine.* **13** (5):346–51.

3   Rosenstock L *et al.* (1991) Chronic central nervous system effects of acute organophosphate pesticide intoxication. *Lancet.* **338**:223–7.

4   Stephens R *et al.* (1995) Neuropsychological effects of long term exposure to organophosphates in sheep dip. *Lancet.* **345**:1135–9.

5   Mearns J *et al.* (1994) Psychological effects of organophosphate pesticides: a review and call for research by psychologists. *Journal of Clinical Psychology.* **50**(2):286–94.

6   Ohtsuka Y *et al.* (1995) Smoking promotes insidious and chronic farmer's lung disease and deteriorates the clinical outcome. *Internal Medicine.* **34**(10):966–71.

7   Kowsaka H *et al.* (1993) Two year follow up on the protective value

of dust masks against farmer's lung disease. *Internal Medicine.* **2**:106–11.

8   Will RG *et al.* (1996) A new variant of Creutzfeldt-Jakob disease in the UK. *Lancet.* **347**:921–5.

9   Thomas DR and Salmon RL (1997) *Zoonotic Illness in Farmworkers and their Families: clinical presentation and extent: a prospective collaborative study.* (Project No. 1/HPD/126/308/90). Health and Safety Executive, London.

10 Welsby P (1990) Lyme disease. *The Practitioner.* **234** (8 June).

11 Kirton SM and Pennington TH (1995) The diagnosis of Lyme disease. *Journal of the Society of Medicine* **88**:248–50.

12 Baird AG, Gillies JCM, Bone FJ *et al.* (1989) Prevalence of antibodies indicating Lyme disease in farmers in Wigtownshire. *BMJ.* **299**:836–7.

13 Shapiro ED, Gerber MA, Halobird MD *et al.* (1992) A controlled trial of anti-microbial prophylaxis for Lyme disease after tick bites. *New England Journal of Medicine* **327**:1769–73.

14 Salisbury DM and Begg NT (eds) (1996) *Immunisation Against Infectious Disease.* HMSO, London.

Further reading

Bannister BA, Begg NT and Gillespie SH (1996) *Infectious Diseases.* Blackwell Science, Oxford.

Bell JC, Palmer SR and Payne JM (1988) *The Zoonoses: infections transmitted from animal to man.* Edward Arnold, London.

Benenson AS (1995) *Control of Communicable Diseases Manual*, 16th ed. American Public Health Association, Washington.

Isselbacher KJ *et al.* (1994) *Harrison's Principles of Internal Medicine*, 13th ed. McGraw Hill, New York.

Stanford CF (1991) *Health for the Farmer.* Farming Press, Ipswich.

Weatherall DJ, Ledingham JG and Warrell DA (1995) *Oxford Textbook of Medicine*, 3rd ed. OUP, Oxford.

Acknowledgements

I am hugely indebted to Nicol Black, Daniel Thomas and RMM Smith for their help on zoonoses, Suzanne Ellingham for her help with literature searches, and Derek Blades for his guidance and overall support.

3
Animal diseases

Neil Frame

Introduction

In the UK in 1996 there were approximately 12 million cattle, 41 million sheep and 7 million pigs. Many people's lives are inextricably linked with these animals – the farm labour force in the UK numbers more than 600 000 people. Most animal diseases are predisposed by poor knowledge, poor management and intensive farming methods. Early identification and diagnosis of veterinary problems and owner cooperation are crucial to successful treatment.

There is considerable overlap between veterinary medicine and human medicine. This chapter describes animal husbandry and some diseases common in animals. It includes lay terms commonly used by patients in GPs' consulting rooms. An understanding of patients' occupations helps health workers not only to appreciate health needs, but also to 'speak the same language'. Some diseases, e.g. zoonoses, may have a direct effect on patients' health, while others may affect mental wellbeing, particularly because of their financial consequences.

Sheep

Sheep are kept mainly for their fleece (wool) and meat (mutton and lamb), although there are increasing numbers of milking flocks where, as in dairy cattle, the production of offspring is a means to milk production.

Sheep farms are categorised according to their height above sea level into lowland, upland or hill farms. Sheep are bred to suit the terrain and altitude at which they are kept. Hill breeds, such as Scottish Blackface,

Swaledale and Herdwick, are extremely hardy and the ewes are attentive mothers. Ewes may be crossed with lowland tups (male breeding sheep), such as Cheviot or Border Leicester, to produce more fertile and productive offspring. Young female lambs (gimmers) are sold to upland farms for breeding. Breeds such as Suffolk or Texel, which are less robust but which have good feed conversion, are kept on lowland farms.

Tups are turned out with ewes and hoggs (females in their first breeding season) in the autumn after the ewes have been 'flushed' with good grass to stimulate ovulation. 'Sponging' the ewes (pre-tupping with progesterone vaginal implants) or running 'teasers' (vasectomised tups) with the ewes prior to tupping also stimulates ovulation and helps to ensure a tight lambing period. The majority of the ewes should conceive within 6 weeks, i.e. two oestrus cycles. Coloured 'raddle' dyes may be attached to the tups' briskets (chests) by a harness to mark the ewes they have served. Those ewes that have been mounted by the tup can be identified by the telltale coloured dye transferred on to their backs. The dye colour is changed after 3 weeks.

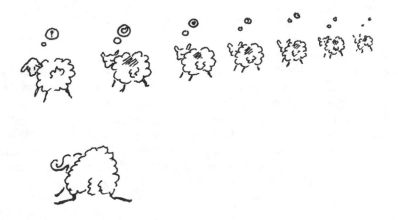

The sheep gestation period is 5 months. Twinning is desirable, except in hill flocks where there may be insufficient food for a ewe to raise two lambs. Triplets require excellent husbandry and much labour to ensure their survival. They account for 15% of lambs but 45% of neonatal mortality.

Abortion ('throw') is endemic in many sheep flocks. An infectious agent is the usual cause of an abortion rate in excess of 1%. The two main abortigenic organisms in sheep are *Toxoplasma gondii* and *Chlamydia psittaci*, which causes enzootic abortion of ewes (EAE). Both Toxoplasma and Chlamydia infections are dangerous to pregnant women (see Chapter 2). Although awareness of the dangers of pregnant women being involved with sheep around lambing time is increasing, it is still not unusual to find premature newborn lambs being warmed in the farm kitchen. Amniotic fluid contains a heavy burden of contagious organisms, which readily vaporise from a drying fleece.

Both Toxoplasma and Chlamydia attack the placenta rather than the ewe or foetus, and lambs may be born alive, but weak or premature. Vaccines against these organisms are available and effective. *Listeria monocytogenes*, Salmonella spp. (particularly *typhimurium* and *dublin*) and Campylobacter spp. may also cause ovine (i.e. sheep) abortion.[1]

Lambing may occur indoors or outdoors depending on the time of year. It is a period of concentrated activity on the farm. Lowland farms may aim to lamb soon after Christmas, while hill farms commonly lamb in April. Caesarean section may be necessary because of foeto-maternal oversize or incomplete dilation of the cervix (ringwomb).

Unlike humans, domestic animals confer little immunity through the placenta, immunoglobulins being instead absorbed from the colostrum. The neonate lamb is most capable of such absorption during the first 4 hours of life, therefore it is imperative to ensure that small, weak lambs receive adequate colostrum soon after birth. Newborn lambs are particularly susceptible to disease if colostral uptake is poor.

E. coli septicaemia in lambs under 72 hours of age becomes more prevalent at the end of lambing, with increasing faecal contamination of the lambing shed or pasture. 'Watery-mouth', 'rattle-belly' and 'lamb scour' (diarrhoea) are all descriptive lay terms for the symptoms. Many farm workers have a reasonable understanding of terms such as endotoxaemia, septicaemia and metabolic acidosis. They may also understand the principles of fluid therapy and the use of hypertonic intravenous solutions.

Gram-positive bacteria (especially *Actinomyces pyogenes*) can gain entry via the navel (navel-ill) causing infective arthritis (joint-ill).

During late pregnancy, pregnant ewes may exhibit neurological symptoms caused by pregnancy toxaemia (twin-lamb disease). In lowland breeds this may be complicated by fatty liver syndrome. Other common neurological diseases include scrapie, the ovine equivalent of CJD in humans and BSE in cattle. Staggers is a descriptive term for magnesium deficiency. Listeria is a soil-borne organism ingested by sheep and cattle from big bale silage, which can cause both abortion and meningitis (circling disease). A parasitic (coenurus) cyst in the brain causes 'gid' or 'sturdy'. Hypocalcaemia ('milk fever') results in progressive ataxia and recumbency.[2]

Some dermatological conditions, such as sheep scab caused by the mite *Psoroptes ovis*, cause such intense pruritus they may initially be mistaken for a neurological condition. Recent reduction in the use of organophosphorus sheep dips has led to a re-emergence of this parasite. Despite the availability of an excellent vaccine, orf, a poxvirus, is still prevalent in sheep and therefore in sheep farmers and their families.[3]

Pigs

Most of Britain's pig rearing takes place indoors in intensive farming systems. However, recent much-needed welfare legislation and concerns about endemic diseases are leading to the return of many farmers to outdoor breeding. Outdoor arcks for hardier breeds of pigs (which 10 years ago had almost been extinct), where a sow and her piglets can stay in a loose family group until weaning, are becoming more common again.

A sow's gestation period is 3 months, 3 weeks and 3 days. Parturition is usually an uncomplicated procedure, particularly in fitter outdoor breeds. A sow can produce two litters each year. Between 13 and 18 piglets are born at approximately 5-minute intervals. Within seconds of birth the newborn piglets stand and walk towards the sow's udder (or an artificial heat source).

Diseases of the newborn, such as *E. coli* enteritis and septicaemia and streptococcal meningitis, are common in intensive systems. Iron deficiency anaemia is treated by iron injections administered shortly after birth.

Young pigs are intelligent, inquisitive creatures. Lack of environmental stimulation can lead to behavioural vices, such as tail biting.

Breeding boars can weigh up to 500 kg. Artificial insemination is not used to the same extent as it is in the dairy industry. Pig farmers determine whether a sow is in season by leaning on its back in a somewhat undignified manner. If the sow will 'brim' or 'stand' for the farmer, it should do the same for the boar.

Birthing problems include vaginal or uterine prolapse and metritis-mastitis-agalactiae syndrome or 'farrowing fever', a rapidly developing, life-threatening septicaemia. Treatment must be prompt to save the sow.

Pig farmers try to achieve 'minimal disease status', but problems such as enzootic pneumonia caused by *Mycoplasma hyopneumoniae* are difficult to eliminate. Sometimes it is necessary to cull all the sows and give a house a period of rest. However, even if replacement gilts (young sows) are obtained from so-called 'disease-free status' herds, infections such as enzootic pneumonia often return within a year or two.

Britain is currently free of classic swine fever, a serious pig disease currently prevalent in some European countries. It will have enormous welfare and economic significance if it finds its way into British herds.

Cattle

Cattle in Britain are grass-grazed during the summer months and generally loose-housed in a cubicle system and fed silage in the winter. Large amounts of concentrates are fed to dairy cows to boost milk production. Most dairy herds consist of the modern Holstein cow, which at peak yield will produce 50 litres of milk every day, and over 10 000 litres during each 10–month lactation.

The bovine gestation period is 9 months. In both dairy and beef herds the farmer's aim is to attain a calving index of 365 days, i.e. a calf born by each cow every 12 months. To achieve this, a cow should conceive 90 days after calving. This is the optimum interval for maximum milk output and calf production without detriment to the cow. Like sheep and horses, cows ovulate approximately every 21 days and display oestrus behaviour at this time. Rectal palpation or ultrasound per rectum 24–28 days post conception can confirm pregnancy. Poor ovulation and absent oestrus behaviour occur commonly when a cow is 'milking off its back', i.e. its food intake is inadequate.

Cows are 'dried off ', i.e. stopped milking, two months prior to calving. Routine intra-mammary antibiotic therapy ('tubing') is used in the dry period to prevent mastitis. Once the cows have calved, the cycle begins again. Obstetric problems include malpresentation or uterine torsion, both of which may be corrected under epidural anaesthesia. Foeto-maternal oversize is managed by Caesarean section using a flank approach, preferably under paravertebral anaesthesia with the mother standing.

Viral enteritis ('scour'), commonly caused by a rotavirus or coronavirus, is particularly prevalent in the first 14 days of life and can cause death if fluid and electrolyte therapy is not initiated rapidly. Intestinal absorption is severely limited by virus damage to intestinal villi and calves may take many days to recuperate.

Other causes of 'scour' include *Cryptosporidium* infection, which is becoming increasingly common in suckler calves and may contaminate human water sources if contaminated slurry is spread on the land. *Salmonella* and *E. coli* spp. are also common causes. They too may infect humans. *Salmonella typhimurium* 204c is probably the most commonly encountered strain in calves and is presenting difficulties because of multiple drug resistance.[4]

In the autumn and winter, calves less than 4 months of age are particularly susceptible to pneumonia. In dairy calves, pneumonia is usually caused by respiratory syncytial virus (RSV) or parainfluenza virus (PI3). Vaccines against these viruses are used routinely, but the response is variable because of interference from maternal antibodies acquired from colostrum and the weak antigenicity of the vaccine.[5]

In beef calves pneumonia may be viral but is often bacterial, caused by *Pasteurella haemolytica*, *Mycoplasma bovis* or, increasingly, *Haemophilus somnus*.

Copper deficiency during pregnancy causes locomotor problems in the newborn ('swayback'), due to lack of myelination of nerve sheaths. Muscular weakness and paresis in calves and lambs may be caused by selenium deficiency ('white muscle disease'). Better understanding of nutrition has now made these trace element deficiency diseases much less common.

Parasite diseases in young cattle (e.g. the respiratory disease 'husk' caused by *Dictyocaulus viviparus*) have also become less common. However, acquired resistance to antihelmintic therapy is increasing and so this favourable situation may change.

Outbreaks of trichophyton ringworm, lice and mange (caused by sarcoptic or psoroptic mites) are usually associated with poor nutrition. Ticks (*Ixodes ricinus*) are common in parts of the country and may be vectors of disease such as 'louping ill' in sheep (caused by *Cytoecetes phagocytophilia*) and 'tick-borne fever' (caused by *Ehrlichia ovis*). Lyme disease (*Borrelia burgdorferi*) is not commonly recognised in domestic animals, perhaps partly due to the lack of the classic skin rash seen in man.

Heifers calve for the first time between 24 and 30 months of age. Unlike sheep flocks, abortion epidemics in cattle are now rare, mainly because of compulsory eradication of *Brucella abortus* ('contagious abortion'). However, *Leptospira hardjo* is still a common cause of abortion and precipitous drop in milk yield in affected cows ('milk-drop syndrome', 'flat bag').[6] Many farm workers have contracted leptospirosis from handling aborted material or from milking in a modern herring-bone parlour. Working at udder level in a sunken pit allows urine to splash directly into the dairyman's conjunctivae.

Hypocalcaemia ('milk fever') in the periparturient period can quickly progress from ataxia through recumbency to death by respiratory failure. Hypomagnesaemia ('grass staggers') can cause cardiac arrest and death even more quickly.

Calving can cause birth tract damage and lead to peritonitis, as can undiagnosed retained foetal membranes. Another problem of the periparturient period that can rapidly lead to death is toxaemic mastitis, usually caused by *E. coli*. Treatment must be rapid and intense, otherwise the toxins cause lasting parenchymatous organ damage. It is not unusual to have to administer 60–80 litres of intravenous fluid during the first 12 hours of treatment.

Viral diseases can cause high morbidity and serious economic loss. Farmers are familiar with the shortened descriptions of these viruses, for example infectious bovine rhino-tracheitis (IBR) and bovine viral diarrhoea (BVD). Expensive vaccines help to control these diseases.

BSE is a relatively new infectious disease. It is caused by an infectious, proteinaceous particle (a prion) ingested from feed contaminated by sheep brain (from sheep with scrapie) or cattle brain. The incidence of the disease is falling rapidly. However, many questions remain unanswered, not least the question of vertical transmission (firmly established in the scrapie model) and the full risk to which the human population has been exposed.

Primary acetonaemia, when milk production outstrips energy intake, is known as 'slow fever'. Apart from the classic ketone breath, some bizarre neurological manifestations can arise, including obsessional self-licking and roaring like a bull.

Cows and sheep have four stomachs and the fourth stomach, the acid-producing abomasum, may displace from its usual right flank position to become entrapped between the left flank and the rumen (first stomach). In the condition known to farmers as 'twisted stomach', there is no entrapment of blood supply, unlike in the less common 'right torsioned abomasum'. Here the omental attachment of the abomasum tears, allowing rotation. Surgical intervention is corrective in both conditions and many dairy farms will experience several such operations each winter.[7]

Cows eat some 40 kg of silage plus up to 10 kg of cereal-based ration ('straights') every day. Under poor management they are in a constant state of metabolic acidosis and at risk of a variety of conditions, ranging from abomasal stomach ulcers to laminitis (an inflammatory process involving the sensitive laminae of the feet). Many other infectious feet problems, e.g. 'foul of the feet' and 'lure', are predisposed by poor horn growth following laminitis.

Many cows are slaughtered because they have chronic feet problems. Infertility and recurrent mastitis are the other major reasons for culling. However, preventative veterinary medicine programmes have made enormous progress in minimising these chronic problems.

Horses

While cattle owners focus on veterinary problems of feet, udder and genital tract, horse owners' attention is centred largely on wind and limb. This is because horses are largely kept for athletic pursuits and anything, however slight, adversely affecting oxygen exchange or locomotion can result in poor performance.

Horses, particularly young horses kept in large groups, can be affected by viruses of the upper respiratory tract ('the cough'), but effective vaccines for equine flu virus and equine herpes virus have reduced the incidence greatly. Regular flu vaccination is compulsory for horses racing under Jockey Club Rules.

Much attention is paid to the presence of an inspiratory noise ('roaring') while the horse is exercising. This is due to dysfunction of the left recurrent laryngeal nerve and leads to paralysis of the left arytenoid cartilage. This hereditary dysfunction is common in hunter types and surgery to replace the left crico-arytenoid muscle with a prosthetic ligament ('tie back') is usually successful, although it may cause dysphagia.

As many as 10% of Britain's horses are sensitised to the fungal spore *Microsporum faenii*, leading to the respiratory condition incorrectly known as 'broken-winded'. This is a misleading term because, unlike farmers' lung in humans, there is practically no alveolar involvement. The symptoms of coughing and exercise intolerance are due to bronchospasm, goblet cell metaplasia and excess mucus production and the situation is totally reversible.[8] Management may include removing the horse from the allergen, e.g. by putting it out to graze on green grass, and administration of inhaled sodium cromoglycate, which is more dramatically effective than it is in humans.

Most lameness is centred on the distal limb or foot, predisposed by poor foot care, shoeing and conformational problems. Young thoroughbreds are predisposed to osteochondritis dessicans (OCD) lesions, damage to the digital flexor tendons, periostitis of the metacarpus ('bucked shins') and spontaneous fractures of the first and second phalynx ('split pastern') caused by excessive exercise on immature limbs.

Hunter types are predisposed by breed, weight and poor foot care to proliferative and degenerative osteoarthritic conditions, e.g. 'navicular', a degenerative condition of the distal sesamoid; 'spavin', a progressive arthritic condition of the intertarsal and tarso-metatarsal joints; and 'ringbone', an exuberant arthritis of the interphalangeal joints.

Native ponies are predisposed by well-meaning overfeeding to laminitis. Excessive carbohydrate intake can lead to a rapid build-up of lactic acid in the large bowel, death of gut commensals and severe metabolic acidosis with endotoxaemia. This situation leads to serum exudation at the laminae or 'white line' of the foot. The ensuing pressure can cause permanent damage to the foot ('foundered') with rotation or downward displacement ('sinker') of the pedal bone.[9]

Horses are prone to bouts of abdominal 'colic'. They are monogastric and fermentation takes place in the large bowel. The anatomical arrangement of the gut, verminous aneurysms of the mesenteric arteries, poor dentition and feeding are all predispositions for colic. As well as alleviating pain, the veterinarian's task is to quickly differentiate medical from surgical colic, e.g. intussusception, where urgent surgery is essential.[10]

Some colics do not involve the bowel. Tears to the broad ligament in the parturient mare, bladder calculi and 'grass sickness', a disease of the autonomic nervous system, are the most common examples.

Exotics

Farmers have been encouraged to diversify, and all manner of non-indigenous species now grace our landscape. Ostriches, farmed for their feathers and low cholesterol meat, are increasing in numbers. Adults are hardy and can cope with all weathers. Egg laying is restricted to 5 months of the year, unlike in warmer climes where they lay all year.

Camelids, mainly alpacas and llamas, are a pleasant addition to the farmscape. They have few veterinary problems and breed well. They are solely kept for their hair, an extremely valuable 'fibre' that is sheared annually.

Conclusion

People who work with animals are familiar with birth, life, death, disease and suffering. This affects the way they regard their own health and mortality and that of their families. Many will have seen or assisted in invasive procedures such as bronchial alveolar lavage, paracentesis, cerebrospinal fluid collection and surgical procedures, such as Caesarean sections or colic surgery.[11] All this combines to help make such people phlegmatic and patient, tolerant and understanding.

References

1 Drost M and Thomas GA (1996) Infectious causes of infertility and abortion. In: BP Smith *Large Animal Internal Medicine*, 2nd edn. CV Mosby, St Louis, pp. 65–94.
2 Scott PR (1993) A field study of ovine listerial meningoencephalitis with particular reference to cerebrospinal fluid analysis as an aid to diagnosis and prognosis. *British Veterinary Journal*. **149**:165–70.
3 Fadock VA (1984) Parasitic skin diseases of large animals. *Veterinary Clinics of North America*. **6**:3–26.
4 Snodgrass DR, Terzelo HR, Sherwood D *et al.* (1986) Aetiology of diarrhoea in young calves. *Veterinary Record*. **119**:31–4.
5 Baker JC (1986) Bovine respiratory syncytial virus: pathogenesis, clinical signs, diagnosis, treatment and prevention. *Compend Cont Educ Pract Vet* **8**:F31–8.
6 Songer JG and Thierman AB (1985) Leptospirosis. *Journal of the American Veterinary Medicine Association*. **193**:1250–4.
7 Guard C (1996) Abomasal displacement and volvulus. In: BP Smith *Large Animal Internal Medicine*, 2nd edn. CV Mosby, St Louis. p. 792.
8 Cook WR (1976) The diagnosis of respiratory unsoundness in the horse. *Veterinary Record*. **77**:516–28.
9 Adams OR (1987) *Lameness in Horses*, 4th edn. Lea & Febiger, Philadelphia, pp. 486–99.
10 Murray JM (1992) Alimentary tract disease. In: NE Robinson *Current Therapy in Equine Medicine*, 3rd edn. WB Saunders, Philadelphia, pp. 190–223.
11 Frame NW and Scott PR (1996) *Ancillary Diagnostic Aids for Bovine Practitioners*. XIX World Buiatrics Conference, Edinburgh, 8 July.

Glossary

BROKEN-WINDED   allergy to fungal spores in horses causing small airway constriction.

BUCKED SHINS   periostitis of the metacarpal bones in young horses as they adjust to training.

CIRCLING DISEASE   meningitis in ruminants, usually caused by *Listeria monocytogenes*.

CONTAGIOUS ABORTION   abortion in cattle caused by *Brucella abortus*.

DRYING OFF   infusion of antibacterial drugs into the udder at the end of lactation, usually about 2 months prior to calving.

E. COLI MASTITIS   mastitis causing acute endotoxaemia.

FLAT BAG   sudden drop in milk yield often associated with *Leptospira hardjo.*

FOUL (LURE)   interdigital infection in cattle caused by *A. pyogenes.*

FOUNDERED   anatomical changes in the horse's foot as a sequel to laminitis.

GID (STURDY)   symptoms in sheep associated with a space-occupying lesion in the brain.

GIMMER   young female sheep who has yet to produce a lamb.

GRASS SICKNESS   autonomic nervous disorder in horses, of unknown aetiology, causing invariably fatal colic-like symptoms.

HEIFER   female cow who has not yet produced a calf.

HOGG   a male or female sheep, older than a lamb but still in its first year.

HUSK   respiratory disease in young grazing cattle associated with lung worm.

JOINT-ILL   bacterial infection of the joints in young animals.

LAMINITIS   inflammation of the laminae of a horny foot, e.g. in cows or horses.

LOUPING ILL   a nervous disorder in animals caused by a tick-borne virus.

MILK DROP   precipitous drop in milk yield usually associated with *Leptospira hardjo* infection.

MILK FEVER   nervous symptoms, usually in periparturient cows, associated with hypocalcaemia.

NAVEL-ILL   ingress of bacteria at birth through the umbilicus. May lead to a generalised septicaemia.

NAVICULAR   degeneration of the distal sesamoid bone in the horse's foot.

RATTLE-BELLY   symptom of *E. coli* septicaemia in neonatal lambs.

RING-BONE   proliferative osteoarthritis involving phalangeal bone of horses.

RING-WOMB   incomplete dilation of the cervix during second stage labour.

ROARING   inspiratory noise in horses caused by laryngeal hemiplegia.

SCOUR   diarrhoea.

SINKER   anatomical displacement of the distal phalynx caused by equine laminitis.

SLOW FEVER   primary acetonaemia in lactating cows.

SPAVIN   a lay term for pathological change involving the equine tarsus.

SPLIT PASTERN   a fracture of the first or second phalangeal bone in the horse.

SPONGING   using progesterone-impregnated vaginal implants in sheep to synchronise oestrus.

STAGGERS   acute neurological signs associated with hypomagnesae-mia in ruminants.

SWAY-BACK   copper deficiency in ruminants.

TEASERS   vasectomised male sheep used to help synchronise oestrus in ewes.

THE COUGH   upper respiratory signs in horses of viral origin, usually influenza or herpes virus.

THROW   abortion.

TIE-BACK   corrective surgery for laryngeal hemiplegia.

TUBING   insertion of intramammary drug or the passing of a stomach tube.

TUP   male, breeding sheep.

TWIN LAMB DISEASE   pregnancy toxaemia in ewes.

TWISTED STOMACH   displacement requiring correction of the abo-masum in ruminants.

WATERY MOUTH   *E. coli* septicaemia in lambs.

WHITE LINE   division between horn wall and sole of the foot.

WHITE MUSCLE DISEASE   muscular dystrophy associated with vitamin E or selenium deficiency.

4
Emergencies

Jim Cox

Trauma

Until recently, the first person to be called to the scene of a rural accident, whether on the road, farm, fell or elsewhere, was the local doctor or nurse. More recently, in the event of a serious accident, it has become normal for members of the public to dial 999 and call for an ambulance. Nevertheless, rural practitioners are still more likely than their urban counterparts to be called upon to clean and suture wounds, remove foreign bodies and generally patch up the wounded.

Most urban doctors and nurses no longer respond to accidents. Ambulance paramedics and technicians are now the professionals best equipped to provide the service the public has come to expect. There are, of course, exceptions. In particular, doctors who are members of BASICS (British Association for Immediate Care) work alongside the uniformed emergency services in a voluntary capacity. They also provide medical incident officers and other doctors at the scenes of major accidents.

Rural ambulance services

Rural ambulances are now normally crewed by paramedics who are well trained in pre-hospital care. Unlike most GPs and community nurses, their skills in resuscitation and the management of trauma have been assessed and they are required to recertify at regular intervals. The effectiveness of paramedic interventions in trauma patients remains unproven.

In 1974 the Department of Health specified that, in 95% of emergency calls, a fully equipped and staffed ambulance should respond to a 999 call within a specified time period. These 'ORCON' standards require a response within 14 minutes in urban areas, 19 minutes in rural areas and 21 minutes in sparsely populated parts of Wales, Scotland and Northern Ireland (Table 4.1). New targets published by the Government will require an even faster response to 'Category A' calls, whether or not they come from a rural area (Table 4.2).

Table 4.1 Ambulance response times

Current standard	
Urban areas	95% within 14 minutes
Rural areas	95% within 19 minutes
Sparsely populated areas (Scotland, Wales and Northern Ireland)	95% within 21 minutes
Proposed standard for 'Category A' calls (urban and rural)	
By 2001	75% within 8 minutes
Long-term goal	90% within 8 minutes

Table 4.2 Ambulance 'Category A' calls

1 Adults with chest pain associated with any of the following: pallor, cyanosis, shortness of breath, sweating, nausea or vomiting; but specifically excluding those for whom the pain is intensified by breathing.
2 Individuals who are unconscious, fitting or unresponsive for any cause.
3 Individuals with severe breathing problems who are unable to speak whole sentences.
4 Individuals who have suffered trauma with penetrating injuries to the head or trunk.
5 Any individuals recognised as having anaphylactic shock.
6 Women with severe obstetric haemorrhage.
7 Children under the age of two.

Urban practitioners can choose to opt out of trauma care if they wish. This is not the case for those who practise in rural areas, who are much more likely to be first on the scene of an accident. In isolated areas, they are likely to be called by members of the public and they will be expected to 'do something'. It therefore behoves those who intend to work in a rural area to be prepared!

What opportunities exist for those who live in or visit rural areas to damage themselves?

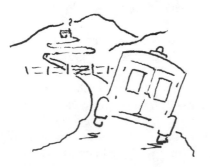

Agricultural accidents

Although farms are much less labour intensive than in the past, they are more mechanised. Most of the machinery is heavy and powerful and some of it is used in hostile conditions, such as on sloping or wet ground in rain, snow and/or mist. Tractors and four-wheel drive motorbikes turn over, limbs get trapped in machinery and people fall off things or get run over.

Animals and their management are also dangerous. The dangers of bulls are well known, but cows may also cause injury. A cow may weigh up to one ton and, particularly when they have calves, they may become aggressive and kick, butt or trample humans.

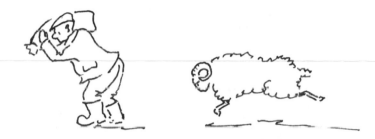

Farmers and vets attempting to inject animals frequently inject themselves with contaminated needles.

Other agricultural hazards include slurry pits – underground, anoxic, offensive lakes of excreta. (I can say from personal experience that one needs a strong stomach to resuscitate a victim of near drowning in a slurry pit.) Farmers use and abuse sharp instruments and noxious chemicals, e.g. herbicides, grain-drying agents and sheep dip fluids. They also have access to rifles and shotguns for vermin control and sometimes sport. Shotgun injuries can be a messy form of suicide.

Road traffic accidents

Although the injuries sustained in rural road traffic accidents are similar to those sustained in towns, access can be restricted by narrow roads, and definitive treatment may be delayed because of the distance to hospital. The patient's condition must be stabilised if it is going to take a long time to get to hospital. The 'golden hour' – the first hour after injury where treatment can have a major impact on outcome – may be over before the patient reaches the hospital.

Fish farming

Fish farming, a relatively new rural industry, has its own occupational health problems.[1] Not only can farm workers fall into the water and suffer hypothermia or drowning, but also they may become entangled in nets when diving. When clearing out dead fish, divers may make repeated descents and ascents ('yo-yo diving'). Because standard decompression tables do not allow for this sort of activity, it is difficult to predict how many descents and ascents they can make safely, and decompression sickness has been reported.[2]

Fish foodstuffs attract rats, creating a risk of leptospirosis, and the use of organophosphate pesticides to treat lice can lead to poisoning. Needlestick injuries can be serious. Self-injection of oil-based salmon vaccines against the bacterial infection *Aeromonas salmonitica* can cause vascular spasm and tissue necrosis. Injuries should be explored under local or general anaesthetic and flushed out with saline as soon as possible.

Training

How should a doctor or nurse who intends to practise in a rural area prepare? Most will sleep more easily if they have appropriate training and equipment to deal with the sorts of emergencies that may crop up unexpectedly.

First of all, be prepared for day-to-day minor trauma. If necessary, brush up on your knowledge and skills in wound management, including suturing and the use of Steri-strips and Histoacryl glue.

Many GPs will have spent 6 months or more working in an accident and emergency department as part of their vocational training for general practice. This is enormously valuable, particularly in preparation for dealing with patients who have suffered trauma who present at your surgery. You may, however, be less well prepared for the circumstances of pre-hospital care, where patients may be in inaccessible situations and doctors do not have the benefit of the staff or equipment of A & E departments. If you are going to work in an isolated area you should at least attend a pre-hospital care course. Contact BASICS Education (Tel: 01473 218407) or the Royal College of Surgeons of Edinburgh (Tel: 0131 527 1600) for more information. Although focused on management in hospital, Advanced Trauma Life Support (ATLS) courses are also excellent. The 'gold standard' qualification is the Diploma in Immediate Medical Care of the Royal College of Surgeons of Edinburgh (Dip IMC RCS Ed), soon to be available to paramedics and nurses, as well as to doctors.

Equipment

Calls to accidents can come at any time and without warning. It is therefore necessary to carry basic resuscitation and trauma treatment equipment in your car at all times. If, when the call comes in, you are miles from your surgery it would be unsatisfactory to have to go back to pick it up before travelling to the incident.

Minimum equipment carried in the car should include:

- A. Airway management with protection of the cervical spine

  - rigid cervical collars (e.g. NecLoc, Stifneck),
  - Guedel airways
  - nasopharyngeal airways
  - laryngoscope and endotracheal tubes
  - aspirator to clear vomitus, etc., from the airway (e.g. Vitalograph Emergency Aspirator)
  - cricothyroidotomy equipment (e.g. Mini-trach II).

- B. Breathing

  - bag and mask (with oxygen reservoir)
  - oxygen
  - tension pneumothorax equipment (e.g. Cook Emergency Pneumothorax Set)
  - Asherman seal or paraffin gauze and tape for open chest wounds.

- C. Circulation

  - at least 3 litres of Hartmann's solution
  - giving sets and wide-bore IV cannulae.

- Splints

  - traction splint for fractured femur
  - armlock splints for keeping the elbow extended when an IV cannula has been inserted into the antecubital fossa.

- Protective clothing (very important)
  - Wellington boots
  - fluorescent jacket
  - protective helmet, preferably with a visor
  - green beacon.

Depending upon his or her training and experience, every person is likely to carry a slightly different kit. The above is simply a guide.

Communications

Whether a call comes from a member of the public to the emergency services or to the doctors' surgery, it is important that those attending can communicate with each other and with the receiving A & E department. In Chapter 6, Philip Spencer discusses pagers, mobile telephones and two-way radios.

Don't panic

Some people work in rural areas because they enjoy the challenges of relative isolation. Even if you are there to enjoy a quiet life and avoid the stresses and strains of urban living, you can make an effective contribution to pre-hospital care by following the basic principles of 'ABC'.

A Airway management with protection of the cervical spine

Make sure the patient's airway is patent and secure. If there is any possibility of neck injury, the cervical spine should be stabilised manually, then secured by a rigid cervical collar and neck blocks on a spinal board. Ensure that the airway is clear by using a jaw-thrust manoeuvre. Where appropriate, insert an oropharyngeal, nasopharyngeal or endotracheal airway.

B Breathing

Ensure that the patient is breathing adequately. If necessary, assist ventilation with a bag and mask (always with an oxygen reservoir) and high-concentration oxygen. Treat tension pneumothorax by inserting a suitable needle (such as the one supplied in a Cook Emergency Pneumothorax Set) through the second intercostal space in the mid-clavicular line. Seal open chest wounds with an Asherman seal or paraffin gauze taped on three sides only. Support flail chests and broken ribs with manual support and by lying patients on the side of the injury.

C Circulation and haemorrhage control

Control haemorrhage by direct pressure on the wound. If the patient is shocked or travel to hospital may be prolonged or if in any doubt, always insert a large-bore intravenous cannula (gauge 14 (brown) or gauge 16 (grey)) and either flush it with normal saline or start an infusion of Hartmann's solution. Do not over-transfuse.

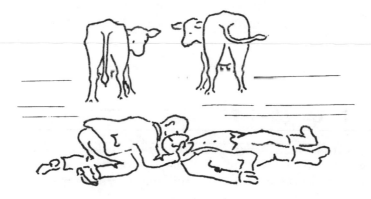

Pain control

Pain relief in the pre-hospital situation is still often inadequate. Much pain can be relieved by splinting broken bones and through the use of Entonox (50% nitrous oxide and 50% oxygen). If necessary, do not be afraid to administer an intravenous opiate such as diamorphine.

Triage

A doctor can be particularly useful at the scene of an accident where there are several people with serious injuries or where there is prolonged entrapment of casualties. In the circumstances, try not to be drawn into the care of individual patients, but take an overview of the situation. You can assess priorities for immediate treatment, suggest to members of the emergency services where they are best employed, advise about the requirement for additional resources and report back to the receiving hospital indicating what they should expect.

Priorities can change rapidly. For example, a patient with a compromised airway is of immediate priority until the airway is secured. Other patients may then become higher priority. Transfer of the first patient may be delayed, provided that the patient's condition is not deteriorating. Look for life-threatening problems in the order A B C. As well as preparing participants for the role of medical incident officer at major incidents, courses such as MIMMS (Major Incident Medical Management and Support) are extremely valuable in helping partici-pants to understand and apply the principles of triage.

Medical emergencies

The rural practitioner must be more resourceful than his urban colleagues. If a patient collapses or dies, the doctor or nurse is just as likely to be called as a paramedic ambulance. Vocational training for general practice or community nursing should provide adequate preparation for such events. However, because of the distances involved, there may be a significant delay in transferring patients to secondary hospital care, and decisions about treatment should take this into account.

Intravenous cannulae

If in doubt, insert an intravenous cannula before transferring a patient to hospital. Apart from giving you something to do while you are waiting for the ambulance, it provides ready access for drugs and fluids if the patient's condition deteriorates. Flush it with normal saline, which is just as good as heparin.

Cardiac monitors

A cardiac monitor (preferably with a defibrillator attached) can make management of ill patients much easier. You can monitor pulse rate (which rises if the patient is becoming shocked) and cardiac rhythm (which may warn of trouble ahead). Most will sound an audible warning if the patient goes into ventricular fibrillation while you are looking the other way or writing a hospital letter. Most usefully, if your patient has dozed off after a generous dose of diamorphine, you don't have to wake him or her up to reassure yourself that he or she is still alive.

Thrombolysis

Thrombolytic or 'clotbuster' therapy administered within 12 hours of the onset of a myocardial infarction (MI or heart attack) significantly reduces the risk of the patient dying.[3] The sooner it is given, the more effective it is. The British Heart Foundation recommends that thrombolysis should be administered as soon as possible to all patients with good evidence of an MI, provided there are no contraindications.

The 'GREAT' study in the Grampian Region of Scotland showed that early thrombolysis given in a rural community by GPs reduced mortality by 15% at 2 years.[4] The European 'EMIP' study also demonstrated the feasibility and safety of pre-hospital thrombolysis.[5] In both these studies the drug used was anistreplase. It is likely that lives could be saved by a policy of community thrombolysis administered by GPs or paramedics, particularly for those patients with long travel times to hospital.

The thrombolytic streptokinase is cheap and does not need to be refrigerated. However, streptokinase antibodies may persist for 2 years or longer, and other thrombolytics, such as anistreplase or retoplase, may be more suitable alternatives.

The main risks of thrombolysis are untoward bleeding (including stroke), arrhythmias, inappropriate treatment (e.g. in aortic dissection) and allergic reaction after repeated administration. Provided that administration follows a standard protocol and patients are closely monitored, benefits clearly outweigh risks.[6]

Box 4.1: Example thrombolysis protocol

- Consider thrombolysis in all patients with chest pain *and* ECG evidence of recent myocardial infarction

- Monitor the patient's condition with a cardiac monitor

- Insert an intravenous cannula and give metoclopramide and diamorphine

- Administer glyceryl trinitrate by spray or tablet

- Give aspirin 150–300 mg

- Record 12-lead ECG and blood pressure

- If there is clinical suspicion *and* ECG evidence of recent myocardial infarction *and* there are no contraindications, begin to administer thrombolysis, carefully monitoring cardiac rhythm and blood pressure

---

Box 4.2: Contraindications to thrombolysis

- Stroke or subarachnoid haemorrhage within past 6 months

- Active peptic ulcer (chronic dyspepsia is not a contraindication)

- Gastrointestinal bleed within previous 2 months

- Major trauma, dental extraction or surgery within previous 2 weeks

- Proliferative retinopathy

- Systolic blood pressure > 200 mm Hg or < 90 mm Hg

- Diastolic blood pressure > 120 mm Hg

- Heart block likely to require a pacemaker

- Prolonged cardiac resuscitation during this episode

- Bleeding disorder or on anticoagulants

- Menstruation, pregnancy or childbirth within past 6 weeks

- Unconscious patient

- Acute pancreatitis

References

1 Douglas JDM (1995) Salmon farming: occupational health in a new rural industry. *Occupational Medicine.* **45**:89–92.
2 Douglas JDM and Milne AH (1991) Decompression sickness in fish farm workers: a new occupational hazard. *BMJ.* **302**:1244–5.
3 ISIS-2 (Second International Study of Infarct Survival) Collaborative Group (1988) Randomised trial of intravenous streptokinase, oral aspirin, both or neither among 17187 cases of acute myocardial infarction. *Lancet.* **ii**:349–60.
4 Vale L, Silcock R and Rawles J (1997) An economic evaluation of thrombolysis in a remote rural community. *BMJ.* **314**:570–2.
5 European Myocardial Infarction Project Group (1993) Prehospital thrombolytic therapy in patients with suspected acute myocardial infarction. *New England Journal of Medicine.* **329**:383–9.
6 Petch MC (1990) Dangers of thrombolysis. *BMJ.* **300**:483–4

Further reading

Colquhoun MC, Handley AJ and Evans TR (eds) (1995) *ABC of Resuscitation.* BMJ Publishing Group, London.
Skinner D, Driscoll P and Earlam R (eds) (1991) *ABC of Major Trauma.* BMJ Publishing Group, London.

5
Dispensing

David Baker

Introduction

Only 15% of GPs dispense medicines to their patients and, because of the regulations that govern dispensing, most of them practise in rural areas. The law governing dispensing in NHS general practice is enshrined in the NHS (Pharmaceutical Services) Regulations 1992. The act of dispensing as such takes place under the Medicines Act 1968.

As many readers will be aware, there has been ill feeling between rural doctors and pharmacists over the right to dispense medicines. However, patients are usually very satisfied with the service provided by dispensing practices. In many remote and isolated areas where there is no pharmacy, the GP's surgery is the obvious place from which they can obtain their medicines. Morton-Jones and Pringle in 1993[1] suggested that dispensing practices have higher prescribing costs than non-dispensing practices, mainly because of their lower use of generic drugs. However, removal of six outlying practices (five dispensing and one prescribing) from their figures would have made most of the 'dispensing excess' disappear. In dispensing practices, nearly every item is dispensed, but prescriptions given to patients to take to pharmacies are not always 'cashed'. This factor, too, may have had a significant effect on their results. There is a need for further study of the effects on costs per patient to the NHS of 'non-cashing' of prescriptions and substitution of over-the-counter items.

Who can dispense?

- Pharmacists.

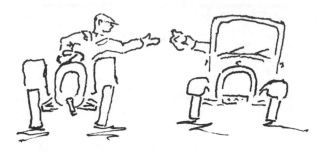

- Doctors who have been given permission to dispense by their health authority under Regulation 20 of the NHS (Pharmaceutical Services) Regulations 1992. The actual regulations are complicated in the extreme, and have kept lawyers in business for years, but the heart of the law is enshrined in Regulation 20, reproduced below. It is anomalous, but if there is no pharmacy available, a health authority may actually require a doctor to start dispensing to his patients. This has not happened in recent times, but the power is still there.

'20(1) Where a patient –

(a) satisfies a Health Authority that he would have serious difficulty in obtaining any necessary drugs or appliances from a pharmacy by reason of distance or inadequacy of means of communication; or

(b) is resident in a controlled locality, at a distance of more than one mile from any pharmacy, and one of the conditions specified in paragraph (2) is satisfied in his case

he may at any time request in writing the doctor on whose list he is included to provide him with pharmaceutical services.'

The dispensary

Under the 'Cost Rent Scheme', which enables health authorities to subsidise new GP premises by paying a rent based on their building costs, a dispensing practice is entitled to additional rent for a dispensary. In effect, they can build larger premises than a non-dispensing practice. The regulations allow 14 m^2 if there are one or two doctors and 23 m^2 if there are three or four. For larger practices, the regulations become more flexible, allowing enough space for the purpose in proportion to the number of patients and doctors. Even in the smaller practices, the permitted size is just about adequate.

Security considerations

It goes without saying that the dispensary should be at least as secure as other parts of the surgery building. Ideally, it should also be capable of being separately secured. Insurance companies are particularly concerned about dispensaries with more than £1000 worth of stock, and most practices will have at least ten times as much.

The Misuse of Drugs Act 1971 and subsequent regulations require that controlled drugs (morphine, diamorphine, pethidine, etc.) and others on special schedules (temazepam, etc.) must be secured in a locked cabinet, which, along with the controlled drugs register, may be inspected by a Home Office inspector or Department of Health medical officer at any time.

Destruction of controlled drugs

Schedule 2 drugs (those that must be recorded in the controlled drugs register, i.e. opioids and amphetamines) can only be destroyed in the presence of an 'authorised person'. A record must be made of the quantity destroyed and the date, and the authorised person must also sign the controlled drugs register. The most convenient authorised person is usually a police officer. The list of authorised persons includes Home Office inspectors, Department of Health medical officers and supervisors of midwives, but not usually GPs or their staff.

Payment

Payment for dispensing is complicated and made up of the following components.

- Reimbursement of the basic price according to the Drug Tariff (a small book regularly circulated to all GPs). Practices are deemed to have received a certain level of discount from their suppliers, and this is deducted on a sliding scale (currently up to 9.57%) from the amount paid to the practice. The scale is calculated by periodic surveys of the discounts available to dispensing practices.

- An 'on-cost' allowance (i.e. profit) of 10.5% of the net ingredient cost of the drug dispensed.

- A 'container allowance' of 3.8p per prescription.

- A 'dispensing fee' on a sliding scale, depending on the number of prescriptions dispensed, from 82.5p to £1.05.

- Reimbursement of Value Added Tax (VAT).

At present, dispensing payments are included in GPs' intended average net remuneration (IANR). Thus, if dispensing doctors receive more drug reimbursement than they have actually paid, all GPs will be deemed to have been overpaid for that part of their contract, and fees and allowances will be reduced in the next round of labyrinthine calculations. There are moves within the profession to remove dispensing from the pool, which would solve this dilemma.

VAT

Practices with a turnover of more than £50 000 on supplies subject to VAT are obliged to register with Customs & Excise for VAT. It is also tempting for smaller dispensing practices to register for VAT and gain tax reimbursement for non-dispensing items. In my view this temptation should be resisted because of the bureaucracy involved.

Once a practice has registered, not only does paperwork increase beyond measure, but also, as the rules are written, there could be serious damage to dispensary profits. This anomaly happens because of an interpretation of the rules by Customs & Excise whereby personally administered items, such as vaccines and, curiously, insulins, are deemed to be dispensed not as zero-rated pharmaceutical items but as part of medical treatment which is VAT exempt. This means that the PPA will not refund your VAT because the practice is registered, and Customs & Excise will not refund your VAT because it pertains to an exempt transaction. Thus the practice is 17.5% worse off on all these personally administered items.

Computer use

Most, if not all, dispensing practices are computerised. Computing aids dispensing probably more than it does other aspects of general practice. However, not all software companies offer dispensing modules, and there is great variability in approach by those that do, with some dispensing packages much easier to use than others.

When choosing a new package, consider the following factors.

- The drug dictionary – how comprehensive is it? How often will the company update it?

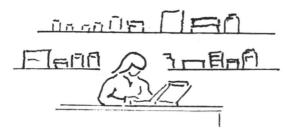

- Is it a commercial package or customised by the company so that only they can modify it?
- Does it allow Read-coded entry?
- How easy is generic substitution?
- Does it provide a secure audit trail to track individual products (to comply with product liability legislation) and the actions of all computer users (professional liability)?
- Does it warn of all potential drug interactions?
- Does it warn prescribers of patients' allergies?
- Does it warn of oversupply or undersupply of medicines to patients?
- Does it link prescriptions with disease history to prevent, for example, prescribing and dispensing a beta-blocker to an asthmatic?
- Will it print both prescriptions and labels in the pharmacy?
- Does it allow automatic stock control and ordering?

Formularies

There is, in fact, little difference in developing a formulary in a dispensing practice compared with a totally prescribing practice. It is easier to have a consistent prescribing policy in a dispensing practice because it has control over what is dispensed against any given prescription and it will be aware of the differences in quality and price between suppliers.

Ordering

Drug supplies for the dispensary can be obtained from a variety of wholesale sources. Although using a single wholesale supplier is not unusual, most practices use more than one method to obtain their supplies.

Box 5.1: Advantages and disadvantages of using a sole supplier

Advantages

- Ease of administration

- Single monthly account

- Can build long-term business relationship

- Large turnover can attract a larger discount

Disadvantages

- Possible difficulty in taking up manufacturers' special offers

- Out-of-stock items may be difficult to get from another supplier

- If the wholesaler gets into difficulty, so does the practice

---

Direct accounts with manufacturers

It can be useful and financially advantageous to have direct accounts with a number of manufacturers. This method of buying is becoming less common for routine purchases, but is still useful for specialist items such as 'flu and other vaccines. The so-called branded generic houses tend to offer good financial deals, but it has to be said that on occasions the reliability of supply can be questionable.

Having decided on your supplier or suppliers it is essential to implement effective stock control. There is no point in having vast stocks of the newest thing for hypertension if you only have one patient on it, and the local cardiologist only gave it to him because nothing else worked. Conversely, it is not good regularly to run out of frequently used drugs such as analgesics or antibiotics. Because ease of obtaining medicines is one of the perceived strengths of a dispensing practice, patients will not thank you if they have to return to the dispensary to collect their routine medication.

The act of dispensing

At present, doctors do not have to use qualified staff to carry out the act of dispensing. However, it is obviously essential that staff are trained for the tasks they perform, and ideally they should have undergone some kind of formal training. Historically, this training has been provided in an ad hoc fashion in-house, but in the last few years schemes have been developed through health authorities, colleges and private educational organisations.

It is also possible (and some would say desirable) to employ a qualified pharmacist to run a dispensary. However, the pharmacist would only be able to act as an agent of the doctor. If he were to act as a pharmacist, the practice would no longer be dispensing and would only be able to dispense when the pharmacist was on the premises and able to supervise the act of dispensing. For reasons not always based on logic, unlike doctors, pharmacists have to be present when medicines are dispensed. That is the law and we have to live with it.

Prescription flow

The FP10 is a valuable document. It is the patient's passport to medication and the dispensing doctor's invoice for payment. The validation of the form is the doctor's signature on it. Except in emergency, no medication should be issued (dispensed) without a prescription already signed telling the dispenser what, how and how much to give.

Whereas in a prescribing practice the patient will almost always be given his or her FP10 or will arrange its collection by the pharmacist, in a dispensing practice, it is quite usual for the prescription form to be printed, signed and dispensed without the patient ever seeing it.

Now most practices are computerised, a useful compromise is to print acute prescriptions at the point of consultation but to print repeat prescriptions centrally. In both cases it is reasonable to have the dispensing label printed in the dispensary.

However the printing is accomplished, checks to ensure the right drug is given to the right patient at the right time must be rigorous. Both the dispenser and another member of staff should initial all items dispensed.

Prescription charges

At present, there is no requirement on dispensing doctors to obtain patients' signatures on the reverse of the FP10, but it is likely to become a requirement in the near future. There will, however, be a number of concessions to dispensing practices, and it is possible that only non-age exemptions will have to be countersigned, and that items delivered to outlying collection points, such as post offices, will be exempted. A further probable change in prescription charge collection policy will mean that practices will be deemed to have collected prescription charges on all items for which exemption has not been claimed. They will be liable for any shortfall. (At present the practice is only required to submit charges collected.)

Endorsing and other housekeeping items

The amount of money reimbursed by the PPA for a given item dispensed can vary widely, depending on the endorsement made on the FP10 form. For example, if 28 atenolol tabs 100 mg were dispensed (1997 prices):

(1) No endorsement: paid at tariff price	£1.48
(2) Endorsed with manufacturer's name (e.g. CP Pharmaceuticals)	£6.00
(3) Endorsed as proprietary (Tenormin or manufacturer = Zeneca)	£6.81

It is obvious from this that endorsing correctly is essential. If you have bought Totamol or Tenormin and fail to endorse your FP10 accordingly, you will make a hefty loss of up to £5.33 on each prescription. It goes without saying that to endorse a generically bought prescription as a proprietary brand would be fraudulent.

Substances such as ranitidine (Zantac) that are available only as one or two branded products present an anomaly (Drug Tariff Category C). In the absence of any endorsement, the Zantac price will be paid even though a cheaper alternative may have been dispensed. The prescription will also be counted as generically prescribed and dispensed even though it may be Zantac that was given.

Although it has been said elsewhere that a record should be kept of batch numbers and suppliers for product liability claims, it is probably sufficient to keep invoices and a record of which brand of medication was dispensed. Only if there were no way of passing the liability back up the supply chain towards the manufacturer would product liability become a problem for dispensing practices. In any event, product liability records must be kept for at least 11 years.

Ethics of dispensing

Because dispensing doctors control two parts of the chain of supply of medicines to patients, they should aim to be whiter than white on the ethical front. The following rules should be applied.

In order, the drug chosen must be:

1 Good for the patient.

2 Good for the NHS as a whole.

3 Then and only then, good for the profitability of the practice.

The future of dispensing

The government is moving towards enabling nurses to prescribe under 'group protocols'.[2] The details remain to be seen, but nurse prescribing would formalise what actually happens in most practices, particularly in respect of dressings and immunisations.

Dispensing by GPs is under great threat. There is a view that its days are numbered. While I have little doubt that the nature of dispensing practice will change over the next 10 years, and that doctors will work much closer with pharmacists, I hope and believe that the service so appreciated by dispensing patients, particularly those in remote and isolated areas, will continue.

References

1 Morton-Jones TJ and Pringle MAL (1993) Prescribing costs in dispensing practices. *BMJ.* **306**:1244–6
2 Crown J (1997) *Review of Prescribing, Supply and Administration of Medicines: a report on the supply and administration of medicines under group protocol.* Department of Health, London.

6
Communications

Philip Spencer

Introduction

Communication is important, but geography can make it difficult in rural areas. Current developments in information technology promise solutions to many longstanding problems.

In an urban setting, it is difficult for people working in large primary healthcare teams to share information. Barriers to communication with patients include language and cultural differences. In contrast, partnerships and list sizes in rural areas tend to be smaller and cultural differences within the population less diverse, making communication easier. Nevertheless, several logistical obstacles impede access to information and good communication with patients, secondary care, the emergency services and within the primary healthcare team itself. A sparse and scattered population, difficult terrain, adverse weather conditions, distance from the surgery and hospital, and out-of-hours rotas all conspire to challenge good communication.

Communication within the primary health care team

Although each professional group may keep its own record about the same patient, medical records provide a vital method of communication between doctors, nurses and other health professionals. They are also a legal record and an aide-mémoire. Branch surgeries and long distances to patients' homes impede access to records, threatening well-informed patient care and increasing the isolation in which staff find themselves

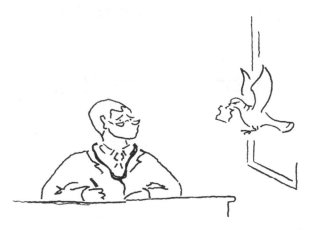

working. Communication systems are increasingly important in rural health, as primary healthcare teams grow in size and complexity.

Computers can store, recall and process huge amounts of information reliably and accurately, offering many advantages over paper systems. They can prompt staff to further action in disease management, repeat prescribing and screening programmes. They can warn of drug interactions and contraindications, assist in audit, and facilitate accounting and management of practice finances. A terminal can be installed in a branch surgery, giving access to the main surgery computer. Laptop terminals with modems allow direct access to the practice computer from patients' homes via their telephone lines or mobile phones.

Mobile telephones are now a feature of most practices. Analogue telephone messages can be picked up by electronic eavesdroppers, but digital messages cannot easily be intercepted and give a better-quality signal with less interference. Coverage remains partial in many rural areas, rendering mobile phones inadequate as a sole means of contact, particularly in emergencies. Satellite telephones give better coverage, even in mountainous areas, but the cost remains prohibitively high. Radiopagers achieve the widest coverage in many remote or hilly areas but only allow messages to pass one way.

Rural GPs often work closely with the ambulance service. Rural dwellers often contact their GP before calling an ambulance to the scene of an accident or medical emergency, and some doctors are active members of BASICS (British Association for Immediate Care), a voluntary organisation that helps to provide medical care at the scene of accidents and emergencies. To improve coordination and cooperation between the two services, BASICS doctors usually have a car radio on an ambulance frequency

Communicating with patients

Published evidence bears out what common sense suggests: good communication improves outcome for both patients and health professionals. Conversely, poor communication skills often result in failure to elicit patients' ideas, concerns and expectations, and lead to dissatisfaction, missed diagnoses and wasted time. Face-to-face consultations are the essence of general practice, but patients often establish indirect contact by telephone or letter. Such contact does not permit non-verbal communication through body language as a means of assessing a patient's thoughts and feelings.

The telephone is the most common means of indirect contact. It has obvious advantages for both doctor and patient in rural areas where distance from the surgery and lack of public transport limit patients' access to healthcare. Studies suggest that patients would value easier access to their doctor by telephone.[1] Although many callers simply request information such as test results, a diagnosis might be made or treatment arranged.[2] In most cases where patients telephone their doctor, they would have arranged an appointment if telephone advice had not been forthcoming, and as many as 13% might have requested a home visit.[2,3] It is a paradox that despite the clear advantages, practices often do not facilitate telephone access.[4] In one study, 43% of patients were reassured by telephone advice, but in only 26% of cases did the doctor feel that reassurance had been given. Perhaps doctors feel less confident and comfortable about telephone consultations than their patients.[2]

The telephone can also restrict patients' access to their doctor or nurse. Insufficient incoming telephone lines, hostile receptionists or a lack of familiarity with, or availability of, a telephone to the patient may all be factors. The wording and tone of pre-recorded answerphone messages may encourage or discourage callers and influence whether or not they pursue their call.[5]

Telemedicine: patients–primary care

Telecommunications technology allows the transmission of video images by conventional telephone line. Telemedicine is the use of audiovisual links in medicine. Although image quality has improved considerably, equipment costs remain high preventing their widespread use. Additional information given by a visual image clearly adds to that of a conventional telephone consultation. Applications include links with patients who are unable to travel, particularly the chronically sick and terminally ill, who live many miles from the surgery but do not feel that their problem justifies troubling the doctor to make a house call. Such systems are now being evaluated in a general practice setting. It may be that some patients will find the equipment intimidating or inhibiting, making them reticent about contacting their doctor.

Communication between primary care and secondary care

Factors contributing to the problem of poor communication between general practice and hospitals include differences in their respective roles, patterns of morbidity encountered and different styles of working. It is particularly important for health professionals who work many miles from their local hospital to develop a mutually supportive relationship with secondary care staff.

Communication with hospital staff occurs on many levels, e.g. informally at clinical meetings, over the telephone, by letter and by fax. Each method has its own strengths and weaknesses. Verbal communication helps to establish a rapport, but there may be no record of what has been communicated. Telephone or written advice reduces referral rates, saving time and expense.[6] Telephone calls usually interrupt one or other party unless time is specifically set aside for taking calls. Referral and hospital discharge letters often lack information[7] and contain inaccuracies[8,9] Although letters to hospitals normally arrive before or with the patient, a common complaint about discharge letters is their delay in being sent or failing to arrive at all.[10,11] Many of these problems are compounded in very isolated, e.g. island, practices where there may be considerable delay in letters being delivered and it is difficult to visit and meet with hospital colleagues.

Hospitals and practices are increasingly using fax machines to send referral letters, discharge letters and laboratory results, thereby avoiding the delay incurred by using conventional mail services. Faxes can also be used to send raw clinical data, e.g. ECGs to be viewed by a cardiologist, public health circulars and warnings of NHS press releases.

Communication between laboratories and practices is often through computer links. Results are sent directly to the practice computer, where they can be viewed and, if necessary, acted upon without delay. In theory at least, electronic storage of results in laboratories and practices avoids duplication of paper information in hospital notes, laboratory records and practice records.

It is a relatively small step to transfer electronically referral and discharge letters in the form of electronic mail (e-mail). Most general practice computer software includes the facility to generate standardised letters, including information about medical history, medication, allergies and so on, using the practice's computerised patient records with additional free text to explain the referral. The letter arrives at the receiving hospital soon after the press of a button. A similar system for discharge letters could mean that they arrived with the GP before the patient had reached home.

Telemedicine: primary care–secondary and tertiary care

Potential uses of telemedicine include obtaining a consultant's opinion while the patient is in the GP's surgery or remote interviewing and history taking, enabling at least a visual examination of the patient to be conducted. As well as real-time macroscopic images, the system could transmit endoscopic views or radiographic images, such as ultrasound pictures. Such systems have been evaluated in isolated areas, including Wales and rural Norway, for the provision of pathology, radiology, dermatology and cardiology services.[12] Another application, more commonly used in business circles, is videoconferencing, which uses the same process to enable groups of people to link up for management or educational purposes.

The advantages of telemedicine are clear. It allows a consultation to take place without the expense, time and inconvenience of the parties meeting. Consultations can take place across continents or where access to healthcare is limited or impossible, such as in remote parts of the world, at sea or even in space. In the context of primary care, telemedicine could do away with the necessity for some outpatient referrals, particularly in specialities such as dermatology. However, lack of physical contact limits the examination process and contributes to depersonalisation. There are also legal and ethical issues, including shortcomings such as confidentiality, responsibility and liability for clinical errors, all of which may be further complicated if national boundaries are crossed. There is surprisingly little evidence about cost-effectiveness. Those who live in the developed world and who already have access to medical services may benefit from telemedicine before more needy people in the Third World.

The NHS-net

The NHS is developing its own computer network across the entire country, the NHS-net. The aim is to provide a communal database and electronic messaging service encompassing the NHS as a whole, including health authorities, trusts and general practices. Provided that security and confidentiality can be assured, there is scope for information exchange with parties outside the NHS via the Internet, with a gateway or 'firewall' preventing unlawful access to the system from outside. Potential uses include:

- patient registration and item of service payments without paperwork
- hospital referrals and discharge details exchanged via e-mail
- practices booking outpatient appointments directly from their surgery
- practices obtaining accurate information about hospital waiting times
- transport services booked directly from the surgery
- direct access to laboratory and radiology records
- on-line access to guidelines, protocols and clinical reference data
- e-mail connections within the network
- e-mail connections to the rest of the world via the Internet
- noticeboards for sharing information locally and nationally
- telemedicine and videoconferencing.

These benefits have to be balanced against the massive investment costs and potential threat to patient confidentiality that would undermine such a system.

Accessing information

To practise evidence-based medicine and reach the ever-higher standards expected of GPs and nurses, it becomes increasingly import-ant to have access to dependable sources of information and best evidence. Literature searches are now easy through sources such as MEDLINE, which is available on the Internet or on CD-ROM. Many reference books such as the *British National Formulary* or *Oxford Textbook of Medicine* are also available on CD-ROM.

The Internet

The Internet provides access to international databases through a personal computer with the necessary software, modem and telephone line to an Internet provider (a company with a permanent connection to the Internet that charges for access). Users each have their own Internet address and have access to services including e-mail, the WorldWide Web, newsgroups and file transfer services.

The WorldWide Web enables users to navigate their way towards information posted by other users. Any organisation, group of people or individual can set up a website and offer information about themselves or the service that they provide. A website is a noticeboard on which users can place text as a means of sharing information. This helps to bring together thoughts and ideas and offers an opportunity for users to air their views, ask questions and participate in discussions. The Royal College of General Practitioners' rural discussion forum is at: http://www.rcgp.org.uk/forums/rural/wwwboard.htm.

Part of the philosophy of the Internet is that any user should be at liberty to set up a website. It is important, therefore, to remember that information gleaned from the Internet may not be evidence-based, accurate or user-friendly. Because authors are often untraceable and unaccountable there is even scope for the widespread dissemination of deliberately misleading or deceptive information.

An interesting consideration is the impact of information on the doctor–patient interaction. Medical information used to remain firmly in the domain of doctors, nurses and other health professionals, being largely confined to journals and medical textbooks. Patients were only as well informed as their doctors allowed, giving doctors considerable power over their patients, securing their 'Aesculapian' authority.

For Internet users there is now a wealth of medical information available. It may be misunderstood, misinterpreted or plain wrong. This gives scope for conflict. It may raise patients' expectations, increase pressure on doctors to use treatments that have not been properly evaluated and challenge the nation's healthcare budget.

The Internet can connect the most isolated of practices to a massive range of information and services. Education is no longer dependent on proximity to a postgraduate centre or university library. Communication is no longer constrained by postal delivery times. Participation in debate and the opportunity to pose questions to like-minded parties are no longer dependent on attending meetings, which are all too often inaccessible. Lectures can be transmitted and received live. The Internet does not negate the need for good medical libraries, nor can it substitute for face-to-face communication, but it goes a long way towards helping to reduce isolation.

Implications of computerisation

In view of society's massive investment in information technology, and our increasing dependence on it, it is important to remain objective about both its benefits and its detrimental consequences, particularly the effect on quality of patient care.

Many patients harbour concerns about loss of confidentiality and intimacy.[14] They are reluctant to interrupt a doctor engaged on the computer. This concern may affect the disclosure of information by patients and the flow of information from doctor to the patient.[15] On the positive side, computers can remind users about potential drug interactions and contraindications, overdue screening procedures, clinical guidelines and protocols. They encourage health promotion activity, cheaper prescribing, increased uptake of immunisations and better coverage of screening procedures. But they also lead to longer consultations and less attention to the social aspects of patients' problems,[16] and there is a danger that consultations become computer centred and task oriented, neglecting the patient's agenda.

Computer-assisted practice management and administration may lead to better-run practices with less wasted time, money and manpower, leaving doctors free to concentrate on patient care. It is equally well recognised that the process of computerisation or changing systems can be expensive, time consuming and frustrating.

Confidentiality

Confidentiality is an ethical requirement and crucial to the doctor–patient relationship. Sensitive medical and personal information stored on practice computers would be of considerable financial interest to insurance companies, employers, police, the media and those with criminal intent. Increased communication between computers, through

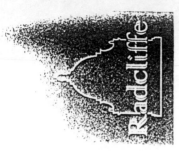

Radcliffe Medical Press Ltd
18 Marcham Road
Abingdon, Oxon
OX14 1AA, UK

Tel: +44 (0)1235 528820
Fax: +44 (0)1235 528830

ERRATUM –

RURAL HEALTHCARE
Edited by Jim Cox and Iain Mungall

Please note the following amendment on the colour plate section between pages 88–89.

- Plate 4 caption should read Ringworm

- Plate 5 caption should read *Erythema chronicum migrans of* Lyme disease

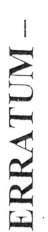

With Compliments

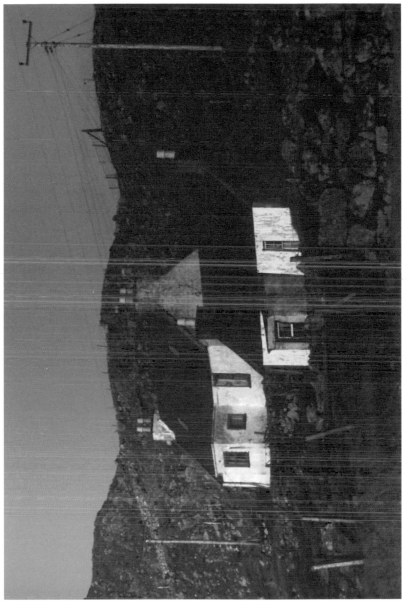

1 Living in the country: one example

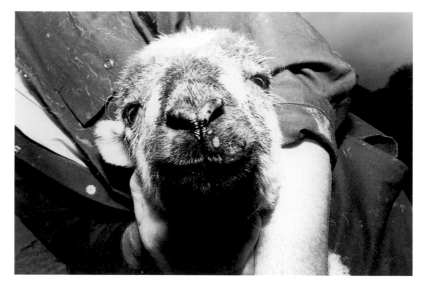

2 Orf

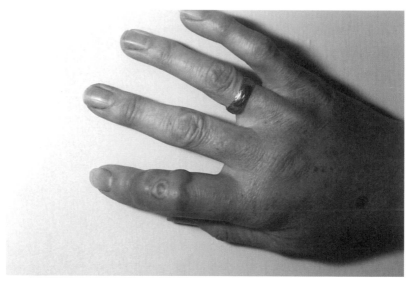

3 Orf

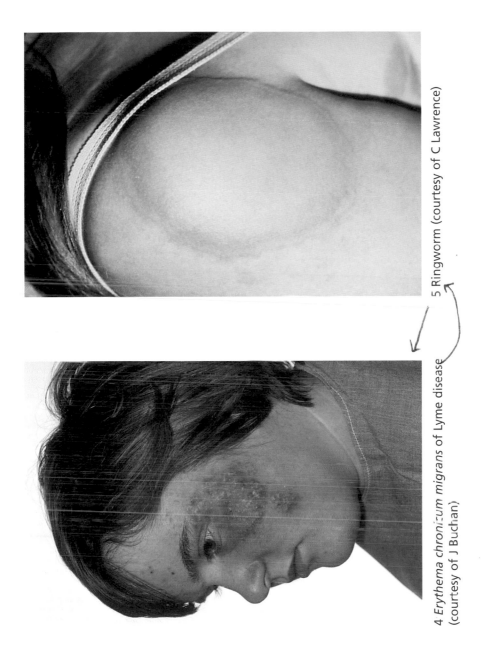

4 *Erythema chronicum migrans* of Lyme disease (courtesy of J Buchan)

5 Ringworm (courtesy of C Lawrence)

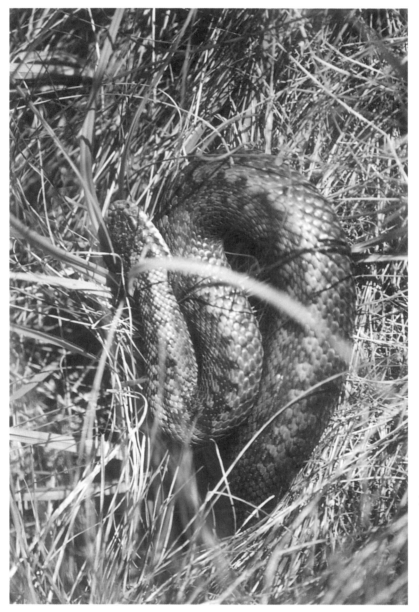

6 The common adder

networks such as the Internet or NHS-net, makes breaches of data security and fraudulent modification of records more likely. The use of passwords, etc. does not stop the determined hacker. Because of these considerations, the British Medical Association has reservations about the security of the NHS-net.[17]

Quality of information

The ease and speed with which information can be sent has led to an escalation in the quantity of irrelevant information to which we are all subjected, with the consequent dilution of important and useful information. The quality of information has not increased in line with its quantity. The scope for broadcasting inadvertently or deliberately misleading, corruptive, deceptive or incorrect information over the Internet is a serious consideration. Internet users should be aware that information may not be generally accepted or properly researched. It may represent an unusual personal view.

Reliability

The complexity and sophistication of modern computer systems may lead people to mistrust them. A faulty system can have very damaging consequences for those who depend on it. Some problems, such as power failures, can be anticipated by installing generators and regularly backing up data. Other problems are less predictable. A mistake by a computer operator in Virginia, USA, resulted in millions of e-mail messages around the world failing to reach their destinations (*The Guardian*, 19 July 1997). Many computer users approach the new millennium with uncertainty as to whether their computers, telephones and fax machines will work on 1 January 2000. Computer viruses may enter through software e-mailed or loaded on to a computer, resulting in corrupted programs and data.

Cost

As the cost of microchip technology falls, equipment becomes more and more sophisticated. Pressure to keep upgrading equipment means that computing is likely to remain a major financial commitment for general practices.

Medical hazards of display screen equipment

Eye problems, epilepsy, skin problems from static build-up of dust, reproductive difficulties, general malaise and repetitive strain injury, e.g. tenosynovitis, have all been reported. The evidence for most remains controversial at best.

Summary and conclusions

Technological advances go some way towards reducing the isolation of practices. However, the benefits must be weighed up against their cost in terms of finance, implications for confidentiality and depersonalisation, and their impact on the doctor–patient relationship.

References

1 Allen D, Leavey R and Marks B (1988) Survey of patients' satisfaction with access to general practitioners. *Journal of the College of General Practitioners*. **38**:163–5.

2 Nagle J, McMahon K, Barbour M *et al.* (1992) Evaluation of the use and usefulness of telephone consultations in one general practice. *British Journal of General Practice*. **42**:190–3.

3 Marsh G, Horne R and Channing D (1987) A study of telephone advice in managing out-of-hours calls. *Journal of the College of General Practitioners*. **37**:301–4.

4 Hallam L (1993) Access to general practice and general practitioners by telephone: the patient's view. *British Journal of General Practice*. **43**:331–5.

5 Benett I (1992) Pre-recorded answerphone messages: influence on patients' feelings and behaviour in out of hours requests for visits. *British Journal of General Practice*. **42**:373–6.

6 Hartog M. (1988) Medical outpatients. *Journal of the College of Physicians*. **22**:51.

7 Jacobs L and Pringle M (1990) Referral letters and replies from orthopaedic departments: opportunities missed. *BMJ*. **301**:470–3.

8 Gilchrist W, Lee Y, Tam H *et al.* (1987) Prospective study of drug reporting by general practitioners for an elderly population referred to a geriatric service. *BMJ*. **294**:289–90.

9 Price D, Cooke J, Singleton S *et al.* (1986) Doctors unawareness of the

drugs their patients are taking: a major cause of overprescribing. *BMJ.* **292**:99–100.

10   Penney T (1988) Delayed communication between hospitals and general practitioners: where does the problem lie? *BMJ.* **297**:28–9.

11   Grundmeijer H (1996) General practitioners and specialists: why do they communicate so badly? *European Journal of General Practice.* **2**:53–4.

12   Elford D. (1997) Telemedicine in Northern Norway. *Journal of Telemedicine and Telecare.* **3**:1–22.

13   Impicciatore P, Pandolfini C, Casella N *et al.* (1997) Reliability of health information for the public on the world wide web: systematic survey of advice on managing fever in children at home. *BMJ.* **314**:1875–81.

14   Rethans J-J, Hoppener P, Wolfs G *et al.* (1988) Do personal computers make doctors less personal? *BMJ.* **296**:1446–8.

15   Greatbatch D, Heath C, Campion P *et al.* (1995) How do desktop computers affect the doctor–patient interaction? *Family Practice.* **12**:32–6.

16   Sullivan F and Mitchell E (1995) Has general practitioner computing made a difference to patient care? *BMJ.* **311**:848–52.

17   Anderson R (1996) Clinical system security: interim guidelines. *BMJ.* **312**:109–11.

7
Teamwork

Antoinette Ward

A professional person starting work in a rural area will already have experience of working as a member of a team. Doctors, nurses, midwives and health visitors have all trained in hospitals, where teamwork is part of the natural order. Social workers and paramedical workers are organised in teams. So why a chapter on teamwork? What is different about teamwork in rural practice?

The aim of this chapter is not to reiterate theories about teamwork. It is to suggest practical guidelines for effective teamwork for the benefit of patients and clients, overcoming problems posed by geography, etc. It also includes some exercises to enable professionals to audit their own effectiveness and that of their team.

Members of the PHCT and their roles: implications for rural practice

Peter and James Pritchard define a team as 'a group of people who make different contributions towards a common goal'.[1] Common goals in primary healthcare include not only benefit for patients but also professional satisfaction and personal happiness for health and social work professionals. Each works autonomously and yet as a member of a team. Understanding each other's roles and perspective, and the constraints imposed by having different professional backgrounds, employers and management structures, helps team members to work together effectively.

The primary healthcare team (PHCT) usually consists of one or more GPs, their employed staff (practice nurses, receptionists, dispensers, practice manager, secretary and, increasingly, nurse practitioner) and attached professionals (community nurses, midwives, health visitors, community psychiatric nurses, etc.), who are usually employed by health trusts. In some areas, social workers are also attached to the team and some practices employ physiotherapists, chiropodists, pharmacists, dieticians, etc.

Figure 7.1 illustrates a typical team, but it must be emphasised that core teams vary in their membership. In a very rural area, the roles of nurse, midwife and health visitor may be combined in one person, a 'triple worker'. Attached staff may be responsible for the patients of one practice only or they may be assigned to a geographical area, liaising with several GP practices on a patient-by-patient basis. These factors have a major impact on whether the PHCT is a close-knit functioning unit, or a loose cat's cradle of professionals linked only by individual patients or clients.

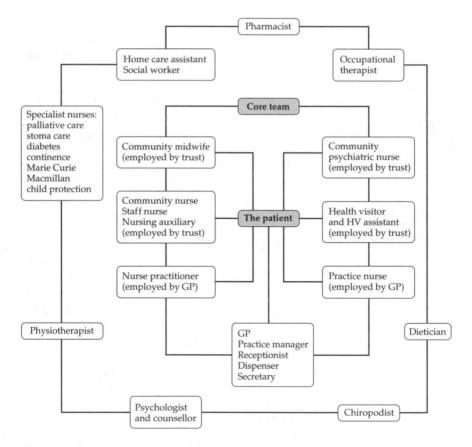

Figure 7.1 Example of a primary healthcare team.

It is a useful exercise for all members of the PHCT to clarify their roles, their specialist and generalist skills, management structures and professional accountability. This exercise leads to better-focused referral and to collaboration in the care and treatment of patients. It also identifies overlap of skills, pointing the way to flexible patterns of working (see 'Innovative Schemes' below), identifies gaps in local service and highlights training and development needs.

Exercise 1

Working in groups of two or three, each member of the team describes his or her perception of the role of another team member in terms of:

- generalist skills

- specialist skills

- employer and management structure

- area of practice, e.g. practice attached or geographical

- professional accountability: to patients, to professional registration body, to employers, to colleagues

- workload, including patient contact and administration. Are there tasks that could be performed better and more cost-effectively by someone else?

Each team member then tells the whole group what they really do and explains where their role is constrained by lack of training, lack of confidence or by management or insurance considerations. Open discussion should then be encouraged

---

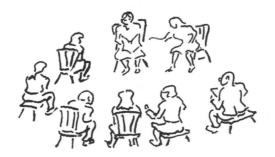

It is important to follow up such an exercise with positive action, involving others, including senior managers, if necessary. This can be daunting. Focusing on patients and their needs and turning 'this would never work here' into 'how can we make this work here?' helps.

Issues specific to rural areas

- Distance affects every aspect of rural working.

- Although employed staff care for all patients in a practice, attached staff may have geographical limits. Patients living towards the periphery of the practice area may be served by nurses, midwives and health visitors attached to other practices.

- Social workers are liable to be based in towns, not in the villages where rural practices are based.

- The practice is likely to be distant from a district general hospital. This increases the likelihood that the surgery will function as at least a 'minor injuries unit' and possibly provide more sophisticated accident and emergency care for local patients. Clinics, e.g. diabetic, respiratory and antenatal, have to be organised so that they are easy for patients to attend. As Cunningham and Sargeant point out, 'the further away professionals are from the district general hospital, the more skilful and self-reliant they need to be'.[2]

- To attend management or educational meetings or make informal, personal contact with fellow professionals is time-consuming and expensive.

- Distance puts pressure on professionals to organise their home visits carefully, and to ensure that the patient will be at home (and not at the day hospital today, for example).

- If the practice is a dispensing practice it is important that employed and attached staff are knowledgeable about and familiar with dispensing procedures, e.g. GPs can only dispense to patients who live within a mile of a chemist if they are temporary residents or if the item is one of a limited list and personally administered, e.g. an injection or sutures. Nurses and midwives have to ensure that all items used for patients are correctly prescribed and dispensed. Nurses are used to a different supply system.

- Rural populations are more stable than urban populations and this is reflected in a slower turnover of staff.

- Staff are more likely to live in the same community as their patients.

This brings both benefits:

- deeper knowledge about patients' background

- continuity of care

- well-established team work because members are not continually changing

- ease of tapping into neighbourhood support

and tensions:

- it is less easy for staff to find other 'near to home' work if they become unhappy with their work or colleagues

- there is less input of fresh ideas and new skills from new team members

- confidentiality can be a minefield. When patients and their families are well known as neighbours and friends, professionals need to maintain an absolute guard on gossip and observe great care about passing on information.

Exercise 2   Checklist for team members

- What effects does distance have on my practice?

- How can I minimise time lost in travelling?

- Am I confident about prescribing and dispensing regulations and procedures?

- Am I careful to avoid gossip and only pass on information with the patient's consent and in his interest?

- How long have I and other members of the team been in post, and what benefits and tensions result?

- Am I, and other members of the team, identifying training and development needs to update skills and knowledge?

Communication and liaison

Liaising with colleagues is fraught with difficulty at the best of times. By the nature of their work, team members are often in contact with their patients and should not be disturbed unless the need is urgent. This accepted barrier to communication is compounded if professionals work from different premises and visit patients over a wide area.

Nevertheless, teams in rural areas can achieve excellent collaboration and receive very positive feedback from their patients as a result. How can this be done?

Teams can be described as being 'intrinsic', 'functional' or 'full'.[3]

Intrinsic teams

The intrinsic team serves an individual patient and identifies itself. For example, for a pregnant woman and her family it will probably consist of the midwife, GP, health visitor and receptionist/dispenser, with probable liaison with a consultant obstetrician and hospital midwives. This small team can keep in close contact with each other and with the patient by:

- Use of the telephone, answering services, pagers and mobile telephones. Convenient times and places for making and receiving calls should be agreed. Receptionists can take messages and ensure that calls are returned. Tone of voice is all important. A friendly, welcoming voice will establish communication. A voice sounding annoyed or uninterested may result in the district nurse avoiding contact with that surgery or GP in the future – not a successful liaison.

- Message books, which must be read at agreed intervals (e.g. daily), initialled and acted on promptly. Both the time the message was received and the time it was read should be recorded.

- Meeting at the patient's home is a most effective way of both keeping travel to a minimum (because colleagues are visiting anyway) and fully involving patients and their families in care plans.

- Providing prompt feedback to each other – an essential ingredient of teamworking. Feedback ensures that everyone is in the picture and the patient is not confused by conflicting advice. It provides the basis for joint planning and, if an inappropriate referral has been made, an opportunity for clarification of roles.

- Compromise. Wherever more than one person is involved in giving care and treatment, conflict may arise. Indeed, the patient and family may not agree with each other or with the doctor or nurse. Compromise is an art – some would say the art of persuading someone to accept your view, but thinking that it was their idea all along! In reality, compromise means explaining a point of view, listening to others, knowing when it is important to press a point and when best to withdraw, and accepting the outcome of the discussion and working with the decision. A closer relationship with patient and colleagues will result.

- Shared records or agreed access to each other's records, including recording of decisions, care and treatment.

Functional teams

Members of functional teams are identified by the subject in question, e.g. immunisations (health visitor, practice nurse and GP), records and computerisation (the whole team), a case conference (the relevant members of the team). The practice manager may organise meetings to which relevant members of the team should be invited, including the more peripheral members who may also serve other practices. Whereas an intrinsic team consists of the professionals directly involved in caring for an individual patient, a functional team addresses broader policies. An intrinsic team might provide terminal care for one dying patient and his family, but a functional team might include more people involved with a number of patients and consider changes in policy, e.g. provision of 'hospice at home' or new drugs.

Full teams

No matter how successful intrinsic and functional teams are, the full primary healthcare team should still meet regularly, say at least four to six times a year. Agenda items may include: the practice's plans for the future, continuing professional development and training (including regular resuscitation revision), multidisciplinary research projects or team-building exercises. Consider inviting patient representatives.

Meetings should be planned and should have a clear purpose. They are popular if they are productive. If they are not, members of the team will vote with their feet. Their workloads are too heavy to waste time at purposeless meetings.

Small, rural teams often have a regular weekly or fortnightly meeting which combines functional team and full team meetings. If this is the case, the whole agenda will not always be relevant to everyone, but as one midwife put it, 'I may find some of the meeting a bit tedious but I would still rather be there. I get to know everyone and I feel I'm one of the team. My manager sees me as a part of the midwifery team at the hospital but I see myself as part of the primary healthcare team. The meetings are too important to miss.'

There is no substitute for meeting in person, but those who cannot attend can still be included. Aids to successful meetings include:

- Keeping to time.

- Advance notification of the meeting with a written agenda.

- Invitations to members of the team to submit points for discussion, whether or not they are able to attend in person.

- The chairperson should make sure that everyone has the opportunity to contribute, not just the vocal members.

- Speakers may be invited to update people's knowledge and skills or to stimulate discussion.

- The chairperson should sum up each meeting, and clarify responsibilities.

- Ensure that minutes of the meeting are sent to all relevant members of the PHCT, not just those able to attend. (Minutes are not needed when the meeting is an informal get-together to enable professionals to discuss progress with patients' treatment and give each other feedback.)

Videoconferencing may enable far-flung PHCT members to meet without incurring travel/time costs.

Exercise 3   Communication and liaison

Arrange a team meeting to discuss the following questions.

- Is the patient at the centre of our teamworking?
- How easy is it for patients to contact each member of the team?
- How long does it take to respond to messages left with receptionists?
- How easily, how often and how effectively do intrinsic teams meet to plan care with the patient and carers?
- How quickly do team members act on referrals?
- How effectively do team members give feedback to each other?
- How often and how effectively do teams meet to plan for the future?
- How do teams identify their educational needs?
- How frequent and how effective are multidisciplinary educational activities?
- How frequently does the full team meet? Are meetings well attended? Is there a clear agenda? Are minutes circulated to all members?
- How well do we listen to, and learn from, new members of the team and visitors?
- What is the induction programme for new members of the team?

Innovative schemes

Flexible working; skill mixing

Where once there was the district nurse, and in rural areas often the triple worker (nurse, midwife and health visitor in one person), there are now community nurses, nursing or healthcare assistants, practice nurses, nurse practitioners and health visitors. Skill mixing has sometimes been dictated by the need to save money and employ nurses on lower pay grades. The increase in numbers of practice nurses has highlighted the value of general nurses with a broad range of skills who can work in close collaboration with GP colleagues and who have a commitment to only one practice team.

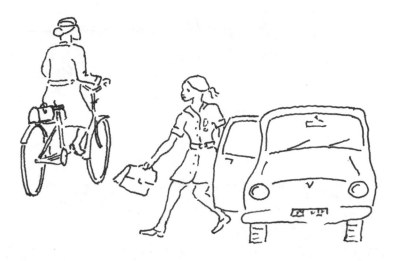

Over recent years, as team members have collaborated more and got to know and trust each other, there have been both formal and informal moves towards removing barriers, both contractual and personal, that cause overlap in nurses' work. It is often appropriate for a 'key nurse' to be identified for a particular patient and for that nurse to manage all the care within her skills. So if a community nurse is responsible for a patient who is chronically ill and over 75 years of age, she will undertake routine over-75 health screening for that patient in addition to her normal duties. The practice nurse who would otherwise have visited to do the over-75 health check does not need to visit. Similarly, if a health visitor is visiting a family, she might give Grandma her routine vitamin B12 injection instead of the community nurse making a call. These examples of flexible working result in greater continuity of care for the patient, and help nurses and health visitors to retain their generalist skills. Such a scheme depends on careful collaboration and communication, but saves both time and money while benefiting the patient.

Rather than contract with a health trust for community staff, commissioning groups of GPs may employ nurses, midwives and health visitors to work in both the surgery and the community.

Other ideas for integrated teams bringing community nurses, practice nurses, health visitors and sometimes midwives into one management structure are being piloted under the Primary Care Act 1997. These pilots will provide valuable information on how community healthcare can be developed in the future

Healthy villages

The Brockenhurst Healthy Village project[4,5] employs a community coordinator, working 18 hours a week, to help people of all ages to make full use of local activities and facilities, and so benefit their health and overall sense of wellbeing. The coordinator collates information about local facilities and meets clients to discuss the possibility of their using the various clubs, societies, organisations and resources available in the community. The project attempts to meet more than simply physical and medical needs, and is an excellent example of a successful alliance between health, education, social services and local authorities. The idea builds on normal village activities and develops the concept of team working to include the wider rural community.

Telephone reassurance: a social support intervention

A community assessment in the USA[6] highlighted lack of transport and routine social contact as well as inadequate links between natural and formal support systems for elderly people on Mount Desert Island, Maine. The elderly people were participants in planning a scheme in which a volunteer telephones elderly people once a day at a specific time. He enquires as to the person's wellbeing and needs, and passes on to the appropriate service any request for help, e.g. snow-shovelling, meal delivery or nursing care. If the telephone is not answered, a designated contact person is notified and makes a personal visit. An important factor in the success of the project is that the elderly people themselves helped to set it up. This scheme is one of many across the USA and is attractive to volunteers because they do not need to leave their homes to be of service.

In the UK, community alarm systems have become a valuable and reassuring safety feature for isolated or housebound people (and their families). The 'telephone reassurance project' provides daily social contact and a caring relationship as well.

Conclusion

Primary healthcare teams bring a wealth of skill and experience to their communities, but their effectiveness depends on sound relationships between professionals and the people they serve. Because of distance from services, people in rural areas have particular problems in gaining access to the full range of health and social care. By listening to patients and working with them as well as for them, utilising each other's knowledge and skills to the full, and using modern means of communication, PHCT members can significantly reduce rural disadvantage and offer high standards of service, treatment and care.

References

1 Pritchard P and Pritchard J (1994) *Teamwork for Primary and Shared Care*. Oxford Medical Publications, Oxford, p. 13.
2 Cunningham W and Sargeant J (1995) Teamwork In rural practice. In: J Cox (ed) (1995) *Rural General Practice in the United Kingdom*. Occasional paper 71. Royal College of General Practitioners, London, p. 20.
3 Pritchard P and Pritchard J (1994) *Teamwork for Primary and Shared Care*. Oxford Medical Publications, Oxford, pp. 17–19.
4 Browne D (1994) Brockenhurst Healthy Village Project. *Southampton Medical Journal*. **3**:36–40.
5 Browne D (1995) Healthy villages. In: J Cox (ed) *Rural General Practice in the United Kingdom*. Occasional paper 71. Royal College of General Practitioners, London, pp. 30–2.
6 Cozzi-Burr H (1992) Telephone reassurance. In: P Winstead-Fry, TP Churchill and RV Shippee-Rice (eds) *Rural Health Nursing*. National League for Nursing Press, New York.

8

Access to care

Ian Watt

Introduction

If health services have any value, then access to them must be important. While the quality of healthcare can be described in a number of dimensions – Maxwell[1] for example identified six (access to services, relevance to need, effectiveness, equity, social acceptability and efficiency) – access may be argued to be the one most influenced by rurality. In large part this stems from the fact that rural dwellers often have to travel greater distances than their urban counterparts to attend health facilities, particularly as service provision becomes increasingly centralised. However, geographic factors are not the only influences, and a variety of social, cultural and economic factors also affect access to healthcare. This chapter discusses the problems posed by impaired access on the health and healthcare of rural populations and describes the responses that have been developed to cope with them.

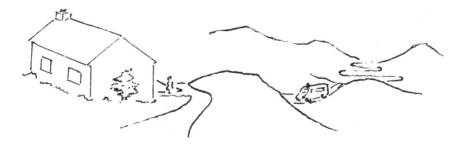

Access to primary care

Evidence exists to show that distance from a general practice surgery is negatively related to consultation rates. The term often given to this phenomenon is 'distance decay'. In general, a consultation rate lower than expected may be taken to indicate some hindrance to access, although this may not be the sole explanation. What is not clear from the studies that have considered distance decay is the degree to which decreasing use of primary care with increasing distance represents unmet need, rather than a reduction of utilisation surplus to need.

Elements of primary care other than general practice can also be influenced by rurality. For example, family planning services in urban areas are often provided by teams other than a person's own GP. If some individuals are reluctant to consult their own family doctor, for example teenage girls requesting contraception, then some rural people may be deterred from seeking help, because there is no easily accessible alternative. Lack of alternative sources of provision may result in general practice backed primary healthcare teams undertaking extra work. For example, one study[2] found that only 10.2% of rural and suburban children were registered for immunisations with a child health clinic as opposed to 61.6% of inner city children. Finally, some researchers have actually found better service provision in rural areas in specific circumstances and localities, for example community and social provision for older people (health visitors, district nurses, meals-on-wheels).

Access to hospital care

Distance decay has been shown to occur for hospital as well as GP consultations. For example, a study in East Anglia[3] showed a decrease in the ratio of actual to expected hospital outpatients the further people lived from a district general hospital. Evidence from the USA suggests that such distance decay can even occur in relation to more specialised facilities, such as cancer hospitals. The frequency of hospital visiting by a patient's relatives and friends has also been shown to decrease the further a patient lives from the hospital.

As with general hospital services, studies have detailed that the distance from the casualty department is a major factor in variation in utilisation.[4] In part at least, the relative inaccessibility of emergency and trauma services in rural areas is partly addressed by GPs. In some areas, rural GPs play a significant role in the early management of trauma victims, and will frequently deal with minor trauma entirely within the practice.

Does impaired access matter?

Although research is reasonably consistent in demonstrating decreasing utilisation of health services with increasing distance from a health facility, it is less clear about the effect barriers to access may have on health outcomes. A study of the presentation of colorectal cancer in France showed that a lower proportion of rural populations than urban populations were treated in specialised health centres, and a higher percentage were diagnosed at a later stage, especially in women. In addition, among women, a rural environment appeared to confer a worse prognosis. Similar findings have been reported from the USA.

In the UK, however, there has been an assumption that the quality of care provided by the NHS prevents the problems associated with rural health and healthcare in other developed countries. One of the ideals on which the NHS was founded was that of providing a uniform standard of care for all, to ensure, as Bevan said in 1945, 'that an equally good service is available everywhere'. Nevertheless, differential outcomes between rural and urban populations have been demonstrated in the UK. For example, rural patients have been found to be more likely to have advanced diabetic retinopathy than urban patients, although the overall prevalence was the same. A study in Scotland documented higher mortality from asthma in the more rural areas, which also tended to have lower hospital admission rates.

Trauma deaths show a similar pattern, and the relative inaccessibility of accident and emergency services to rural residents has been cited as one explanation. The trend towards increasing centralisation of trauma services has been criticised for paying too much attention to the potential advantages of centralisation and not enough to the extent to which delays in reaching hospital care contribute to preventable deaths. Such a problem could also arise for other services. For example, the administration of thrombolytic therapy following myocardial infarction can markedly reduce the risk of death. However, such benefits are dependent on the treatment being given early after the onset of symptoms.

Despite such studies there is insufficient evidence to clarify whether in the UK, the barriers to access faced by rural populations have an overall detrimental effect on their health. As service provision becomes increasingly centralised, however, the impaired access to healthcare experienced by many rural people has the potential to impact not just on health outcomes but on other areas of quality, such as equity and cost. For example, Norway has a system of healthcare that has concentrated on equity and the removal of financial barriers to use. Despite this, a retrospective cohort study showed that rurality was associated with a decreased referral rate per GP visit after adjusting for health and social factors, which indicates a degree of inequity in access to referral services.[5]

Financial factors can influence equity, and distance is an important determinant of at least two types of cost. The financial costs of travel, by whatever mode, are directly related to distance. The costs of time spent travelling are also influenced by distance. Time has costs in terms of activities foregone, such as paid work, child care and leisure activities. In rural areas, journeys to centralised hospital services are often difficult and many hours can be spent travelling to and from outpatient appointments. However, the costs, both financially and in terms of time, are usually less when travelling by private car than by public transport, points which favour the wealthy, who usually have easier access to private transport.

Transport to hospital in rural areas is particularly difficult in the UK for individuals who do not have access to a car, especially in the light of declining public transport in these areas. In some parts of the UK it is now no longer possible to attend an outpatient appointment in a district general hospital and return home the same day if relying on public transport.

In terms of activities foregone, whereas professional people may be given paid leave to attend a hospital appointment, manual workers are less likely to receive such benefits. A Welsh Consumer Council survey, for example, found that two out of five mothers taking a child to clinic appointments lost pay as a result. The overall effect of this supports the view that it is the poor and those people with low levels of personal mobility in rural communities who face the greatest costs in obtaining access to centralised hospital services. These two groups overlap and have a greater need for healthcare than others. Thus a strategy which some commentators have referred to as 'come and get it', whereby those who need the health service most are expected to come first to join the queue and to stay longest in it, may not be equitable. The costs of joining the queue are not equal.

The move towards centralisation of services is driven by two main concerns. First, a belief that concentration of healthcare provision improves the quality of care, and second, that economies of scale are offered by single large centralised units over multiple smaller units of provision. However, a recent review of the research evidence[6] on the impact of centralisation demonstrated a number of concerns about the validity of these two assumptions. The authors concluded that, for those proposing centralisation of services, 'the burden of proof must be with those who propose change to quantify the expected costs and benefits, to demonstrate the process by which benefits will be realised in practice, and to explain the way in which efficiency gains will be assured and monitored'.

Responses to problems of access

A number of different solutions have been developed in an attempt to help rural people overcome the difficulties posed by distance and other factors in accessing healthcare. Although not developed to deal with rural problems per se, perhaps one of the most important 'solutions' is that of a well-functioning and comprehensive primary healthcare service. The importance of primary healthcare in helping to overcome barriers to access and provide good outcomes at less cost is becoming increasingly recognised. A study in rural Australia, for example, suggested that since the number of patients self-presenting to hospital fell away more quickly than the number of referred patients, GPs may have a mitigating effect against distance by providing an additional impetus for patients who might otherwise be reluctant to travel.

More specific responses to the problems posed by access for rural populations include the following.

Branch surgeries and home visiting

Studies in UK primary care have failed to show that home visiting rates are higher in rural areas to compensate for low surgery consultation rates. Branch surgeries may increase access to general practice, although the recent tendency has been for them to be closed down. A survey of branch surgeries in rural parts of Norfolk found that, despite often being poorly equipped, they seemed to improve the access to primary care for many, especially for those people who would normally be expected to have a high demand for medical care, such as elderly people. In one study,[7] researchers found that:

- The majority had poor facilities and were held in private houses or village halls, and only about one fifth were held in purpose-built premises.

- Doctors using village halls/private houses reported seeing greater proportions of elderly people, females, working class people and people without cars at the branch surgery than at the main surgery. Purpose-built branch surgeries were reported to have the same clientele as the main surgery.

- Villages with branch surgeries had markedly higher consultation rates than villages with no surgeries. In villages with no surgery facilities, telephone consultations were slightly increased and home visits by the GP slightly fewer.

Unfortunately branch surgeries may be unpopular with GPs because of the poor level of care they feel they are able to provide in them. It is not clear whether this perceived poor quality of care affects outcome in any way or is compensated for by improved access. Another possible reason for the unpopularity of branch surgeries may be that some GPs find them inconvenient to work in, especially as they have not been shown to reduce GP workload.

Mobile provision

Mobile service provision has long been used to try and overcome problems of access. The provision of a mobile branch surgery, for example, resulted in increased consultation rates for village residents in East Anglia. Mobile provision is now widely used for screening services. Over a quarter of respondents in a survey of users of a mobile mother and baby clinic stated that it would be impossible or difficult for them to travel elsewhere. The average distance travelled by those using the clinic was between 0 and 0.5 miles, whereas without it 73% would have had to travel more than 5 miles to their GP.[8] While mobile provision may improve access and therefore equity for rural populations, it is staff-intensive and often seen as less efficient than static provision.

Community hospitals

Community hospitals, sometimes referred to as 'cottage hospitals', have long ameliorated the problems of access to secondary care. The popularity of community hospitals with health service planners has waxed and waned over many years, representing, in part, the tension between centralisation and access to local services. The impetus for much of the recent push towards centralisation of hospital services can be traced back to the 1962 Hospital Plan for England and Wales. It led to the closure of many cottage hospitals, so that by the end of the 1960s only 300 were functioning. The past 15 years have seen an upsurge in their numbers, although opinions on their value still vary, as does the range of services they provide. Studies have found costs per inpatient day to be lower in some community hospitals than their local district general hospital. Obviously this will be affected by the nature and severity of illnesses treated and procedures undertaken. Unfortunately little research has been undertaken to look at how different hospitals compare across the same range of procedures for a similar case mix of patients.

These issues are discussed at greater length in Chapter 12.

Telemedicine

Advances in technology now mean that it is relatively straightforward to transmit images from remote healthcare facilities for assessment in centralised specialised units. This has seen rural practitioners increasingly use a range of interventions including faxing ECGs to the local cardiologist; transmitting X-ray images from community radiology facilities for prompt specialist reporting; video consultations between the practitioner/patient in the rural setting and the specialist in the district general hospital. The new technologies offer many exciting possibilities to help overcome problems of access for rural healthcare. However, the cost-effectiveness of many telemedicine services has not been adequately evaluated, and there is a danger that people will be seduced by the technology for little gain in healthcare quality.

Funding premiums for rural health services

It is often argued that to overcome the problems of access in rural areas requires additional funding to be made available. This is because there is evidence that the direct costs of providing services in rural areas tend to be higher than in urban areas. The reasons for this include:

- additional travel costs
- additional telecommunication costs
- the extra costs of providing mobile and outreach services
- the extra costs of accessing training and other support.

In the UK, the NHS does not have a consistent policy about whether to explicitly take rurality into account when allocating resources. Even when rurality is considered, the basis of the weightings is often unclear and inconsistent. Inclusion may be more for political reasons than meeting possible excess costs of providing healthcare to rural populations. Scotland and Wales use a rural weighting when allocating resources to community healthcare, but England does not, despite the fact that it has many large rural areas. Rurality is taken into account throughout the UK, albeit in a small way, when funding general practice but not at all in allocating resources for hospital services. This inconsistency in policy is reflected by disagreements among academics in this field. Nevertheless, there is a strong case to be made that if high-quality rural health services are to be provided, some form of rural premium should be built into funding allocations.

Conclusion

Rural communities almost universally encounter problems accessing high-quality healthcare. The impact of such access problems is unclear although it seems likely that in at least some circumstances, health outcomes can be adversely affected. Within rural populations such disadvantage is not uniformly experienced and affects some groups (such as the poor, the elderly and others with low levels of personal mobility) more than others. The ways in which healthcare is delivered in rural areas reflect the priority given, either explicitly or implicitly, to differing dimensions of quality. For example, current financial pressures in the NHS often lead to efficiency and economy receiving higher priority than concerns over access and equity. Such trade-offs are political decisions, and one author has defined remoteness as 'where there are problems of access which it has not been thought worthwhile to overcome'.

References

1   Maxwell RJ (1984) Quality assessment in health. *BMJ*. **288**:1470–2.
2   Li J and Taylor B (1991) Comparison of immunisation rates in general practice and child health clinics. *BMJ*. **303**:1035–8.
3   Haynes RM and Bentham CG (1979) Accessibility and the use of hospitals in rural areas. *Area* **11**:186–91.
4   McKee CM, Gleadhill DN and Watson JD (1990) Accident and

emergency attendance rates:variation among patients from different general practices. *British Journal of General Practice.* **40**:150–3.

5 Fylkesnes K, Johnson R and Forde OH (1992) The Tromso Study: factors affecting patient-initiated and provider-initiated use of healthcare services. *Sociology of Health and Illness* **14**:275–92.

6 Ferguson B, Posnett J and Sheldon TA (1997) *Concentration and Choice in the Provision of Hospital Services* (summary report). CRD Report 8. NHS Centre for Reviews and Dissemination, York.

7 Fearn R, Haynes RM and Bentham CG (1984) Role of branch surgeries in a rural area. *Journal of the Royal College of General Practitioners.* **34**:488–91.

8 Langley M and Pithouse A (1990) Keep on moving. *Health Services Journal.* **100**:1184–5.

9
Rural poverty, deprivation and health

Jim Cox

In general, rural dwellers are healthier than their urban counterparts. They live longer and their morbidity rates are lower. There are, however, two important problems in interpreting the statistics, which can be deceptive. First, rural societies are diverse.[1,2] Scattered among the relatively wealthy landowners, commuters, managers and professional people are other rural dwellers living on very low incomes. They may be neither obvious to visitors nor readily visible in routine statistics. Advantaged and disadvantaged people, in terms of both income and health, live side by side. Second, morbidity rates reflect, in part, the way the population uses medical services, but people who live furthest from doctors' surgeries and hospitals are least likely to seek medical attention. Urban dwellers are more likely than rural dwellers to consult their doctors for comparable problems. These differences are most significant for people aged 16–64 and elderly women. So low morbidity rates may not mean low morbidity.

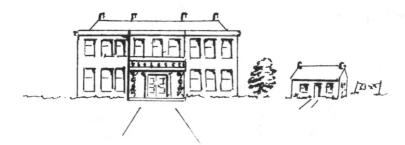

The relationship between wealth and health

The link between poverty and ill health is well known. Dickens described it and the relationship was emphasised in 1982 by the Black Report.[3] Wealth is the most important driver of health, and the gap between poor and wealthy people is becoming wider both within the UK and worldwide.[4] Unskilled men have a mortality three times that of professional men. There is a strong relationship between national census indicators of poverty and premature mortality.[5] If additional resources are to be channelled towards deprived or poor people, it is important that the rural poor are not forgotten.

Wealth and poverty in rural areas

Because of the diversity of rural societies, it is necessary to look at very small units, i.e. individual people and their families, when considering socioeconomic status. Whereas in cities it may be reasonably accurate to make generalised observations about a street or electoral ward, in the country an affluent landowner or commuter and his poor, socially isolated and underprivileged neighbour may be the only residents for miles around.

Twenty per cent of the rural population of England and 25% of rural households live in 'absolute poverty' (on an income of less than 140% of supplementary benefit entitlement). Importantly, elderly people are worst affected. Thirty five per cent of rural households in poverty are occupied by elderly people living alone. In rural Scotland in 1994, 49% of heads of households had annual incomes below £7800 (half the median Scottish wage). In some remote areas, such as the Outer Hebrides, almost the whole population was on 'poverty' income.[6]

Definition of rurality

There is no universal definition of rurality. A village in the southeast of England might be a town in the Highlands or the Lake District. The definition depends on the purpose. For example, a GP receives rural practice payments if at least 20% of his patients live more than 3 miles from his main surgery. Other definitions are based on population density or sparsity (e.g. Carstairs and Morris, Phillimore and Reading), remoteness from urban centres (e.g. Williams and Lloyd, Haynes and

Bentham) or subjective assessment (e.g. Ritchie *et al.*).[7] The subject is discussed thoroughly by Nicky Rousseau in the Royal College of General Practitioners' Occasional Paper on Rural Practice in the United Kingdom.[8]

Deprivation indices

The 1990 contract for British GPs included extra payments for providing services to patients in deprived areas, as defined by the Jarman underprivileged area index (UPA 8). The Jarman score was derived from comments of GPs and organisations in London and has a strong urban bias. For example, access to healthcare is excluded. Although other indices correlate well with each other and with health indices such as standard mortality ratios, they fail to reflect the characteristics of rural deprivation. They do not always correlate in rural areas.[7] Just as there is no generally accepted definition of rurality in the UK, so there is no suitable index of rural deprivation either.

The Townsend index includes car ownership, an expensive necessity in isolated areas, as a measure of wealth (Table 9.1).

Table 9.1 Variables used in deprivation indices[7]

	Townsend index	Jarman index	Carstairs index
Old people living alone		×	
Single-parent households		×	
Unemployed people	×	×	×
People who have moved house		×	
Children under five		×	
Overcrowded households	×	×	×
Ethnic minority households		×	
Car ownership	×		×
Home ownership	×		
Low social class		×	×

Disadvantage or 'social exclusion'

Townsend describes poverty as 'financial inability to participate in the everyday styles-of-living of the majority'. The European Union's broader, dynamic concept of 'social exclusion' may be more helpful. It shifts the focus from income and expenditure to multidimensional disadvantage, relating the individual to the society in which he or she lives. Despite an increase in the size of many villages, there has been a decline in rural services such as shops, schools, banks, police stations and pubs. People without their own transport and those with mobility problems have increasing difficulty in gaining access to services and are likely to use those local services that remain.[9] They spend more per item at village stores than those who can drive to supermarkets. The rural rich can economise in ways that their poorer neighbours cannot.

These differences extend to health and social services. There has been a trend towards larger, more centralised doctors' surgeries with closure of branch surgeries. The range of services may have improved in quality and quantity, but they have become less accessible. Some services, such as day care or support for 'carers' of elderly or chronically ill people, are simply not available in isolated areas.

Employment

Employment trends help to explain the reasons for such low incomes. The number of people employed in agriculture is decreasing. The trend is towards insecure, low-paid, often part-time or seasonal work with limited potential for career progression, for example in tourism. Only 38% of women in rural development areas are in paid employment, compared to a British average of 45.5%. Rural dwellers are less likely to register as unemployed and more likely to migrate in search of work. Those who are in work are less likely to be members of trades unions.

Homelessness

Contrary to popular belief, there is a substantial rural homelessness problem.[10,11] More than 46 000 people in England alone, 11.6% of the country's homeless, are in rural areas. Homeless people, as defined in the Housing Act 1985, are most commonly families with young children, women expecting babies and those vulnerable through age, disability or illness who can no longer live with parents, relatives or friends. There is a shortage of available, low-cost housing. The popularity of second homes and retirement homes has led to inflated property prices, unattainable by young people. Rented accommodation may only be available during the winter, out of the tourist season. The situation was compounded by the sale of council houses, which reduced the stock of low-cost housing available for rent.[11]

Transport

Although lack of car ownership features as a characteristic of deprivation in the Townsend index, lack of rural public transport since the privatisation of bus services means that 77% of rural households have a car compared with an English average of 68%. Independent transport is an expensive necessity in remote areas, compounding the poverty of low-income families. Running a car on subsistence income is not easy, but it may be essential to get to shops, markets or services. The problem will become even worse as direct and indirect taxes on motoring are increased.

The popular image of poor, rural dwellers being uncomplaining seems to be true. Many compare their situation with the harsher conditions of the past rather than with the current lifestyles of the majority. Although our knowledge of rural health need is limited, it is both logical and justifiable to assume that poverty and poor health are associated in rural areas, just as they are in our towns and cities.[12-14] Poverty exists in rural areas and is an important indicator of health and disease. Rural health workers should be aware of the importance of poverty and deprivation and look out for those who are affected. They may not be obvious.

References

1 Shucksmith M, Roberts D, Scott D, Chapman P and Conway E (1996) *Disadvantage in Rural Areas*. Rural Development Commission, Salisbury.
2 ACRE (1994) *Rural Life: facts and figures*. ACRE, Cirencester.
3 Townsend P and Davidson N (1982) *Inequalities in Health: the Black report*. Penguin, Harmondsworth.
4 Haines A and Smith R (1997) Working together to reduce poverty damage. *BMJ* **314**:529–30.
5 Joseph Rowntree Foundation (1997) *Death in Britain: how local mortality rates have changed: 1950s to 1990s*. Joseph Rowntree Foundation., York.
6 Joseph Rowntree Foundation (1994) *Disadvantage in Rural Scotland*. Social Policy Research 62. Joseph Rowntree Foundation, York.
7 Rousseau N, McColl E and Eccles M (1994) *Primary Care in Rural Areas: issues of equity and resource management – a literature review*. Centre for Health Services Research, Newcastle upon Tyne.
8 Cox J (ed) (1995) *Rural General Practice in the United Kingdom*.

Occasional paper 71. Royal College of General Practitioners, London.

9 Archbishop's Commission on Rural Areas (1990) *Faith in the Countryside*. Churchman Publishing Ltd, Worthing.

10 Rural Development Commission (1994) *Homelessness in Rural England Update to 1992/93*. Rural Development Commission, London.

11 Lambert C *et al.* (1992) *Homelessness in Rural Areas*. Rural Development Commission, London.

12 Cox J (1994) Rural general practice. *British Journal of General Practice.* **44**:388.

13 Watt IS, Franks AJ and Sheldon TA (1993) Rural health and healthcare. *BMJ.* **306**:1358–9.

14 Watt IS, Franks AJ and Sheldon TA (1994) Health and healthcare of rural populations in the UK: is it better or worse? *Journal of Epidemiology and Community Health.* **48**:16–21.

10
Continuing professional development

John Wynn-Jones

We are experiencing a period of rapid and extensive change in the delivery and administration of primary healthcare in the UK, and this process shows no sign of slowing down. The success of any reforms will depend on the ability of the workforce to assimilate new ideas and adapt their working practices to meet the challenge. Continuing professional development (CPD) will enable them to do this, and this chapter describes many of the various ideas for maintaining professional competence in rural areas in the UK and abroad.

Increasingly, primary healthcare is being provided by teams who come together from different professional backgrounds and educational experiences. Arguably, CPD – a lifelong process after the completion of formal qualifications – is by far the most important element of training for healthcare professionals and yet it is still relatively poorly resourced and the least formalised. Traditional educational activities, such as the didactic lecture format favoured for so long, are slowly giving way to newer forms of education, often much more interactive and problem based.

Rural practitioners have always been disadvantaged because distance from education centres, isolation and lack of cover have tended to exclude them from traditional CPD activities.[1-7] However, current moves towards self-directed learning are particularly appropriate for rural professionals, although they do not provide direct contact with colleagues, which has always been one of the advantages of meetings held in training departments, postgraduate centres, etc.[8,9]

Many different learning styles have been described.[10-12] For each person the appropriate style is influenced by several factors: personality, preference, the learning format and the context. Successful CPD, therefore, must be flexible and include a selection of learning formats based on the principles of adult learning.[13-17] Excessive workload in primary care has been shown to be one of the major barriers to effective professional development.[10, 11, 18, 19] Educational innovators must recognise this fact. It is also important that both the process of CPD and its outcomes are evaluated properly.[5, 10] These outcomes can be competence or performance or indeed measured improvement in patients' health. There is clearly a close link between audit and CPD.[8]

CPD will be one of the keys to effective rural healthcare in the future, ensuring that practitioners can provide up-to-date care for their patients and communities.[20] CPD not only facilitates professional contacts between isolated practitioners, but also social contacts between their families. Learning together helps to build networks, which foster self-help and mutual support. To ensure that rural practice continues to attract high-quality applicants, retain established practitioners and does not end up as a backwater, rural practitioners must have access to relevant and affordable continuing education.[21] The availability and accessibility of CPD[22] will influence the recruitment of young practitioners who see rural practice as a career option. The World Organisation of Family Doctors (WONCA) policy document on training for rural practice identifies CPD as a crucial element in the future of rural health throughout the world.[2] The perceived needs of rural practitioners, as seen by urban-based academics and pharmaceutical executives, may be very different from their actual needs.[1] CPD must be locally based where possible and rural practitioners should be involved in every stage of planning.[5, 22-6]

Exposure to rural practice during undergraduate and subsequent vocational training encourages fully qualified practitioners to enter rural practice.[6] The same individuals and practices are often involved in providing several strands of professional training. Linking of undergraduate, vocational training and CPD is not only desirable in rural areas, but essential to ensure that resources and people are used efficiently and opportunities maximised. Students and GP registrars help to stimulate established practitioners and ensure that they begin to meet their own educational needs through their roles as tutors, preceptors and mentors.[1]

Multidisciplinary educational activities, especially within individual practices, ensure that teaching resources are used effectively and that as many professionals as possible can benefit. Evidence suggests that practice-based activities are more effective than traditional forms of CPD in changing GP performance.[13] It is also possible that these activities contribute to closer teamwork. Learning together encourages closer working together through greater understanding and cooperation (see Chapter 7). Shared experiences and knowledge also help professionals to develop their own local guidelines and protocols.

However, multidisciplinary learning also raises a number of problems. Professional groups have their own separate agendas and accreditation criteria for CPD. It is important that tutors and trainers from each discipline liaise at an early stage to ensure that courses and activities are accredited for each professional group taking part. A multidisciplinary format is only suitable for a proportion of perceived CPD needs and each professional organisation still needs to provide training that is exclusive to its own professional group.

Rural practitioners provide a wide range of services that include many skills not normally associated with urban practice.[1, 19, 25, 27] These include the management of minor injuries, obstetrics, minor surgery, and immediate care at road traffic accidents and life-threatening emergencies. GPs also often staff community hospitals in their roles as clinical assistants and hospital practitioners.[28] Tutors and CPD providers need to be aware of these needs when organising continuing education in rural areas.[24]

Rural CPD tutors and preceptors should be appointed from, or have experience of, rural healthcare needs. Nominally, they can be based centrally, for example in postgraduate centres, but they should have a peripatetic, community-based role, assessing local needs, facilitating educational activities and stimulating self-directed learning. Rural medical societies and organisations that provide CPD have an important role in ensuring that practitioners have access to relevant education.[8]

The Montgomeryshire Medical Society started as a small peripatetic society in Mid-Wales, providing practice-based, multidisciplinary education organised by local practitioners. It now has a national and international reputation through its Annual Rural Doctors Conference. This conference was the first of its kind in Europe and attracts GPs from the UK and abroad. A day is now also dedicated to rural nursing issues and 1997 saw the first rural dentists' day. Medical schools with large rural areas within their sphere of influence are at last beginning to address rural issues.[1] The School of Postgraduate Medical and Dental Education at The University of Wales College of Medicine in Cardiff has appointed an Associate Advisor in Rural Primary Care Education and intends to develop a diploma course in rural health in the future.

The Institute of Rural Health in Mid-Wales has recently been established to address issues related to the provision of healthcare in rural areas. The Institute's principal goals are:

- information gathering and dissemination
- education and training
- research
- networking
- use of technology in rural practice.

CPD is inexorably linked to all the goals of the Institute. Rural organisations such as the Institute, the Royal College of General Practitioners Rural Practice Group[29] and EURIPA (European Rural and Isolated Practitioners Association) have an important role in gaining recognition for rural health issues and facilitating rural-based CPD across the UK and Europe.

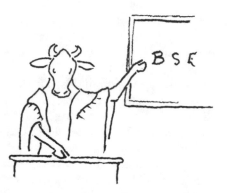

Different models of CPD (a changing scene)

Traditional lectures

Despite the changes that have occurred in the field of CPD, it is disappointing that the traditional lecture still appears to be the most popular form of activity and one of the mainstays of general practice educational activities.[18, 23] Lectures promote a dependent, passive relationship between the lecturer and those attending the session,[26] modelled on the teacher–pupil relationship. Lectures are often delivered in hospitals and there is a danger that too great an emphasis is placed on secondary, hospital-based care.[12]

Evidence from the west of Scotland shows that GPs will travel long distances to attend postgraduate centres.[23, 30] Attendance at lectures gives the isolated rural practitioner the opportunity to meet with colleagues and discuss issues. The importance of face-to-face contact in CPD is often underestimated and is not taken into consideration when evaluating educational activities. Lectures are sometimes given at venues such as hotels and restaurants and many of these are promotional in nature, sponsored and arranged by pharmaceutical companies.[31] Lectures provide a quick and relatively effortless way for practitioners to collect CPD credits such as PGEA (Postgraduate Education Allowance) points for GPs, where the process measures attendance rather than learning. Accreditation can lead to a system where the need to gain points overrides the educational potential of CPD. Evidence exists that the lecture format is popular among many GPs for this reason. But traditional lectures appear to have little value in changing the performance of GPs.[13]

Small group work

Group work is becoming increasingly popular.[32, 33] It allows practitioners to learn from each other and encourages self-directed learning. It also builds bridges between practitioners and practices, improving co-operation and dialogue. Small group activities are less dependent on postgraduate centres and are often held in GP surgeries and community hospitals. Group work is often suited to meeting the needs of limited numbers of individuals with special interests, such as rural practice. Isolated practitioners may, however, still have difficulty getting together on a regular basis. Modern technology, such as audio and video-conferencing, can facilitate contact, irrespective of distance or location. Successful groups include young practitioner groups, audit and evidence-based medicine groups and journal clubs.

Peripatetic groups and societies

Small rural groups and societies are usually organised on a local basis by the practitioners who will benefit directly from them. Issues relevant to local needs are addressed and links are built with local consultants who may otherwise communicate with them only through hospital letters. The traditional hierarchical relationship between consultant and practi-tioner is replaced with a more beneficial association where primary and secondary care share ideas and learn from each other. Meetings take place in doctors' surgeries, community hospitals or sites that are most convenient for the majority of the members. Some medical societies have a long and illustrious past and were usually established as a response to a lack of local postgraduate education. Most societies have a mainly medical membership, but some are gradually becoming multidisciplinary.[8] The advent of information technology is reviving the concept of societies and networks by linking groups with special interests, irrespective of distance or location.

Distance learning programmes

The number of distance learning packages available is increasing.[34] Many universities and academic organisations offer a range of courses with associated qualifications at certificate, diploma or Masters level. The University of Dundee was a pioneer in this field and has a wide range of courses available. The University of Wales College of Medicine now offers a comprehensive range of diploma courses for doctors. Modular nursing courses, which contribute to diplomas and degrees in professional practice, are also available. The University of Glamorgan is currently running a module in 'Recent Advances in Professional Practice' using a video link as part of the course. Many distance learning courses have a residential element, which gives participants the opportunity to share ideas with colleagues. Distance learning courses are often associated with a considerable amount of personal study and work. Most of the work is done outside working hours and places a heavy demand on the individual. Success depends on how well the student is prepared and organised. To minimise drop-outs, access to local tutors and preceptors is essential. Before they embark on such a course, students need to be well counselled to ensure that they know the implications for their personal, family and professional lives.

Self-directed learning, PEPs and personal portfolios

The development of personal education plans (PEPs) and portfolio-based learning makes CPD more relevant to individual practitioners' needs and practice.[23,35,36] PEPs represent specific assignments that practitioners undertake in agreement with their local tutor. The participant identifies areas of need within his or her professional development and, with the help of a local tutor, constructs a learning programme to address those specific needs. The number of PEPs is increasing and this flexibility encourages a range of learning formats, such as reading journals, audit, research, CPD courses, attendance at clinics and other forms of practical work. It is expected that PEPs will continue to grow in number and they may provide a model for formal reaccreditation in the future. PEPs offer rural practitioners an opportunity to extend their education and at the same time receive accreditation for the work they do.

Nurses registered with the United Kingdom Central Council for Nursing, Midwifery and Health Visiting (UKCC) are now required to undertake a minimum of 5 days CPD over 3 years, recorded in a portfolio. All professionals should be encouraged to keep a portfolio, which includes a record of the CPD activities they have undertaken, irrespective of whether they qualify for credits or not.

Reading

Healthcare professionals have access to a wide range of professional literature, ranging from peer-reviewed scientific journals to free publications which provide summaries of recently published research and news. Reading medical journals should always be an important element of a practitioner's professional development. Access to journals is now considerably easier through databases such as MEDLINE and Cinhal, and the growing number of electronic publications and data available on the WorldWide Web and local Intranets. The growth of published medical and health-related information is continuing to accelerate. It is clear that generalist practitioners find it impossible to read it all. Commercial and professional organisations now provide summary services that supply practitioners with an overview of current clinical literature.

Miscellaneous educational material of variable quality is available to practitioners at no or little cost. Much of this is provided by pharmaceutical companies in various formats, including audio and videotapes, software packages, audit programmes and reading material. Some of this can be of help, but it is important that working through this material does not make up the sum total of a professional's educational activities; much of it is promotional and may not give an objective view of the subject.[31] Tutors and educational directors have a responsibility to ensure that CPD activities are objective and encourage the practitioner to learn through a reflective and self-directed process.

Many surgeries have their own libraries, whose upkeep can impose a heavy financial burden. Although an up-to-date library is a prerequisite for training GP registrars, multimedia material in the form of CD-ROMs has extended the choice available and access to the WorldWide Web and services such as MEDLINE has reduced the need for maintaining a traditional library. These developments will help isolated rural practices and practitioners, but links still need to be developed with libraries in postgraduate centres and universities to back up this service with access to journals and the data needed for dissertations, audit and research.[1, 27, 37]

Telematics

Modern telecommunications provide rural practitioners with an invisible bridge, linking them with people, information and organisations, and in doing so minimising the effect of distance and isolation.[8, 22, 27, 38] The Internet provides access to a plethora of health-related sites throughout the world. The number of sites is now so great that it is becoming difficult to pick out the quality sites from the choice currently available. Health-related search engines and directories are available and links on individual web pages help to provide access to most of the important and valuable sites. Intranets are small but secure networks, similar to the Internet, that allow individuals to share confidential and structured information. The NHS Wide Web is an example of a larger Intranet, which will link all NHS healthcare professionals, trusts and authorities throughout the UK. Information provided on the network will be secure and controlled. Smaller Intranets are being established to link GP surgeries with local district general hospitals, allowing the primary and secondary sector to share electronic records and data. The Internet and Intranets can also give practitioners access to distance learning material in the form of multimedia CPD packages. Interactive computer-based learning and communication allows the participant and education provider to link for worthwhile communication and accreditation.[39]

Audio and videoconferencing on a multipoint basis give isolated practitioners the opportunity to participate in educational activities without the need to travel significant distances. Audioconferencing, using a device called 'an audio bridge' which links multiple sites, was pioneered in Australia and Canada, where the vast distances create a barrier to meeting for CPD. Participants can listen to presentations, interact with colleagues and obtain accreditation. Recent work in Mid-Wales on the TEAM Project (Tele Education And Medicine) and in

Northern Queensland, Australia, has extended this work using ISDN (Integrated Services Digital Network) and PC-based videoconferencing to link a number of sites on an interactive video basis. Participants can watch and listen to presentations or participate in a virtual small group. This technology gives rural professionals the opportunity to interact with colleagues anywhere in the world, developing networks irrespective of borders or distance. The telemedicine consultation can in itself become an educational activity. CME credits are given to family physicians in interactive consultations in Georgia, USA, as recognition of this.[40] Telemedicine may also promote two-way learning by helping urban physicians to understand rural needs.

Sabbaticals

The heavy workload experienced by many primary care professionals increases stress and reduces job satisfaction. Practitioners are increasingly experiencing high levels of stress and burnout. Sabbaticals can give the practitioner the opportunity to take time out, learn new skills and achieve long-held ambitions. The self employed status of GPs discourages them from taking time out as they have to fund locum cover, but the Government can reimburse a sizeable proportion of the costs. The culture of the sabbatical is not as well established in rural practice in the UK as it is in North America and Australia. However, it could become an important element in the working life of all practitioners, ensuring that they maintain professional interest through to retirement and at the same time making a wider contribution to the health of the UK population.

CPD in a reformed health service

The recently proposed health service changes outlined in the Government White Papers for England, Wales, Scotland and Northern Ireland are the first reforms in recent years to have emphasised the importance of training and education for health professionals. A recurring theme throughout the White Papers is the concept of integrated teams with access to comprehensive information systems and organisations such as the new Institute of Clinical Excellence. They will work within a framework that is guided by primary care groups which will have responsibility for ensuring that local healthcare professionals have the skills necessary to provide effective and efficient services for patients in the community. This new challenge should ensure that CPD will at last be recognised as one of the fundamental elements of a practitioner's career. The breadth of CPD activities will have to be extended to incorporate training in commissioning, public health and advanced management in order to manage a locally devolved healthcare system.[41]

Conclusion

Rural practice provides professionals with a number of challenges, the range and nature of which will inevitably increase over the next decade. CPD can provide individuals and teams with the opportunity to meet these challenges, cope with change and help to ensure that patients receive the best care that resources allow. Education should aim at encouraging self-directed learning through reflection on personal experiences in practice, while at the same time ensuring that care is based on sound research and evidence. A range of CPD activities is already available to rural practitioners. Traditional forms of CPD, such as lectures at postgraduate centres and training centres, may be denied to rural professionals, but practice-based, multidisciplinary activities may be better. Modern telecommunications can build invisible bridges, linking practitioners to an enormous database and enabling participation in interactive activities.

Rural health professionals need to ensure that their CPD activities are based on the needs of local patients and practitioners. The range of activities provided and situations encountered by rural practitioners must be reflected in the planning of educational activities. Academic organisations such as the Institute of Rural Health and the Royal College of General Practitioners have an important role to play in this process.

The responsibility for CPD provision and accreditation rests with a number of individuals, professional bodies and organisations. Co-ordination and cooperation between these disparate bodies still leave much to be desired. Closer links between the three strands of training (undergraduate, specialist and CPD) would benefit rural practice by maximising the use of resources and improving recruitment and retention. It may be contentious to suggest that a single individual or organisation could coordinate a multidisciplinary rural education and training programme, but this approach could have a significant impact on the development of healthcare in rural areas in the UK.

References

1 Rourke JB (ed) (1995) *Education for Rural Medical Practice: goals and opportunities. An annotated bibliography.* Australian Rural Health Research Institute, Monash University, Victoria, Australia.

2 Working Party on Training for Rural Practice (1995) *Policy on Training for Rural Practice.* World Organisation of Family Doctors (WONCA), Victoria, Australia.

3 Murray TS, Dyker GS, Kelly MH, Gilmour WH and Campbell LM (1993) Demographic characteristics of general practitioners attending educational meetings. *British Journal of General Practice.* **43**:467–9.

4 Owens JC, Steiner J, Hilfiker J and Eversole C (1979) Continuing education for the rural physician. *JAMA.* **241**(12):1261–3.

5 Cudney SA (1991) Making gerontic continuing education accessible for rural nurses. *Journal of Gerontology Nursing.* **17**(7):29–34.

6 Anderson J and Kimber K (1991) Meeting the continuing education needs of nurses in rural settings. *Journal of Continuing Education in Nursing.* **22**(1):29–34

7 Wynn-Jones J (1995) Peripatetic medical societies. In: J Cox (ed) *Rural General Practice in the United Kingdom.* Occasional Paper 71. Royal College of General Practitioners, London.

8 Al-Shehri A, Stanley I and Thomas P (1993) Continuing education for general practice. 2. Systematic learning from experience. *British Journal of General Practice.* **43**:249–53.

9 Gray DP (1988) Continuing education for general practitioners (editorial). *Journal of the Royal College of General Practitioners.* **38**:195–6.

10 Stanley I, Al-Shehri A and Thomas P (1993) Continuing education for general practice. 1. Experience, competence and the media of self directed learning for established general practitioners. *British Journal of General Practice.* **43**:210–14.

11 Lewis AP and Bolden KJ (1989) General practitioners and their learning styles. *Journal of the Royal College of General Practitioners.* **39**:187–9.

12 Royal College of General Practitioners (1993) *Education and Training for General Practice. Policy statement 3.* RCGP, London.

13 Davies AD, Thomson MA, Oxman AD and Haynes RB (1995) Changing physician performance. A systematic review of the effect of continuing medical education strategies. *JAMA.* **274**:700–5.

14 Janes RD and Turner N (1995). Reaccreditation in general practice: how New Zealand approaches the solution. *Canadian Family Physician.* **41**:1733–8

15 Allery LA, Owen PA and Robling MR (1997) Why general practitioners and consultants change their clinical practice: a critical study. *BMJ*. **314**:870–4.

16 Davies DA, Thomson MA, Oxman AD and Haynes RB (1992) Evidence for the effectiveness of CME. A review of 50 randomised controlled trials. *JAMA*. **268**:1111–17.

17 Shirriffs GS (1989) Continuing educational requirements for general practitioners in Grampian. *Journal of the Royal College of General Practitioners*. **39**:190–2.

18 Strasser R (1995) Rural general practice: is it a distinct discipline? *Australian Family Physician*. **24**(5):870–6.

19 Royal College of General Practitioners (1993) *Portfolio-based Learning in General Practice*. Occasional Paper 63. RCGP, London.

20 Forney DF and Evans W (1997) Development of a rural oncology nursing conference: proposal through implementation. *Oncology Nursing Forum*. **24**(3):537–3.

21 Abernethy RD (1990) Continuing medical education for general practitioners in North Devon. *Postgraduate Medical Journal*. **66**:847–8.

22 Rourke JTB and Strasser R (1996) Education for rural practice in Canada and Australia. *Academic Medicine*. **71**(5):464–9.

23 Kelly MH and Murray TS (1994) General practitioners views on continuing medical education. *British Journal of General Practice*. **44**:469–71.

24 Wise AL, Hayes RB, Adkins PB *et al.* (1994) Training for rural practice. *Medical Journal of Australia*. **161**:314–18.

25 Wise AL, Hayes RB, Adkins PB *et al.* (1994) Training for rural general practice. *Medical Journal of Australia*. **161**:315–18.

26 Editorial (1980) Continuing education and general practitioners. *Lancet*. **1**(8183):1397.

27 Rourke JB (ed) (1996) *Education for Rural Medical Practice: goals and opportunities. An annotated bibliography*. Australian Rural Health Research Institute, Monash University, Victoria, Australia.

28 Perry BC, Chrisinger EW, Gordon MJ and Henze WA (1980) A practice-based study of trauma in a rural community. *Journal of Family Practice*. **10**(6):1039–43.

29 Cox J (1994) Rural general practice (editorial). *British Journal of General Practice*. **44**:388–90.

30 Murray TS, Dyker GS and Campbell LM (1992) Characteristics of general practitioners who are high attenders at educational meetings. *British Journal of General Practice*. **42**:157–9.

31 Kelly MH and Murray TS (1996) Motivation of general practitioners

attending postgraduate education. *British Journal of General Practice.* **46**:353–6.

32 Owen PA, Allery LA, Harding KG and Hayes TM (1989) General practitioners' continuing medical education within and outside their practice. *BMJ.* **299**:238–40.

33 Challis M, Mathers NJ, Howe AC and Field NJ (1997) Portfolio-based learning: continuing medical education for general practitioners – a mid-point evaluation. *Medical Education.* **31**:22–6.

34 Editorial (1997) Home study essential for rural nurses. *Australian Nursing Journal.* **5**:5, 20.

35 St Clair C and Brillhart B (1990) Rural nurses as self-directed learners: overcoming obstacles to continuing education. *Journal of Continuing Education in Nursing.* **21**(5):219–23.

36 Challis M, Mathers NJ, Howe AC and Field NJ (1997) Portfolio-based learning: continuing medical education for general practitioners – a mid-point evaluation. *Medical Education.* **31**:22–6.

37 Money P (1986) Continuing medical education for isolated rural general practitioners – a journal project. *Family Practice.* **3**(2):117–19.

38 Cox J (1997) Rural general practice: a personal view of current key issues. *Health Bulletin* (Scottish Office). **55**(5):309–15.

39 Neafsey PJ (1997) Computer-assisted instruction for home study: a new venture for continuing education programs in nursing. *Journal of Continuing Education in Nursing.* **28**(4):164–72.

40 Sanders J, Brucker P and Miller MD (1995) Using telemedicine for continuing education for rural physicians. *Academic Medicine.* **70**:457.

41 Wynn-Jones J (1998) *Working with The White Paper: a vision for rural practice NHS Wales: putting patients first.* The Institute of Rural Health, Gregynog, Wales.

11
Research

Eleri Roderick

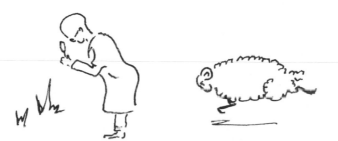

There is a tendency to associate medical research with large institutions such as universities and tertiary care hospitals. This situation is now changing, with more research being commissioned from and carried out in primary care. Because there is a dearth of knowledge about health issues as they affect rural populations, research is particularly important in rural areas. It is facilitated by the formation of research networks and research practices.

Along with the concept of a 'primary care-led NHS', there has been a fundamental change in the way healthcare research is commissioned, organised and funded. As a result of the Culyer Report on research funding in the NHS, primary care researchers can now apply for research support funding along with all other providers of NHS research.[1] The system allows for infrastructure funding rather than individual project funding and recognises that there are costs associated with planning and starting up a programme of research as well as actually carrying out research projects. The bidding process involves providing detailed costings with justification of the costs, and meeting a number of assessment criteria, including quality, ethics and strategic ability. This process is applied equitably to all bidders and is therefore open to rural practitioners as well as academic researchers.

Although rurality is not a barrier to research, there are difficulties to be overcome. These include keeping in touch with other researchers and forging links with academic departments or research networks that may be able to offer support.

To obtain funding, research has to be high quality, provide new knowledge and be generalisable in order to show healthcare benefits. Studies therefore need to be well planned, statistically sound and possibly on quite a large scale to achieve worthwhile results. This does not mean that those in a small rural practice cannot plan a study, but it may mean that the project has to involve several practices.

Why do research?

As a partner in an RCGP research practice, one of the questions colleagues (and the practice accountant) ask me is 'Why do you do research?'. The answers include the personal satisfaction of rising to challenges, broadening knowledge, learning to sift evidence and making informed decisions on patient management. The satisfaction of publishing a paper and seeing one's name in print cannot be overestimated. On the other hand, we are unlikely to get rich through our research activities, which require a great deal of goodwill from partners and practice staff.

Fellowships

Fellowships are personal awards for practitioners wishing to carry out their own research. They are available from several sources, including regional health authorities, charities such as the Clare Wand Fund, the RCGP and the MRC. Details are usually advertised in the medical press. Ideally, an applicant should have developed a research idea as far as an outline protocol. Awards may be for several years and allow the recipient to be freed from clinical work either full or part time. There is often a requirement to undertake a course on research methodology. Working in a rural or isolated practice may make this difficult, but with the availability of distance learning and part-time courses, the problems are not insurmountable.

Research practices

Research practices are NHS general practices where one or more partners and other practice staff have a special interest in and experience of research. The first two in the UK were appointed in 1994 by the RCGP. Since then further practices have been funded both by the College and by the NHS. A survey[2] of the first 14 practices revealed that one was rural, eight were semi-rural and the rest urban or mixed. Funding for a research practice (in the order of £15 000 per annum in 1997) is usually used to fund protected time for a research partner and to finance staff, e.g. a research assistant, to carry out research activities. The schemes usually require a lead partner with previous experience of research and an undertaking that links will be made with an academic department. Rurality need not be a bar to this, given the current availability of information technology and electronic links. The availability of free access to MEDLINE for BMA members means that literature searches can be carried out easily from practices distant from medical libraries. All that is required is a PC, modem and appropriate software. MEDLINE and other medical search services, such as Health on the Net (http://www.hon.ch), Medical Matrix (http://www.medmatrix.org), OMNI (http://www.omni.ac.uk) and Cliniweb (http://www.ohsu.edu/cliniweb), are all available on the Internet.

To make a successful application, some groundwork should be carried out in advance. It is important to identify everyone who is interested in research in the practice, to know what they have done in the past and what they would like to do. A research strategy should then be formulated, building on the strengths of individuals and the practice. For example, it may be wise in the first instance to concentrate efforts on the areas of team members' previous experience. Research should be included in the practice's overall practice business plan or strategy.

Research networks

Research networks are a relatively new development in primary care research in Britain. Most have been formed since 1993. However, they have been around for a long time in the USA and some have developed into large and influential organisations, for example the Ambulatory Sentinel Practice Network of North America (ASPN), based in Denver, Colorado.

The aims of research networks include promoting high-quality research by primary care practitioners, promoting collaborative projects, recruiting practitioners to collect data for larger studies from universities, etc., and promoting research awareness among primary care practitioners.

Some research networks are university department led, e.g. South Thames Research Network (STaRNet), and some are general practice based but with links to academic departments, e.g. the Northern Research Network (NoReN). Research networks play an important role in facilitating research in the isolation of rural practice. For example, the Cumbria Practice Research Group links researchers across a large area of North Cumbria and facilitates collaborative research between geographically distant practices. Advances in information technology improve these links. One research network in Canada, the Upper Peninsular Research Network (UPRNet), has successfully carried out research projects almost entirely through computer networking, a necessity because of the isolation of member practitioners from the network headquarters at Michigan State University.

Membership of research networks brings advantages such as ready-made links with academic departments, to like-minded individuals in the research world and sources of training and expert advice. There is a national forum for organisers of research networks to exchange thoughts and ideas.

The Royal College of General Practitioners Research Network is a different sort of network. Its aims are to foster a research culture in general practice nationally, to establish research training fellowships for general practitioners, to establish research practices, to promote doctoral theses from general practice and to promote strong links between the college and academic organisations concerned with general practice.

The RCGP has a national research adviser who is able, free of charge, to advise GPs about research projects. This is an important service for rural practitioners who have difficulty accessing academic departments directly.

Information about local research networks is available from regional research and development directorates. Information about the Royal College of General Practitioners Research Network is available from the RCGP.

Multidisciplinary research

Research in primary care lends itself to a multidisciplinary approach because of the strengths of the primary care team. Research practices are particularly well placed to develop multidisciplinary projects. The advantages of this approach are the different skills and perspectives that a variety of professionals can bring to a project and the strengthening of the primary care team that occurs when all work together with a common goal. The importance of getting the reception staff on board early in the development of projects cannot be overstated. Their participation in projects is often overlooked, but they may well be carrying out extra tasks, such as ensuring consent forms are signed and finding and filing extra notes. Their goodwill is essential.

Planning and carrying out a research project

This subject merits a whole textbook, but here are a few pointers gleaned from personal experience of carrying out research projects in a rural area. First, make sure the area you want to research is worth knowing about, and that the study hasn't already been done. This requires a systematic review of currently available literature, e.g. by using MEDLINE.

Second, get advice on study design from an expert such as the RCGP National Research Advisor, a member of an academic department of primary care or an experienced researcher recommended by a local research network. In particular, statistical advice is important in planning sample size at an early stage. Consider doing a small pilot study first, especially if you are introducing a new method of doing something or testing a questionnaire, and don't be misled into thinking that it is easy to run off a questionnaire. There are a large number of reliable validated questionnaires available on many topics. It is better to use one of these if it fits your project rather than to construct one of your own which then requires validation. However, if you modify the questions in any way, it will require revalidation. Remember that you may require permission to use certain questionnaires and that there may be a charge for their use.

If you are planning to apply for funding for your project you will also need to apply for ethics of research committee approval. Most sources of funding insist on this. Directories of funding bodies can be obtained from the RCGP and should also be available from NHS research and development directorates. Research networks often have information or directories.

There is little published research on rural health, which is therefore a potentially fruitful research area. Just as much hospital-based research has been extrapolated erroneously to primary care populations, urban research findings cannot necessarily be extrapolated to rural communities. For example, there is evidence that distance of residence from the

GP's surgery is inversely related to the likelihood of that patient consulting the doctor.[3-5] This can lead to delayed treatment for serious disease and may affect prognosis.[6] Access to services is therefore an important factor in healthcare, especially where there is a lack of public transport and distances are great. Some health problems almost exclusively affect rural dwellers, for example the effects of organo-phosphate sheep dips on the health of farmers[7] or access to confidential contraceptive advice for teenagers in rural areas.

These are exciting times, with major changes in public policy bringing a wealth of opportunities for everyone interested in good-quality primary care research. If we are to practise 'evidence-based' healthcare, we must undertake research to ensure that the evidence is valid in rural communities.

References

1   Culyer Report (1994) *Supporting Research and Development in the NHS.* HMSO, London.
2   Smith LFP (1997) Research general practices: what, who and why? *British Journal of General Practice.* **47**:83–6.
3   OPCS and Royal College of General Practitioners (1974) *Morbidity Statistics from General Practice: second national study 1970–71.* HMSO, London.
4   OPCS and Royal College of General Practitioners (1989) *Morbidity Statistics from General Practice: third national study 1981–82.* HMSO, London.
5   OPCS (1995) *Morbidity Statistics from General Practice: fourth national study 1991–92.* HMSO, London.
6   Launoy G, Le Coutour X, Gignoux M *et al.* (1992) Influence of rural environment on diagnosis, treatment and prognosis of colorectal cancer. *Journal of Epidemiology and Community Health.* **46**:365–7
7   Orr A (1994) Effects of organophosphate sheep dips on the health of farmers in one rural practice in Cumbria. (Unpublished)

12
Community hospitals and maternity units

Gordon Baird

Healthcare in rural areas is difficult to provide because the facilities that provide care tend to be inaccessible. This has consequent effects on patients, populations and health professionals. Providing care close to the patient gives better healthcare outcomes than more sophisticated but inaccessible secondary care. The most effective way of providing care to a community is by ensuring equity of access to the most effective medical interventions for the highest possible proportion of the population. In rural areas, limited accessibility (due to geographical constraints) may reduce the number of procedures performed.[1] This has been termed 'the inverse care law'.

The provision of hospital care in a rural area is a compromise between accessibility and quality of care. In developed countries, urban patients can expect easy access to a wide variety of high-quality care. But rural populations cannot reasonably expect rapid access to tertiary facilities, such as neurosurgery, cardiothoracic surgery or neonatal intensive care. Additionally, the management of conditions such as medical and obstetric emergencies which are managed as secondary care in an urban area, e.g. myocardial infarction and complications of labour, cannot always be provided efficiently or effectively in rural areas by specialist services. The gap can be filled by community hospitals, often run by GPs.

Community-based hospitals exist in almost all rural areas from barefoot clinics in the developing world to relatively sophisticated establishments in developed countries such as Australia, Canada, New Zealand and the UK. In the UK, many pre-date the state provision of care and were provided by local communities to fill an otherwise unmet

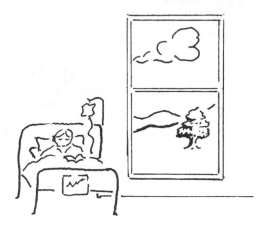

need. While circumstances have changed over the last few decades, with improved transport and an increasing likelihood of needing highly sophisticated secondary care, most rural populations still perceive a need for a local hospital.

Proof of effectiveness of care is hard to produce for several reasons. The randomisation of study groups to test a hypothesis may be regarded as unethical when both carers and the public believe that one intervention is better than another. Variations in case mix, personnel and buildings as well as geographical considerations make valid comparisons almost impossible, and small numbers make statistical analysis impractical. This leads to a dearth of data on the subject. The major asset of a community hospital is being close to the community it serves. Hypothesising about the value of a community hospital may only be properly assessed by its closure – a catch-22 situation.

Community hospitals can provide a surprising range of services. These are outlined in Table 12.1, but the list is by no means exhaustive. Provision of services depends on two things – their need, perceived or

Table 12.1 Services provided by community hospitals

Acute services	Diagnostic	Therapy	Chronic care	Mental health
Medicine	Radiology	Physiotherapy	Rehabilitation	Acute psychiatry
A&E	Haematology	Occupational therapy	Geriatrics	Psychogeriatrics
Obstetrics	Biochemistry	Speech therapy	Respite care	Dementia
Surgery	Blood transfusion		Terminal care	
Anaesthetics				

real, and the enthusiasm or at least willingness of professional groups to provide them. The evolution of many similar local hospitals throughout the world suggests that they fill a need.

Consideration of community hospitals raises several questions.

- Is quality compromised?
- What levels of experience, expertise and training are necessary?
- How can plans help to ensure that services are provided and maintained?
- What can be done to support those working in isolated units?

Is quality compromised?

The simple answer to this question is that the quality of service may be lower than that provided in a district general hospital. Inadequate facilities, lack of experience, expertise and training, and the absence of resident staff all lead to an apparent lack of quality. Balancing this, limited scope for medical intervention may have positive effects. For example, the use of antiarrhythmics in coronary care units is associated with excess mortality[2] and the routine use of electronic foetal monitoring in labour is associated with an increased rate of operative delivery.[3,4] Substitution of GPs for junior doctors in A&E departments reduces unnecessary investigations.[5]

Quality of care can be measured by comparing results with other hospitals. But one must also consider the trauma and delay associated with travel and the effect on morale and wellbeing of social and family isolation when in a distant hospital. Quality measured purely by comparison with a major centre is unfair if these factors, not experienced by urban populations, are not considered.[6] The effect on morale of those who are seriously ill cannot be measured, nor can the reduction in motivation that is so important in long illnesses, such as major injury or stroke. The temptation to use direct comparison should be resisted unless all aspects of care are included. The need to be flexible and adaptable can often be interpreted as disorganisation or lack of focus by those who work in environments with the luxury to be able to specialise in one particular area with others supplying complementary aspects of care.

It is worth looking at some specific areas where there are qualitative differences in rural hospitals.

Accident & emergency (A&E)

Where there is a community hospital there is usually an A&E department, run by GPs. The nature of the work done blurs distinctions between primary and secondary care. In the event of major accident or illness, mature and balanced decisions about stabilisation or transfer have to be made. Community hospital staff must be aware of indications for transfer, the best mode of transport and the support required during transfer, as well as the facilities available in the referring hospital. The GP is best placed to make such decisions.

Medicine

There are a number of medical conditions for which time to treatment forms an important aspect of care. In myocardial infarction (MI), the risk of cardiac arrhythmia or arrest is greatest within the first hour, and studies performed before the advent of thrombolysis showed that management of uncomplicated MI at home was not associated with adverse outcome.[7,8] A reasonable assumption is that the travel or transfer to a strange environment can cause harm equal to the benefits accrued.

The advent of thrombolysis has discouraged home management of MI. For rural populations alternatives include pre-hospital thrombolysis (*see* Chapter 4) or administration in a community hospital.

For cerebrovascular accidents, the disturbance caused by a long ambulance journey has potential for harm in the acute phase of an illness, which currently has no specific treatment. This may change if studies on the use of thrombolysis in thrombotic stroke show benefit, but the requirement for urgent CAT imaging will limit the availability of this intervention to rural patients. The most important factor in recovery is patient motivation, best achieved close to home.

Other common medical conditions such as self-poisoning, status epilepticus, asthma and gastrointestinal haemorrhage can often be safely managed under the care of a GP.

Geriatrics

Elderly people have specific problems, often with a significant social element. Their reduced tolerance to invasive investigations and surgical procedures, together with a combination of medical and social problems, means that management in a community hospital is likely to be appropriate.

Obstetrics

Obstetrics traditionally provokes terror in the medical practitioner accustomed to the high intervention rates and complications seen in a teaching hospital. The low-risk population managed in GP units does not have the same frequency of complications and the range of skills required to deal with likely emergencies (post-partum haemorrhage, retained placenta, neonatal resuscitation) is easily acquired.[9] Protocols for severe hypertension, post-partum haemorrhage and neonatal resuscitation are simple, effective and well proven and should be provided.[10] Electronic foetal monitoring in labour increases the intervention rate and should not be used routinely in a 'low-tech' unit.[3,4]

The balance between social and medical factors is nowhere more evident than in the provision of maternity care. The issues of choice that have been highlighted in the provision of maternity care in the UK[11] have also highlighted some of the dilemmas associated with rural maternity care. Pregnant women regarded as low risk constitute the minority and, even then, at least 5% of them will have unpredicted problems during delivery. In our study in Stranraer, 12.8% of women in labour who had been booked for delivery in a rural unit run by GPs and midwives had unplanned transfers to a consultant unit and 3.8% had Caesarean sections.[9] Most pregnant women cannot be offered choice without compromising safety and should be offered hospital delivery. A community hospital is often the most effective environment in which to deal with these experiences.

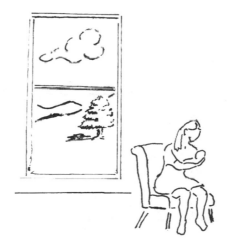

Surgery

A vigorous debate continues as to whether surgery is best performed in major units where procedures are being done frequently or whether the quality of surgery is dependent on the skills of the operator even if the procedure is done infrequently. It is likely that both arguments have an element of truth. There is no doubt that the advent of day surgery and the increase in minimally invasive procedures have great potential to increase the scope of surgery provided close to the patient's home. The cost of equipment may be a limiting factor.

Small units may be less appealing to surgeons, who are less likely to be able to indulge in a speciality because of small populations. Their periods of duty may well not be compatible with family or social life. Many surgeons are now being trained in a subspeciality and this means that a true 'general surgeon' is less likely to be available for such an appointment. Australia and Canada have schemes in place for general training. The Royal Colleges in the UK are looking into the possibility of training specifically for this type of role.

Anaesthetics

The presence of an anaesthetist in a rural setting is probably more important than in any other speciality. Supporting surgical, orthopaedic and obstetric services, whether by specialist or GP, an anaesthetist can be invaluable in the stabilisation of a critically ill patient prior to and during transfer by air or road.

Diagnostic and therapeutic specialities

A realistic range of investigations should be available to a community hospital. Radiology, including fluoroscopy for barium investigations as well as ultrasound and cardiac Doppler imaging, is easily available and can be offered by visiting radiologists or technicians. Laboratory investigations depend on appropriately trained technicians and the availability of equipment. MRI and mammography screening units in mobile vans, which can be attached in a modular way to a docking area within the hospital, have been developed recently. They may make available a wider range of investigations.

The community hospital can be a base for both hospital and

community physiotherapy, occupational therapy, speech therapy and chiropody. This should allow integrated care, both within each service and between professional groups. Where the general practitioner surgery or health centre is attached to the hospital, this encourages very close relationships to develop, with a much more integrated and cohesive approach to care.

Mental health

With the exception of dementia care, the provision of mental health inpatient services is not often a feature of community hospitals. This reflects the importance of anonymity in therapy groups, the amount of time required to properly look after such patients and the social stigma attached to mental illness. Most patients ill enough to need admission also require specialist support.

What levels of experience, expertise and training are necessary?

A period of time in a structured training programme before entering general practice is required throughout the European Union, Australia and Canada. It is hard to see how a 2- or 3-year structured programme can prepare a doctor for a career as diverse as that experienced by rural GPs. Skills and experience must therefore be developed and maintained while in post. A number of excellent courses, often of a multidisciplinary format, are available to develop skills and confidence. ATLS (Advanced Trauma Life Support), ALS (Advanced Life Support), ALSO (Advanced Life Support in Obstetrics) and courses run by BASICS (British Association for Immediate Care) are excellent for developing the appropriate qualities.

One of the reasons often quoted for not wanting to practise in a rural setting is the need to carry out rarely performed (sometimes never before performed) tasks. Courses and guidelines may help. The peer support offered within a hospital setting can be of immeasurable reassurance to a doctor who might otherwise be isolated. The coffee room is one of the most valuable places in the facility, providing support and education as well as a chance to bend a visiting consultant's ear on a difficult case.

A community hospital should also be a focus for formal education. It should have a library, postgraduate facility and information technology for access to remote databases. E-mail, the Internet and video-conferencing promise exciting developments for the future.

How can planning help to ensure that services are provided and maintained?

In the past, many units have developed in an apparently unplanned way in response to local need, perceived or real. The drive towards purchasing or commissioning (as in the UK and New Zealand) has meant an increasing emphasis on the financial aspects of provision of care and a greater need to justify services provided and their cost.

The idea of a basic minimum of care for which clear outcome benefits are definable (such as thrombolysis and maternity care) helps the debate. The GP has an obligation to ensure that costs are considered. For example, the provider of care may ignore the cost of transport. Even purchasers or commissioners may ignore it if the transport cost is not in their budget. The development of elaborate transport arrangements such as helicopters may sound useful, but may not in reality be much more efficient. They can be heavily weather dependent and expensive. The indirect costs, both material and social, of travel in communities without public transport are difficult to quantify but nevertheless important.

Transfer and travel involve risks to patients, relatives and medical and paramedical attendants. In the Scottish islands a road accident caused a perinatal death as well as killing an accompanying midwife, and there have been air crashes involving staff. Such incidents often involve bad weather. Better local services reduce the risks of transfer.

As GPs we have an obligation to inform and educate managers and ensure that financial constraints do not reduce the accessibility of care to our patients.

What can be done to support those working in isolated units?

Hopefully a textbook such as this will provide some encouragement for those who seek support for rural hospitals. The importance of developing standards and skills appropriate to such an environment is central to their future.

The support of the general public for local hospitals can be exceptional. The public, as users and taxpayers, are usually very appreciative of community hospitals. Community hospitals are tangible and reassuring icons for the public and their medical attendants.

Peripatetic services, where the GP performs the day-to-day work of the unit and the consultant offers advice and performs a watching brief, offer support for GPs and nurses. Patients can be worked up by the GP and the case presented to the consultant either as a formal referral, on a ward round or by telephone. In essence the GP acts as junior doctor and the consultant is consulted. The GP may be looking after his own patients or may have an interest in a particular speciality. There is clear evidence in maternity care that the outcomes in such units are no worse than where all patients are dealt with by a consultant unit.[9, 12, 13]

Such a system has problems if the GP is working beyond the limitations of his expertise. This may occur because the most appropriate course of action is dictated by circumstances, for example the performance of a tracheotomy or insertion of a chest drain. More worryingly, it can be due to the doctor overestimating his own ability and performing tasks that are best performed elsewhere, for example the reduction of a fracture that would be better managed by open reduction. The only certainty is that from time to time disasters will occur.

For the system to work, goodwill and a mutual understanding of the conditions under which decisions are made and actions taken are essential. Consultants have an interest in offering the highest level of care to their patients, and for them to have some responsibility for the unit encourages training. The surge of adrenaline (or worse) in the untrained or unprepared GP hospital doctor is a powerful inducement for education and self-improvement. Coffee or lunches undisturbed by requests for information or opinion are rare. The personality of both GPs and consultants is important for such a system to work, but such a system can allow patients to have the best of both worlds.

Conclusion

Whatever system is adopted, it must reflect the needs and aspirations of the community. Such needs may be perceived by the community (such as the need for certain surgical services) or may be dictated by medical advances, e.g. thrombolysis. More debatable is the level of care that should be offered prior to safe and effective transfer to a more sophisticated level of care. Local medical, nursing, laboratory and transport resources must be integrated. The argument over whether it is better to 'swoop and scoop' or 'stay and play' is not yet resolved. It should be a matter of experience and judgement on the day in the light of resources present at the time.

The introduction of trauma centres in the USA has improved outcomes after major trauma and major illness, but requires a transport infrastructure that cannot be expected in rural areas throughout the world. Widespread access to intermediate levels of care in community hospitals and district general hospitals will benefit a greater number of patients than the application of expensive, high-technology medicine to a small number. Rural patients are more likely to die on their way to a trauma centre.

Returning to the accessibility versus quality debate, the community hospital can at best only be an intermediate level of care. It will always be a compromise. The provision of transport is still an important concern. Arrangements for transfer of cases such as those who are critically ill or in advanced labour should be well developed.

Patients, better than doctors, appreciate the balance between the technical superiority of specialist hospital care and the opportunity of being treated near to home. Doctors measure life in tangible chunks of days and months of survival. Patients understand that an additional 30 days in a lonely hospital cannot replace the smile of a grandchild blowing out the birthday candles or the reassurance of a relative or family doctor when terror takes hold. As long as there are communities and doctors able to appreciate the importance of such things, there will be a place for community hospitals. If we accept that the role of doctors, nurses and hospitals is above all to relieve suffering and that loneliness, isolation and fear constitute suffering, then the case for community hospitals is made. The challenge for the future is to be able to prove it.

References

1   Black N, Langham S and Petticrew M (1995) Coronary revascularisation: why do rates vary geographically in the UK? *Journal of Epidemiology and Community Health.* **49**(4):408–12.
2   Garratt C, Ward DE and Camm AJ (1989) Lessons from the cardiac arrhythmia suppression trial. *BMJ.* **299**:805–6
3   Levenko KJ, Cunningham FG, Nelson S *et al.* (1986) A prospective trial of selective and universal electronic fetal monitoring in 34 995 pregnancies. *New England Journal of Medicine.* **315**:615–19
4   McDonald D, Grant A, Sheridan Pereira M *et al.* (1985) The Dublin trial of intrapartum fetal monitoring. *American Journal of Obstetrics and Gynecology.* **152**:524–39.

5 Murphy AW, Bury G, Plunkett PK, Gibney-D, Smith M, Mullan E and Johnson Z (1996) Randomised controlled trial of general practitioner versus usual medical care in an urban accident and emergency department: process, outcome, and comparative cost. *BMJ*. **312**:1135–42.

6 Wall A (1996) Keep it local. *Health Director*. **29 June**:14.

7 Colling A, Dellipiani AW, Donaldson RJ and MacCormack P (1976) Teesside coronary survey: an epidemiological study of acute attacks of myocardial infarction. *BMJ*. **2**:1169–72.

8 Liddell R, Grant J and Rawles J (1990) The management of suspected myocardial infarction by Scottish general practitioners with access to community hospital beds. *British Journal of General Practice*. **40**(337):318–22.

9 Baird AG, Jewell D and Walker JJ (1996) Management of labour in an isolated rural maternity hospital. *BMJ*. **312**:223–6.

10 Department of Health (1994) *Report on Confidential Enquiries into Maternal Deaths: 1988–90*. HMSO, London.

11 Expert Maternity Group (1993) *Changing Childbirth: report of the expert maternity group*. Cumberlege Report. HMSO, London.

12 Jewell D, Young G and Zander L (1992). *The Case for Community Based Maternity Care*. Association for Community-based Maternity Care, Bristol.

13 Rosenblatt RA, Reinken J and Shoemack P (1985) Is obstetrics safe in small hospitals? *Lancet*. **1**:429–33.

Further reading

Cox J (1995) *Rural General Practice in the United Kingdom*. Occasional Paper 71. Royal College of General Practitioners, London.

Ritchie LD (1996) *Community Hospitals in Scotland: promoting progress*. University of Aberdeen, Aberdeen.

Royal College of General Practitioners and Association of General Practitioner Community Hospitals (1990) *Community Hospitals – preparing for the future*. Occasional Paper 43. Royal College of General Practitioners, London.

Skrabanek P (1994) *The Death of Humane Medicine*. The Social Affairs Unit, Dublin.

Working Group Report (1996) *Community Hospitals in Wales: the future*. Welsh Office, Cardiff.

Useful addresses

Community Hospitals Association (Honorary Secretary: Mrs B Moore), Meadow Brow, Broadway Road, Broadway, Ilminster, Somerset TA19 1RG.

Scottish Association of General Practitioner Hospitals (Honorary Secretary: Dr HD Greig), Brechin Health Centre, Infirmary Street, Brechin, Angus DD9 7AN.

13
Branch surgeries

Iain Mungall

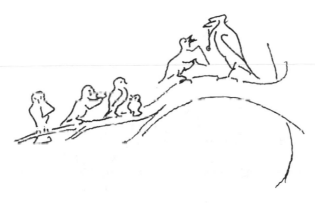

In the UK some medical practices operate from more than one site. Premises other than the main base are referred to as branch surgeries. They are much more common in rural areas but also exist in urban areas. A recent study in Cumbria showed that they were associated more with local population density than with remoteness. No matter how remote, a minimum number of patients is needed to make a branch surgery viable.

Their origins are various and remarkably little has been written about them. They may have been set up to provide services wanted or needed by a remote community, they may be the consequence of a merger between two practices or they may have been set up to raise a practice's profile in a particular area.

There are fewer now than there were a generation ago, and this trend may be continuing.

Branch surgeries vary from being fully staffed and equipped and indistinguishable from main surgeries to being primitive with few amenities. Some have no staff, no records, no telephone and sometimes no water supply. They may be purpose built or take place in patients' living rooms, village halls or public houses. Caravans have been used as mobile branch surgeries. Bentham and Haynes[1] described the introduction of a mobile caravan service serving several rural Norfolk villages, to replace a conventional branch surgery. Consultation rates increased slightly during the first year, but in a village where the mobile surgery was a new facility, consultation rates increased substantially. Patients recognised the limitations of the caravan but welcomed easier access.

In my own practice at Bellingham in Northumberland, with a population of 2800 patients scattered in clusters over approximately 800 square miles, we run four branch surgeries in villages 4, 8, 18 and 19 miles away from the main surgery. Until 1997, we held a surgery at each branch twice weekly. Now we consult twice weekly in the largest village but only weekly at the others. This has released a considerable amount of doctor time. The reduction in service was achieved without complaint following a practice newsletter that laid out the issues while stressing our ongoing commitment to care for remote communities.

Two of the premises are village halls, one is a school and one is a room in a private home. No staff are employed at any of these branch surgeries, where attendance varies from none to 20. Two surgeries have no phone, and examination facilities are primitive. Appointments are not required, although patients are encouraged to inform the main surgery of their intention to visit, so that we can bring records and appropriate equipment, etc. Some patients inform us.

The patients seen are predominantly elderly people, mothers with young children and difficult transport arrangements, the chronically sick and the socially isolated. Many minor illnesses are seen, BPs checked and chests auscultated. Only rarely are procedures carried out and, not uncommonly, patients are advised that they need to make an appointment at the well-equipped main surgery. We take prescriptions to the pharmacist for later delivery. We complete records for unexpected patients later.

Of course, problems abound with lack of immediately available records, literature and IT support, professional support and the full range of equipment, as well as occasional problems with soundproofing, inadequate heating and sometimes no running water. Yet the surgeries are seen as a valuable community support service and the feeling persists that some patients would present later with serious illness and that chronic disease review would suffer if they were to close down.

Most health authorities and health boards do not publish their policy on standards for branch surgeries. To provide accessible services and avoid the public outcry that would follow threatened closure, they quietly approve standards which would not normally be acceptable in main surgeries.

Funding for branch surgeries is identical to that for other GP surgeries, i.e. they may be financed out of the Cost Rent scheme, the Notional Rent scheme or, previously, out of fundholder savings.

Access to care versus quality of care

The availability of branch surgeries, like the availability of home visiting, represents a response to the issue of access to care referred to in Chapter 8. In 1997, patients spent significantly more time travelling to their doctor than they did in 1964.[2] It is likely that, with Government pressure to increase the costs of motoring, the problems of access to care will increase. Circumstances will dictate whether it is the patient or the practitioner who pays the cost.

Access to care is a trade-off against quality of care

- From the patient's perspective, care should be available quickly, conveniently and locally.

- From the perspective of healthcare providers, services should be convenient to provide and efficient. There should be access to full back-up facilities, including equipment, team workers, information, and secondary care services. Health professionals are responsible for providing the highest standards of care, irrespective of the circumstances.

These different perspectives lead to conflict, for which there is no universally correct solution.

No one has argued publicly that different standards of care should be acceptable in different geographical settings. Yet at a time of great financial constraint, the need to justify public expenditure means that very small, remote communities, visited rarely, seldom have the same standards of premises and equipment as standard surgeries elsewhere.

The quality of care available in many branch surgeries is inferior to that provided in main surgeries. Patients have fewer opportunities for team care and can access a more limited range of services.

Closing a branch surgery tends to be a very emotional experience. To be effected successfully, patients need to be involved in discussions and persuaded that the change will represent an improvement for them. The Community Health Council should be involved by the practice itself at an early stage in the process.

McAvoy described the home-visiting rate in a rural general practice during the 12 months before and after five branch surgeries were closed in one practice.[3] He found neither a statistically significant change in the home-visiting rate nor a change in the consulting rate at the main surgery.

Changes in the health of villagers may not become apparent for some time after changes in consulting patterns and reductions in access to care. As there is no scheme to fund patient transport to primary care and public transport in rural areas is often inadequate, those hardest hit would be elderly people, mothers with young children and poor people.

Professional debate on the future of branch surgeries needs to be informed by well-conducted studies quantifying the effects of poor access to medical care and the costs of providing optimum standards of care in different geographical settings.[4] Only then is it possible to make informed decisions about the advantages and disadvantages of closing branch surgeries. For the moment the pressure to reduce health service spending is likely to mean that branch surgeries continue to close down.

References

1 Bentham G and Haynes R (1992) Evaluation of a mobile branch surgery in a rural area. *Journal of Social Science and Medicine.* **34**(1): 97–102.
2 Cartwright A and Anderson R (1981) *General Practice Revisited: a second study of patients and their doctors.* Tavistock, London.
3 McAvoy BR (1985) Does closing branch surgeries affect home visiting? *BMJ.* **290**: 120–2.
4 Rousseau N and McColl E (1997) *Equity and Access in Rural Primary Care: an exploratory study in Northumberland and Cumbria.* Centre for Health Services Research, University of Newcastle upon Tyne.

14
Inducement practitioners, associates and the doctors' retainer scheme

Laura Marshall

Inducement scheme

The inducement scheme is rumoured to have its origins in improving the health of recruits for the British Army.

Anon

In 1912, a committee was appointed to examine the adequacy of the medical services existing in the Highlands and Islands of Scotland. The Dewar Committee[1] reported on Christmas Eve 1912 that the combination of social, economic and geographical difficulties in the Highlands and Islands demanded exceptional treatment. In general, medical care was poor, but it was thought that if doctors could be guaranteed a reasonable income, with adequate nursing and hospital services, well-trained practitioners would be attracted to the area to work. Within 8 months of the report, the Highlands and Islands Medical Service Fund was introduced. In the early years the Fund provided for a minimum income of £300 per annum. In 1947, the last year of the Fund, the minimum was set at £800. By that time there were 150 doctors in the area contracted under the Fund.

The inducement scheme followed on from this and has been incorporated into the NHS and expanded and developed to meet our present-day needs.

The scheme exists to ensure the provision of general medical services in areas where a GP's presence is deemed to be essential but where there are insufficient patients to provide the doctor with adequate income from the generation of fees and allowances.[2] The intention is that an inducement doctor should neither be advantaged nor disadvantaged when compared to other GPs in comparable practices who are not eligible to participate in the scheme.

Any practice can apply for inducement status if their net profit does not come up to the yardstick set annually by the management executive following the publication of the report by the Doctors' and Dentists' Pay Review Body. The yardstick is usually decided by the end of March each year. At present (August 1997) it is set at 81.4% of the national average income for GPs.

Practices with more than one partner may also be eligible for inducement status, especially if their notional list figures allow the deployment of additional partners to deal with the workload of the practice (see Example 1). Currently practices can apply for additional partners if this notional list exceeds 1500 patients per doctor. The notional list is determined by a number of factors, such as temporary resident numbers, mileage within the practice, additional work, e.g. mountain rescue, red cross, coastguard or casualty work. The decision to allow an extra partner is decided by the Medical Practices' Committee and the Secretary of State on recommendation by the health board.

The Secretary of State is involved in deciding which practices are eligible for inducement status and is responsible for determining three outcomes:

- whether a practice is deemed essential

- the minimum income that a practitioner should receive

- the right of appeal against a health board's interpretation of, and application of, the Statement of Fees and Allowances.

The health boards carry out the day-to-day administration of the scheme.

Before 1990 and the new contract, there were 75 inducement practices and 90 inducement practitioners. There are now over 100 inducement practices and 130 inducement practitioners. An inducement practice is a small business and is therefore no different from the rest of general practice. It is not a salaried service and detailed practice accounts must be maintained. The unique distinction is in the supplementary payment, which brings the practitioners' profits up to an agreed percentage of the average net remuneration of the profession as a whole.

The supplementary payment is calculated by deducting certain agreed expenses from the normal practice income of Basic Practice Allowance, capitation fees, supplementary allowances and items of service fees.

Certain allowances, for example PGEA and seniority, are not included in the calculation and are paid in addition to the final inducement income.

The inducement scheme includes small practices of 530 patients, e.g. Carbost (see Example 2), and larger five-partner practices with a list size of over 4000, e.g. Aviemore.

Example 1   Aviemore

A five-partner practice in central Northern Scotland situated below the Cairngorm mountains. It is a major tourist destination with a potential of 25 000 temporary residents a year. Practice population 4100. Practice area 800 square miles. Training practice. The practice is involved with mountain rescue, ski patrol and casualty sessions. Greatest patient–surgery distance 29 miles. The notional list allows five partners to be employed, reflecting the increased workload the practice undertakes.

Example 2   Carbost Surgery

A single-handed practice on the west coast of the Isle of Skye. The Cuillins are part of the geographical practice area of over 300 square miles. Practice population 530. Distance from nearest practice 15 miles. Fully computerised. Dispensing. The doctor on call is available 24 hours a day as the practice is too geographically isolated to allow cross-cover. Mobile phones do not work in the area so communication is difficult. The practice has an Associate GP to allow cover for holidays and study leave.

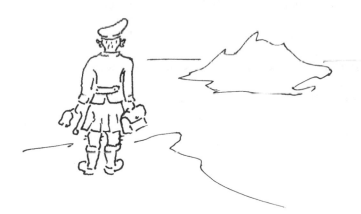

Box 14.1: Advantages and disadvantages of the inducement scheme

Advantages

- ensures medical provision in rural areas
- encourages a comprehensive patient care service
- maintains the viability of small communities
- offers additional employment in isolated areas
- ensures a regular income

Disadvantages

- clinical isolation – small patient numbers, few colleagues to discuss medical problems with or for support
- cash flow – inducement practices may have expenses that at the end of the year are not deemed to be eligible for reimbursement. If these expenses are large inducement doctors can become financially compromised
- no financial incentive to do additional work as any extra money is absorbed into the scheme
- out-of-hours cover is usually poor due to geographical isolation

---

Despite the need for certain aspects of the inducement scheme to be re-examined, it has been successful in maintaining a general practice service in rural isolated areas. In 1995 the Scottish Health Services Advisory Council[3] reviewed the scheme and found it to be well regarded by professionals and patients alike and to be the most suitable for the geographical area covered. In maintaining these essential services small communities are encouraged to remain and develop and a way of life is kept viable.

Further information about the inducement scheme can be obtained through the Secretary of General Medical Services, Committee of the Scottish BMA (Tel. 0131 662 4820).

The Associate scheme

The Associate scheme was manna from heaven.

Single-handed GP, Isle of Lewis, 1990

The Associate scheme was established in 1990, one of the positive developments in a year of controversial change.[4] It acknowledged that single-handed practitioners in isolated areas were in a unique position of permanent, 24–hour on-call availability for 52 weeks of the year. They were clinically and geographically isolated from colleagues and had difficulties obtaining regular time off for study leave and holidays. The scheme was a recognition of the stress involved in being constantly on call.

The Associate scheme allows the deployment of an extra doctor between two single-handed principals, although Associates may also work part-time and be attached to one practice only. Posts are primarily in rural areas of Britain with most being in the Highlands and Islands of Scotland.

To qualify for the allowance to enable a GP to employ an Associate, the GP must be single-handed and fulfil the following criteria:

- be in receipt of rural practice payments or an inducement payment

- be the sole practitioner on an island or practice more than 10 miles from the next GP's main surgery or district general hospital.

Doctors who are employed as Associates must satisfy the vocational training regulations and be eligible to apply for inclusion on the list of an FHSA or health board.

The scheme enables three doctors to work for two thirds of the year each. Though this sounds comfortable, most Associates work for practices where, given their great isolation and the distances involved, on-call cooperative cover is not possible. The Associate and the two principals still have extensive single-handed on-call commitment equating to continuous 24-hour on-call for 34 weeks per year. The remaining 17 weeks is taken as study leave and holiday. How this time off is arranged is flexible. Some practices work in week-long blocks, often up to 6 weeks on-call with similar periods of leave. Others work a system where each doctor has a few days off each week, with increasing flexibility around holiday periods.

The Associate GP is employed by the practitioners, but his or her salary is reimbursed by the local health board. The salary is detailed in the Registrars' section of the Statement of Fees and Allowances ('Red Book'). Associates are entitled to a car allowance, PGEA, reimbursement of a percentage of medical defence fees, removal expenses, distant islands allowance (for those eligible) and an incremental progression of pay for four years. However, they are not eligible for seniority payments or out-of-hours payments.

Recruitment

The Associate scheme was originally aimed at doctors who had just completed their vocational training and were keen to experience rural, isolated practice before committing themselves to a full-time partnership. It was also thought that GPs nearing retirement in a busy partnership might wish to experience a rural practice for their last few working years. For these doctors, however, a disadvantage is their loss of seniority payments, which may adversely affect pension rights as well as resulting in a fall in salary of up to £5000 per year.

By incorporating job-share and part-time positions it also provides a flexible career option for a wide sector of GPs. A 1996 study of incumbent Associates revealed that 78% were over 35 years of age, 65% were women and 61% were in post for more than two years.[4]

Many Associates originate from the so-called 'Generation X' group, that is those doctors who qualify and then disappear to work and travel abroad. The scheme allows re-entry back into general practice in Britain without having to be instantly aware of all the changes in legislation and business that have occurred in the interim. Generation X doctors can learn about these developments by experience as they manage a single-handed practice, and through talking to their employing GP.

The 1996 study showed that 65% of Associates were women, many of whom had been in post for several years, some since the inception of the scheme in 1990. The scheme allows women doctors access to employment in rural areas where their partner is already employed. It is a welcome alternative to the doctors' retainer scheme. The job itself is challenging and allows all medical problems to be dealt with. It prevents women doctors being sidelined into childcare and obstetrics and gynaecology and allows them to use the skills they developed in their training. This in turn boosts women's confidence in difficult clinical situations, making them happier to remain in isolated practice. The local communities also benefit by having a choice of doctors to consult.

Box 14.2: Advantages and disadvantages of the Associate scheme

Advantages

- chance to experience rural practice before making a long-term commitment

- decreased practice management, with a focus on clinical skills

- flexible arrangements compatible with childcare, partners and other work, etc.

- maintenance of superannuation contributions, PGEA

Disadvantages

- status – the scheme is remunerated under the Registrars' section of the Red Book and this is often reflected in how they are perceived, i.e. as senior registrars, not qualified GPs

- seniority payments – these are accrued on a 1 year for 2 years worked basis, and then only after the Associate has become a principal on a health board list

- out of hours – a full-time Associate GP is on call for 112 hours per week and yet is not eligible for out-of-hours money

- salaried – under schedule E not schedule D, therefore no self-employment tax advantages

- housing – if you are working between two practices that are widely separated you may require two houses, which can mean frequent moves. (There are additional subsistence payments if this is the case)

The future

The disadvantages are being addressed by the National Society of Associates in their policy document, which is being presented to the Scottish General Medical Services Committee and has been supported by Local Medical Committees. It is hoped that the title of Associates will be changed to Associate Principals with a zero list. This will ensure seniority payments on a one-for-one basis and not deter pre-retirement GP principals from joining the scheme. It will also improve the out-of-hours remuneration.

General medicine has hugely varying challenges and benefits depending on where it is practised. The Associate scheme allows diversity and challenge within the profession. It could be considered by an urban GP wishing to take a year's sabbatical and work in a rural area, and vice versa. Actually experiencing the jobs that others only perceive improves communication within general practice and shows us what a varied profession we have. Change can bring refreshment and a renewed sense of vision on your return.

The Associate scheme has been very successful in alleviating the difficult demands of continuous on-call, single-handed practice. The scheme has been well received by both employing GP principals and the Associates they employ. For further information contact the National Society of Associates. Contact telephone numbers are available from the Postgraduate Centre in Inverness (Tel: 01463 704000).

Associates – Tae Be or Not Tae Be

In 1990 Associates came tae be,
They share the workload an' set GPs free.
They work for twa years to hae ane year accrued,
In advising the contract, the Red Book wis shrewd.
They bring fresh ideas frae all o'er the world,
Active in communities, at dances they've birled,
They dae the on-call for twa thirds o' the year,
But 'oot o' hours' money tae them does nae appear.
Instead their GPs (who work hard also)
Are meant to part wi' ane third o' their dough.
We dinnae feel that this is quite fair,
In fact it makes oor hairts quite sair,
But the time has come for change tae arise,
Or we fear Associates may meet their demise.
As fewer trainees enter the vocational scheme.
The fewer GPs will head straight for the cream,
An' for principal positions they will reach,
The Associate concept will sadly be beached.
An' the stress and the strain of on-call will return,
Tae single-handed GPs the late candle will burn.
Tak heed this warning afore it's too late –
It's Associate Principals we need to create.

The doctors' retainer scheme

The doctors' retainer scheme[6] was established in 1972 to allow doctors who couldn't practice full time to be able to keep working and maintain their skills.[7,8] It has recently been changed as the benefits of the scheme have been recognised and the disadvantages addressed.

A survey of doctors in Scotland who were working or had worked as retainers revealed that they valued the scheme despite its limitations and inconsistencies.[9] Nearly half the doctors in the survey claimed they would have left medicine if the scheme had not existed.

The present scheme

The scheme is aimed at doctors less than 55 years old who, for 'well-founded personal reasons', are unable to practise full time. It has been particularly useful to women with heavy domestic commitments.[10] Though aimed at doctors of any field of medicine, over 90% of doctors on the scheme are in general practice, the majority being women. There are approximately 700 doctors employed as retainers.

The scheme is administered through area health boards that receive an earmarked sum each year for retainers. Doctors on the scheme receive a small annual retainer fee (£290 in August 1997) from the health board or authority, and the practice they work for receives a small sum (£47.75 per session) towards the cost of employing the retainer. It is up to individuals to negotiate any further payments with the practice. Doctors can only stay on the scheme for a limited period of time, but at present this can vary from 2 to 15 years depending on the health board or authority.

Once accepted on to the scheme, the doctor must work at least 12 sessions per year, but not more than four per week, and maintain registration with the GMC and a medical defence organisation. They must also continue their professional development by attending at least seven educational sessions each year, take one professional journal, and see the clinical tutor annually.

Box 14.3: Advantages and disadvantages of the doctors' retainer scheme

Advantages

- the flexible nature of employment
- being able to practise regularly and maintain skills
- time for other commitments, e.g. family, children, illness
- regular income
- being able to maintain contact with professional colleagues

Disadvantages

- lack of publicity and information about the scheme
- low income compared to expensive overheads, i.e. GMC registration, MDU subscription
- no PGEA to cover educational commitments
- educational nature of the scheme often ambiguous
- sessional work is not automatically superannuable and time spent in the scheme may constitute a break in service

The future

There has been much discussion regarding the doctors' retainer scheme and the GPC has recently agreed improvements with the Department of Health.[11] It is hoped that the scheme will regain its educational focus and it has been proposed that the retained doctor should be allowed access to a range of professional work centred on patient consultations. They should have protected time for the lead principal to discuss consultations and concerns and there should be opportunities to learn about other aspects of general practice. The practice involved will be paid via funds channelled through the regional postgraduate dean's budget. It will be seen as a non-core activity by practices that can offer the appropriate skills and resources to the retained doctor. The practice will support the career progression of the retained doctor under a contract with the regional director of general practice education.

Any practice employing a retained doctor will have the advantage of an extra fully trained GP for a number of sessions per week over a continuous period of years. They will enjoy the stimulation and challenge that having a retained doctor involves.

In 1992 the Advisory Committee on Medical Establishment recommended that doctors on the scheme should be allowed to work for four sessions per week and do controlled short-term locum work.[12] The number of sessions undertaken by retained doctors has now been increased to four per week. It is anticipated that this will increase the confidence of the doctors employed and allow more involvement with the practice. It is intended that the attachment will be time limited to encourage the return to more regular work in due course.

As registrars in all specialities look for more flexible working arrangements the scheme will remain a useful low-commitment option for doctors at appropriate times in their careers.

References

1 *The Birsary Report.* (1967) Cmnd 3257. HMSO, Edinburgh (referring to The Dewar Committee Report of Highlands & Islands Medical Services Committee. Cd6559 and CdC920, 1912).

2 Scottish Office (1992–93) *The Scottish Office Inducement Payment Scheme – notes for the guidance of health boards.* Scottish Office, Edinburgh.

3 The Scottish Office Home and Health Department (1995) *Health Care Services in Remote and Isolated Areas in Scotland.* HMSO, Edinburgh.

4 Marshall L (1997) Associate general practitioners. *BMJ Classified.* **315**:2–3.

5 Steiner E and Mathieson R (1996) *Results from Associate General Practitioner Survey* (Unpublished study)

6 Nanson M and Hastie A (1994) *Nobody's Baby: the doctors' retainer scheme.* Women's Career Advisory Committee, South Thames Region, London.

7 Anon (1993) Background on retainer scheme. In: *Women in General Practice*: task force resource pack. Royal College of General Practitioners, London.

8 Oswald J and Ray R (1994) Looking to the future. *Scottish Medicine.* **13**:6–7.

9 Douglas A and McCann I (1996) Doctors' retainer scheme in Scotland: time for change? *BMJ.* **313**:792–4.

10 Chapman J (1994) *Doctors' Retainer Scheme.* Medical Women's Federation, London.
11 *GMSC Medical Workforce Task Group Report* (1996) BMA, London.
12 Advisory Committee on Medical Establishment (1992) *Part Time Training and Working for Doctors in Scotland.* SHHO, Edinburgh.

Acknowledgements

Thanks go to Dr Sue Tracy, Dr Donald Fraser, Dr Tom Pearce, Dr Gillian Irvine, and Dr MacNichol for their help and information.

Index